NEUROLOGICAL EMERGENCIES
Second edition

NEUROLOGICAL EMERGENCIES

Second edition

Edited by
Richard A C Hughes

Professor of Neurology, UMDS,
London, UK

Editor, *Journal of Neurology,
Neurosurgery, and Psychiatry*

BMJ
Publishing
Group

First published in 1994
Second edition 1997
by the BMJ Publishing Group, BMA House, Tavistock Square,
London WC1H 9JR

British Library Cataloguing in Publication Data

A catalogue record for this book is available
from the British Library

ISBN 0-7279-1104-X

Typeset, printed and bound in Great Britain by
Thanet Press Limited,
Margate, Kent

Contents

INTRODUCTION

Neurological disease accounts for about a fifth of admissions to general hospitals in the United Kingdom and this proportion is likely to be replicated worldwide. Most of these admissions are emergencies and the responsibility for care falls jointly on family practitioners or primary care physicians, accident and emergency doctors, internists, general physicians, and neurologists. In some countries, and the United Kingdom is unfortunately the most obvious example, neurologists are involved late, little, or not at all, and yet they are the only members of this team whose training and skills are focused on the diagnosis and care of patients with diseases of the nervous system.

During 1993 the *Journal of Neurology, Neurosurgery, and Psychiatry* published a series of solicited but peer reviewed articles on neurological emergencies by neurologists, which are now collected in this book. The words "neurological" and "neurologist" have been used broadly and we have chosen as authors the appropriate "neurological" specialist. Neurosurgeons have written about neurosurgical topics, psychiatrists about the interface between neurology and psychiatry, and neurological physicians about "hard core" neurological diseases. To reflect the international character of neurology, our editorial committee, and the articles in the *Journal of Neurology, Neurosurgery, and Psychiatry*, our authors write from both sides of the Atlantic Ocean.

The book is designed for every doctor who deals with neurological emergencies. Each chapter reviews current management and the evidence for its efficacy, and concludes with a brief summary of recommendations that should be a useful *aide-mémoire* in an emergency. The reviews do not shrink from controversy but authors have had to make decisions about best courses of management in the absence of adequate evidence. For instance, Marshall and Mohr's recommendation to use intravenous heparin in small or moderate sized ischaemic strokes reflects common practice in the United States, but the benefits of this treatment have not been proved by individual trials or an overview analysis.[1]

Although a book like this is inevitably targeted at the doctor in training, especially residents in internal medicine, accident and emergency medicine, and neurology (including neurosurgery and psychiatry), we are all perpetual students of medicine. We hope therefore that this work will help the whole profession improve the care of neurological patients when they most need it, in an emergency.

R A C HUGHES

November 1996

1 Sandercock PAG, Belt AGM, Lindley RI, Slattery J. Antithrombotic therapy in acute ischaemic stroke: an overview of the completed randomised trials. *J Neurol Neurosurg Psychiatry* 1993;**56**:17–25.

1 Medical coma

DAVID BATES

The patient in coma who is brought to the hospital casualty department, or seen on the intensive care unit, though not having been exposed to evident trauma, may be harbouring delayed effects of trauma such as a subdural haematoma or meningitis arising from a basal skull fracture. The possibilities of raised intracranial pressure following a parenchymal haematoma in a hypertensive patient, the decompensation of a cerebral tumour, or the collection of pus means that all possible causes of loss of consciousness must be considered by the physician when dealing with a patient in coma. Thus in the diagnosis of medical coma it is not easy to exclude the patient in coma following head injury.

If one excludes patients with a transient loss of consciousness following seizure, syncope, cardiac dysrhythmia or hypoglycaemia and those unresponsive due to impending death, and considers patients who have been unconscious for some 5–6 hours, then 40% of such patients seen in medical practice will have taken some form of sedative drugs with or without alcohol.[1] Of the remainder just over 40% will have suffered a hypoxic ischaemic insult as the result of cardiac arrest or anaesthetic accident, a third will be unconscious as a result of cerebrovascular accidents, either haemorrhage or infarction, and about a quarter will be unconscious as a result of metabolic coma including infection, renal failure, hepatic failure, and complications of diabetes mellitus. If one considers only those cases which are initially regarded as "of unknown aetiology" the proportion of drug overdoses is about 30%, mass lesions about 34%, and diffuse metabolic causes account for 36%.[2]

Few problems are more difficult to manage than the unconscious patient because the potential causes of loss of consciousness are considerable and because the time for diagnosis and effective intervention is relatively short. All alterations in arousal should be regarded as acute and potentially life threatening emergencies until vital functions are stabilised, the underlying cause of the coma is diagnosed, and reversible causes are corrected. Delay in instituting treatment for a patient with raised intracranial pressure may have obvious consequences in terms of pressure coning but, similarly, the unnecessary investigation of patients in metabolic coma with imaging techniques may delay the initiation of appropriate therapy. It is therefore essential for the physician in charge to adopt a systematic approach initially to ensure resuscitation, and then to direct further tests towards producing the most rapid diagnosis and the most appropriate therapy. The development of such a systematic approach demands an understanding of the pathophysiology of consciousness and the ways in which it may be deranged.

Causes of coma

The phenomenon of consciousness depends upon an intact ascending reticular activating substance in the brainstem to act as the alerting or awakening element of consciousness, together with a functioning cerebral cortex of both hemispheres which determines the content of that consciousness. The ascending reticular activating substance is a continuous isodendritic core, extending from the medulla through the pons to the midbrain which is continuous caudally with the reticular intermediate grey lamina of the spinal cord and rostrally with the subthalamus, the hypothalamus, and the thalamus (fig 1).[3] Its functions and interconnections are considerable and its role greater than that of a simple cortical arousal system. There are named nuclei throughout the reticular formation and, although it was originally considered that cortical arousal depended upon projections from the reticular formation via the midline thalamic nuclei to the thalamic reticular nucleus and the cortex, it now seems unlikely that the thalamic reticular nucleus is the final relay and the specific role of the various links from the reticular formation to the thalamus has yet to be identified.

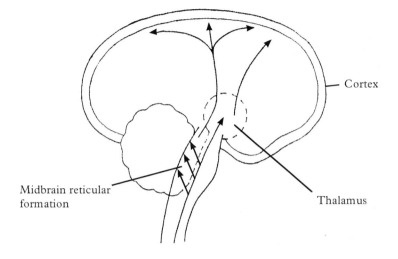

Figure 1—The anatomy of consciousness

Similarly the neurotransmitters involved in this arousal system are not fully determined though it seems likely that, in addition to cholinergic and monoaminergic systems, gamma aminobutyric acid (GABA) may be important in controlling consciousness.[4-6]

It follows from recognition of the anatomy and pharmacology of the ascending reticular activating substance that structural damage to this pathway or chemical derangement of the neurotransmitters involved are mechanisms whereby consciousness may be impaired. Such conditions will occur with focal lesions in the brainstem, mass lesions in the posterior fossa impinging directly on the brainstem, or mass lesions involving the cerebral hemispheres causing tentorial pressure coning and consequently compromising the ascending reticular activating substance either by direct pressure or by a process of ischaemia (fig 2). In addition toxins, including most commonly ingested drugs, may have a significant depressant effect upon the brainstem ascending reticular activating substance and thereby result in loss of consciousness.

3

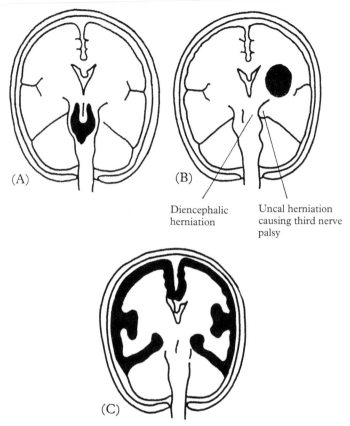

Diencephalic
herniation

Uncal herniation
causing third nerve
palsy

Figure 2—Causes of coma. (A) Focal brainstem lesions; (B) mass lesions;
(C) diffuse cortical pathology

The content of consciousness resides in the cerebral cortex of both hemispheres. Unlike those discrete cortical functions such as language or vision which are focally located within the cortex, the content of consciousness can best be regarded as the amalgam of all cognitive functions. Coma arising from disruption of this cortical activity requires a diffuse pathology such as generalised anoxia or ischaemia, commonly seen after cardiac arrest or anaesthetic accidents, or the effects of presumed cortical vasospasm seen in infective meningitis, or the chemical meningitis following subarachnoid haemorrhage where generalised cortical ischaemia is believed to be the cause of disruption of function.

For the physician attempting to diagnose the cause of coma, consideration must be given to the following.

(1) *Supra- or infratentorial mass lesions.* Typically these will provide evidence of raised intracranial pressure and commonly produce focal signs. Processes such as neoplasm or haematoma, infarction with cerebral oedema, abscess, focal encephalitis, and venous sinus thrombosis should be considered.

(2) *Subtentorial destructive lesions or the local effect of toxin.* These processes will directly damage the ascending reticular activating substance as in brainstem infarction, rhombencephalitis, brainstem demyelination, and the much more common effects of self-poisoning with sedative drugs.

(3) *Diffuse damage to the cerebral cortex.* Bilateral cortical injury is most commonly seen in states of hypoxia and ischaemia but may be mimicked by hypoglycaemia, ketoacidosis, electrolyte abnormalities, bacterial meningitis, viral encephalitis, and diffuse post-infectious encephalomyelitis. It is also the likely pathology of coma following subarachnoid haemorrhage.

Definitions

There is a continuum from the individual in full consciousness to the patient in deep coma. The terminology which is most usually employed derives from the Brain Injuries Committee of the MRC.[7]

(1) *Confusion*—"disturbance of consciousness characterised by impaired capacity to think clearly and to perceive, respond to and remember current stimuli; there is also disorientation." Confusion involves a generalised disturbance of cortical cerebral function which is usually associated with considerable electroencephalographic (EEG) abnormalities. Some authors describe an intervening state between normal consciousness and confusion, that of clouding of consciousness.[2]

(2) *Delirium*—"a state of much disturbed consciousness with motor restlessness, transient hallucinations, disorientation and perhaps delusions."

(3) *Obtundation*—"a disorder of alertness associated with psychomotor retardation."

(4) *Stupor*—"a state in which the patient, though not unconscious, exhibits little or no spontaneous activity." Although the individual appears to be asleep he or she will awaken to vigorous

stimulation but show limited motor activities and usually fail to speak.

(5) *Coma*—"a state of unarousable psychologic unresponsiveness in which the subjects lie with eyes closed and show no psychologically understandable response to external stimulus or inner need." This may be shortened to "a state of unarousable unresponsiveness" which implies both the defect in arousal and in awareness of self or environment manifest as an inability to respond. A more useful assessment of coma is derived from the hierarchical Glasgow Coma Scale[8] in which patients, who fail to show eye opening in response to voice, perform no better than weak flexion in response to pain, and make, at best, only unrecognisable grunting noises in response to pain, are regarded as being in coma. This allows the patients to have an eye opening response of 2 or less, a motor response of 4 or less and verbal response of 2 or less. The sum Glasgow score of 8 should not be regarded as being definitive of coma since the total score can be achieved in several different ways (see page 30).

(6) *Vegetative state.* When the cortex of the cerebral hemispheres of the brain recovers more slowly than the brainstem or when the cortex is irreversibly damaged there may arise a situation in which the patient enters a vegetative state without cognitive function. It may be a transient phase through which patients in coma pass as they recover or deteriorate but, commonly after anoxic injuries to the brain, a state develops in which the brainstem recovers function but the cerebral hemispheres are not capable of recovery. When this occurs the patient enters a "persistent vegetative state" described by Jennett and Plum.[9] Such patients may survive for long periods, on occasion for decades, but never recover outward manifestations of higher mental activity and the condition, which is comparatively newly recognised, relates to the development of modern resuscitative techniques. Other terms have been used in the past to identify similar conditions. These include coma vigil, the apallic syndrome, cerebral death, neocortical death, and total dementia.

(7) *Akinetic mutism* has been defined as a similar condition of unresponsiveness but apparent alertness, as demonstrated by reactive α- and θ-EEG rhythms in response to stimuli. The major difference from the vegetative state, in which there is tone in the muscles and extensor or flexor responses, is that patients with akinetic mutism have flaccid tone and are unresponsive to

peripheral pain. It is thought that this state is due to bilateral frontal lobe lesions, diffuse cortical lesions, or lesions of the deep grey matter.[10]

(8) *The locked-in syndrome.* Feldman[11] described a de-efferented state caused by bilateral ventral pontine lesion involving damage to the corticospinal, corticopontine, and corticobulbar tracts. The patient has total paralysis below the level of the third nerve nuclei and, although able to open, elevate, and depress the eyes, has no horizontal eye movements and no other voluntary eye movement. The diagnosis depends upon the physician being able to recognise that the patient can open the eyes voluntarily and can signal assent or dissent by responding numerically with eye closure. Similar states are occasionally seen in patients with severe polyneuropathy, myasthenia gravis, and after the use of neuro-muscular blocking agents.

(9) *Pseudo-coma.* Rarely, patients, who appear in coma without structural, metabolic, toxic, or psychiatric disorder being appar-ent, can be shown by tests of brainstem function to have intact brainstem activity and corticopontine projections, and not to be in coma.

Resuscitation

Although resuscitation is commonly performed by the casualty officer or the anaesthetist in the intensive care unit, rather than by the neurologist, it is appropriate that the neurologist remembers that, in patients who are unconscious, protection of the airway, respiration, support of the circulation, and provision of an ade-quate supply of glucose are all important in stabilising the patient. It is frequently necessary to intubate the trachea in a patient in coma, not only to ensure an adequate airway but also to prevent the aspiration of vomit. It is also important to note the respiratory rate and pattern before intubation and certainly before instituting mechanical ventilation; because depressed respiration is a fre-quent clue to drug overdose or metabolic disturbance, increased respiration to hypoxia, hypercapnia, or acidosis and fluctuating respiration may indicate a brainstem lesion. The possibility that respiratory failure is the cause of coma should always be consid-ered in a patient with disordered respiration.

Once adequate oxygenation and circulation are ensured and monitored, blood should be withdrawn for the determination of blood glucose, biochemical estimations, and toxicology. It is then reasonable to give a bolus of 25–50 g of dextrose despite the present controversy about the use of intravenous glucose in patients with ischaemic or anoxic brain damage. It can be argued that extra glucose in this situation may augment local lactic acid production by anaerobic glycolysis and potentially worsen ischaemic or anoxic damage. In practice in the situation of ischaemic or anoxic brain damage, and even in the presence of a diabetic ketoacidosis, the administration of such a quantity of glucose will not be immediately harmful and in the hypoglycaemic patient it may well be life saving. A reasonable compromise would be to obtain an early assessment of the level of blood glucose by Dextrostix testing but these are not sufficiently accurate to preclude the need for formal laboratory assessment. When glucose is given in this situation an argument can be made for giving a bolus of thiamine at the same time to prevent precipitation of Wernicke's encephalopathy.[12]

An essential part of resuscitation includes the establishment of baseline blood pressure, pulse, temperature, the establishment of an intravenous line, and the stabilisation of the neck, together with an examination for meningitis. It may be difficult in those patients who have sustained some degree of trauma in their collapse to assess the stability of the neck, but the establishment of an adequate airway certainly takes precedence and the identification of meningism in a febrile patient probably takes precedence over the stabilisation of neck movements. In a comatose, febrile patient with meningism seen outside the hospital environment the intramuscular injection of penicillin before transfer is now recognised to carry a significant advantage.

History

Once the patient is stable it is important to obtain as much information as possible from those who accompanied the patient to hospital or who watched the onset of coma. The circumstances in which consciousness was lost are of vital importance in helping to identify the diagnosis. Generally, coma is likely to present in one of three ways: as the predictable progression of an underlying illness; as an unpredictable event in a patient with a previously known disease; or as a totally unexpected event. Distinctions between these presentations are often achieved by the history of the circumstances in which consciousness was lost. In the first category are patients following focal brainstem infarction who deteriorate or those with known intracranial mass lesions who show similar deterioration. In the second category are patients with recognised cardiac arrhythmia or the known risk factor of sepsis from an intravenous line. In the final category it is important to determine whether there has been a previous history of seizures, trauma, febrile illnesses, or focal neurological disturbances. The history of a sudden collapse in the midst of a busy street or office indicates the need for different investigations from those necessary for the patient who is discovered at home in bed surrounded by empty bottles of sedative tablets.

Examination and monitoring

The third phase of the management of the patient in coma involves a rapid but systematic examination to identify possible causes of the coma.

Temperature

Fever usually indicates infection and, rarely, a brainstem or diencephalic lesion affecting the temperature centres.[13] Most commonly the combination of fever and coma indicates systemic infection such as pneumonia or septicaemia, or a cerebral cause such as meningitis, encephalitis, or abscess. When seizures occur together with fever the possibility of encephalitis or cerebral abscess is greatly increased. Heat stroke may present as a febrile comatose patient when the clue to the diagnosis is in the environment.

Hypothermia is most commonly seen as a complication of an accident or cerebrovascular disease when an elderly patient is discovered, having lain for hours or days in an underheated room. It may also be seen following intoxication with alcohol or barbiturates, with peripheral circulatory failure and, rarely, with profound myxoedema.

Heart rate

A tachyarrhythmia or bradyarrhythmia may be significant in identifying the cause of cerebral hypoperfusion. Irregularity of the pulse always raises the question of atrial fibrillation and associated embolic disease.

Blood pressure

Hypotension might indicate shock, myocardial infarction, septicaemia, or intoxication. It may also indicate diabetes mellitus or Addison's disease. Hypertension is of less help in the diagnosis of the patient in coma as it may be the cause, as in cerebral haemorrhage or hypertensive encephalopathy, but it can also be the result of the cerebral lesion.

Respiration

For those reasons already given, assessment of respiration may be compromised by the needs of resuscitation but, generally, slow and shallow breathing raises the question of drug intoxication. Deep, rapid respiration suggests pneumonia or acidosis which may also occur in brainstem lesions causing central neurogenic hyperventilation.

Integument

The appearance of the skin and mucous membrane may identify anaemia, jaundice, or cyanosis, or raise the possibility of carbon monoxide poisoning. Bruising over the scalp or mastoids, the presence of blood in the external auditory meatus or nostrils will raise the possibility of a basal skull fracture, and bruising elsewhere in the body raises the question of significant trauma. An exanthem may indicate the presence of a viral infection causing meningoencephalitis or meningococcal septicaemia, or raise the question of haemorrhagic disease. Hyperpigmentation raises the possibility of Addison's disease, and the presence of bullous skin lesions is frequently seen in barbiturate intoxication. Evidence of Kaposi's sarcoma, anogenital herpetic lesions, or oral candidiasis would raise the question of an acquired immune deficiency syndrome (AIDS) with the consequent plethora of possible central nervous system diseases.

Breath

The odour of the breath of an unconscious patient may indicate intoxication with alcohol, raise the question of diabetes, or suggest that the cause of coma is uraemic or hepatic.

Cardiovascular

Auscultation and examination of the heart may indicate valvular disease and raise the possibility of endocarditis. Bruits over the carotid vessels may indicate the presence of cerebrovascular disease, and splinter haemorrhages seen in the nail bed would raise the possibility of subacute bacterial endocarditis or collagen vascular diseases.

Abdomen

Examination of the abdomen may reveal signs of trauma or rupture of viscera; hepatomegaly or splenomegaly may indicate the possibility of a portocaval shunt and the findings of polycystic kidneys would raise the possibility of subarachnoid haemorrhage.

Meningism

Examination of the skull and spine is important and the physician should always look for neck stiffness. Kernig's test, in which the resistance to flexion of the thigh with the leg extended is examined, or Brudzinski's test, in which flexing of one thigh is noted to cause flexion of the other thigh, should be performed to help in differentiating neck stiffness, due to meningeal irritation, from that due to a developing tonsillar pressure cone. Positive Kernig's and Brudzinski's tests, together with neck stiffness imply inflammation in the lumbar theca and suggest a diffuse meningitic process. If these tests are negative, however, then the neck stiffness alone is more suggestive of a foraminal pressure cone.[14]

Fundal examination

The presence of papilloedema or fundal haemorrhage, or evidence of emboli, together with the findings of hypertensive, vascular, or diabetic retinopathy is important. The fundal appearances may be diagnostic as in the finding of subhyaloid haemorrhage but more commonly only help to confirm or refute evidence of raised intracranial pressure. The absence of papilloedema does not necessarily mean that there is no increased intracranial pressure.

Neurological examination

The position, posture, and spontaneous movements of the unconscious patient should be noted. The formal neurological examination consists of the elicitation of various reflex responses.[13] The most important aspects of neurological examination are those that define the level of consciousness, identify the activity of the brainstem, and search for evidence of lateralisation (table I).

Level of consciousness

The Glasgow Coma Scale[8] provides the most useful hierarchical assessment of the level of consciousness. The responses to commands, calling the patient's name, and painful stimuli are observed for eye opening, limb movement, and voice. Painful stimuli such as supraorbital pressure for central stimulation and nail bed pressure for peripheral stimulation are useful and reproducible. Eye opening is relatively easy to assess, though the fixed and unresponsive opening of the eyes sometimes seen in deep coma must not be confused with the volitional or reflex opening of the eyes from a closed position in response to stimuli. All four limbs are tested individually for movement and the best response is recorded in assessing the Glasgow Coma Scale but an asymmetry between responses may be of importance in the overall assessment (see below). Patients in lighter grades of coma still retain the ability to vocalise and may grimace and withdraw their limbs from pain. These responses are progressively lost as the coma deepens and it is important to test pain bilaterally in the periphery and cranially as patients may only vocalise or respond to painful stimuli on one side, raising the possibility of hemianaesthesia and providing evidence for a focal lesion. A grimace response to

TABLE I—Neurological assessment of coma

Glasgow Coma Scale	Eye opening
	Motor response
	Verbal response
Brainstem function	Pupillary reactions
	Corneal responses
	Spontaneous eye movements
	Oculocephalic responses
	Oculovestibular responses
	Respiratory pattern
Motor function	Motor response
	Muscle tone
	Tendon reflexes
	Seizures

painful stimulation is believed to indicate intact corticobulbar function[2] but there are patients in coma, particularly after hypoxic ischaemic insults, who show grimace in response to minor peripheral stimulation yet have no associated peripheral motor response. When this situation is seen it always raises the question of a ventral pontine lesion or of a cervical cord injury but more commonly it evolves into a vegetative state and is, generally, a poor prognostic sign.

The level of coma should be documented serially and is one of the most important indicators of the need for further investigation. Thus when the level of consciousness can be seen to be improving there is no need to make urgent decisions but when deterioration occurs then management decisions must be made. It may of course be correct, when the prognosis is recognised to be hopeless, to make a decision not to undertake further investigation or therapy.

Brainstem function

The brainstem reflexes are particularly important in helping to identify those lesions that may affect the reticular activating substance, explain the reason for coma, and potentially help in identifying the viability of the patient. The following reflexes are predominantly related to the eyes and the pattern of respiration.

(1) *Pupillary reactions.* The size, equality and reaction of the pupils to light is recorded. Unilateral dilatation of the pupil with loss of the light response suggests uncal herniation or a posterior communicating artery aneurysm. Midbrain lesions typically cause loss of the light reflex with midposition pupils, whereas pontine lesions cause miosis but a retained light response. Fixed dilatation of the pupils is an indication of central diencephalic herniation and may be differentiated from the fixed dilatation due to atropine-like agents by the use of pilocarpine eye drops, which will cause miosis if the dilatation is the result of loss of parasympathetic innervation but be ineffective if it is pharmacological. A Horner's syndrome may be seen ipsilateral to a lesion in the hypothalamus, thalamus, or brainstem when it will be associated with anhidrosis of the ipsilateral side of the body, but it can also be due to disease affecting the wall of the carotid artery when anhidrosis will only affect the face.[15] Hepatic or renal failure and other forms of metabolic coma may make the light reflexes appear unduly brisk and the pupils therefore relatively small. Most drug

intoxications tend to cause small and sluggishly reactive pupils and a pontine haemorrhage will cause pinpoint pupils due to parasympathetic stimulation.[16]

(2) *Corneal responses.* The corneal reflex is usually retained until coma is very deep. If it is absent in a patient who is in otherwise light coma then the possibility of drug induced coma or of local causes of anaesthesia to the cornea should be considered. The loss of the corneal response when drug overdose is excluded is a poor prognostic sign.

(3) *Spontaneous eye movement.* The resting position of the eyes and the presence of spontaneous eye movements should be noted. Conjugate deviation of the eyes raises the question of an ipsilateral hemisphere or contralateral brainstem lesion. Abnormalities of vertical gaze are less common with a patient in coma but depression of the eyes below the meridian may be seen with damage at the level of the midbrain tectum and in states of metabolic coma. The resting position of the eyes is normally conjugate and central but it may be dysconjugate when there is damage to the oculomotor or abducens nerves within the brainstem or along their paths.

Roving eye movements seen in light coma are similar to those of sleep. They cannot be mimicked and their presence excludes psychogenic unresponsiveness.[13] Periodic alternating gaze or "ping pong" gaze is a repetitive conjugate horizontal ocular deviation which is of uncertain aetiology.[17] Spontaneous nystagmus is rare in coma as it reflects interaction between the oculovestibular system and the cerebral cortex. Retractory nystagmus, in which the eyes jerk irregularly back into the orbit, and convergence nystagmus may be seen with midbrain lesions.[18] Ocular bobbing, an intermittent jerking downward eye movement, is seen with destructive lesions in the low pons and with cerebellar haematoma or hydrocephalus.[19]

(4) *Reflex eye movements.* These are tested by the oculocephalic and oculovestibular responses (fig 3). The oculocephalic or doll's head response is tested by rotating the patient's head from side to side and observing the eyes. In coma with an intact brainstem the eyes will move conjugately and in a direction opposite to the head movement. In a conscious patient such a response can be imitated by deliberate fixation of the eyes but is not common. In patients with pontine depression the oculocephalic response is lost and the eyes remain in the midposition of the head when turned.

The oculovestibular response is more accurate and useful. It is elicited by instilling between 50 and 200 ml of ice cold water into one external auditory meatus. The normal response in the conscious patient is the development of nystagmus with the quick phase away from the side of stimulation. A tonic response with

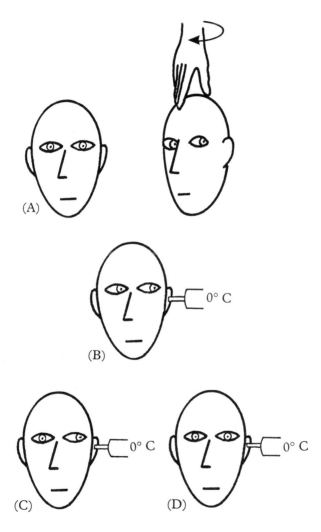

Figure 3—Reflex eye movements. (A) Normal doll's eyes; (B) tonic oculovestibular response; (C) dysconjugate oculovestibular response; (D) absent oculovestibular response

conjugate movement of the eye towards the stimulated side indicates an intact pons and suggests a supratentorial cause for the coma. A dysconjugate response or no response at all indicates brainstem damage or depression. Both ears should be stimulated separately. If unilateral irrigation causes vertical eye movement, the possibility of drug overdose arises because many drugs affect lateral eye movement.

The value of oculovestibular testing in patients without lateralising eye signs is considerable because they identify not only the intactness of the brainstem and corticopontine connections, but also may reveal the presence of an intrinsic brainstem lesion by causing dysconjugate eye posturing. In addition they are the definitive way of identifying patients in psychogenic coma who will show normal nystagmus and frequently be distressed by the manoeuvre.

(5) *Respiration.* Modern techniques of assisted respiration and the need to examine patients in intensive care units where their respiration is controlled complicate the assessment of normal respiratory functions. If, however, the patient is seen before respiration is controlled then the presence of long cycle periodic respiration suggests a relatively high brainstem lesion; central neurogenic hyperventilation implies a lesion at the level of the upper pons; and short cycle periodic respiration, which carries a poor prognosis, is seen with lesions lower in the brainstem. In general the presence of regular, rapid breathing correlates with pulmonary complications and a poor prognosis rather than with the site of neurological disease in patients in coma.[20]

Motor function

As part of the assessment of the Glasgow Coma Scale it may have been appreciated that there is lateralisation in the individual patient which implies a focal cause for the coma. The observation of involuntary movement affecting the face or limbs and asymmetry of reflexes will help to support this possibility. Focal seizures are an important indicator of a focal cause for the coma and the observation of more generalised seizures or of multifocal myoclonus would raise the possibility of a metabolic or ischaemic–anoxic cause for the coma with diffuse cortical irritation. The testing of tone as part of the assessment of muscle function can be useful in the comatose patient where it is possible to detect asymmetry of tone not only in the limbs but also in the face.

16

By this stage of the management of the patient in coma it should be possible to identify those patients who are unconscious with focal signs, those who are unconscious without focal signs but with the presence of meningism, and those who have loss of consciousness without either focal signs or meningism (box).

Investigations of the patient in coma

The relevant investigations to be undertaken in the individual patient will be identified by the differential diagnosis. In general the role of investigation in the patient in coma is to help establish the aetiology of that coma and will vary from simple blood tests through more complex blood tests, examination of the cerebrospinal fluid (CSF), electrophysiological tests, and imaging investigation. Although the EEG has some hierarchical value in the assessment of the depth of coma and has been used to an extent to identify a prognosis of coma,[21][22] its major role is in identifying patients who are in subclinical status epilepticus or have complex partial seizures, because this will significantly alter their

---

Box—Classification of differential diagnosis of coma

Coma without focal or lateralising signs and without meningism
1 Anoxic–ischaemic conditions
2 Metabolic disturbances
3 Intoxications
4 Systemic infections
5 Hyperthermia/Hypothermia
6 Epilepsy

Coma without focal or lateralising signs but with meningeal irritation
1 Subarachnoid haemorrhage
2 Meningitis
3 Encephalitis

Coma with focal brainstem or lateralising cerebral signs
1 Cerebral tumour
2 Cerebral haemorrhage
3 Cerebral infarction
4 Cerebral abscess

17

management.[23] It may also be useful in distinguishing between feigned or psychiatric coma, in which it will be normal, and genuine cerebral disease when it may show diffuse abnormalities or help to identify a focal lesion. The prognostic value of the EEG is probably not as great as that obtained from careful observation of clinical signs.[21]

Evoked potentials, predominantly brainstem evoked potentials, and somatosensory evoked potentials may give information relating to the intactness of brainstem pathways and to the existence of a cortical component. Theoretically the use of brainstem evoked responses could provide evidence for the presence and site of brainstem disease and, as they are relatively unaffected by drug coma, they may provide evidence on the aetiology.[24 25] Regrettably there is as yet little correlation between evoked response studies in coma and prognosis but it seems likely that the use of somatosensory evoked potentials and brainstem auditory evoked potentials will become of value in identifying the prognosis of patients in coma. One technical problem is the need to undertake these recordings in the busy premises of an intensive care unit where considerable other electrical interference is occurring.

Brain imaging techniques including computed tomography (CT) and magnetic resonance imaging (MRI) are important in coma in providing evidence of the diagnosis.[26] CT has a very significant role to play in identifying those patients who have a structural cause for coma, though MRI has not yet been formally evaluated in this respect and there are problems in inserting the patient in coma, together with necessary life support systems, into the field of the MRI scan.

Other, more complex techniques such as intracranial pressure monitoring and cerebral blood flow studies are rarely of help in the diagnosis of medical coma and their role in prognosis is not fully evaluated, although they are likely to be limited by their invasiveness.[27] Measures of biochemical parameters in coma are predominantly diagnostic but some measures such as brain type creatinine kinase and neuron specific enolase in the cerebrospinal fluid may help in determining prognosis.[28]

Diagnostic classification

On clinical grounds patients can be allocated to one of the following three varieties of coma.[29]

Coma with focal signs

Except in those patients in whom an underlying and irreversible terminal disease is recognised, it is obligatory that CT or MRI be undertaken to identify the cause of the coma. This will define whether or not a structural abnormality is present and in many instances give a clue to the underlying nature. If the CT scan is normal then the possibility of a non-structural focal abnormality antedating the onset of coma or being part of the coma, as occasionally happens with hypoglycaemia or hepatic encephalopathy, must be considered. If there is no focal structural abnormality on a CT scan then other investigations including metabolic and CSF examination should be carried out.

Once the image has been obtained the question of more definitive therapy, be it neurosurgical, the reduction of intracranial pressure by the use of steroids and mannitol, the application of a specific antibacterial or antiviral agent, or the use of chemotherapy may be considered.

Coma with meningeal irritation but without physical signs

Patients in this group will usually be suffering from subarachnoid haemorrhage, acute bacterial meningitis, or viral meningoencephalitis. The distinction between infective and non-infective can usually be made on the basis of fever and a lumbar puncture will be expected to reveal the cause. It is a counsel of perfection that, because of the theoretical potential of a collection of pus or of identifying the site of the subarachnoid haemorrhage, CT should be undertaken before lumbar puncture. In practice in many hospitals throughout the United Kingdom, CT of the head is not easily available and the presence of meningism, particularly if associated with fever, raises the possibility of meningitis and indicates the need for an assessment of the CSF.

When CSF examination is undertaken by lumbar puncture it is important to remember that an inadequate lumbar puncture does not preclude the possibility of a pressure cone but may prevent proper assessment of the CSF. Although some authorities still recommend that only a few millilitres of fluid need be obtained for bacterial culture and cell count,[12] in practice once the dura and arachnoid are breached by a lumbar puncture needle the possibility of herniation does not depend solely upon the fluid which is collected but rather upon that which may leak out during subsequent hours. It is therefore important that, when a decision to undertake a lumbar puncture is made, sufficient CSF is obtained to enable an adequate assessment of the cell count, and a Gram stain, and to provide fluid for culture and antibody analyses together with a measure of the total protein and sugar.

In those centres in which CT is available, the detection of blood in the subarachnoid space at CT precludes the need for lumbar puncture but, whether or not lumbar puncture has been carried out to identify the presence of subarachnoid haemorrhage, the patient should then be transferred to a neurosurgical unit, probably be given intravenous nimodipine, and be subjected to angiography and surgery. In general those patients who are in coma from subarachnoid haemorrhage are less of a surgical emergency than those who have higher states of consciousness.

Presence of coma without focal signs or meningism

These patients are likely to have a metabolic or anoxic cause for their coma. One of the commonest causes remains that of drug overdose and it is appropriate to withdraw blood to send to the toxicology laboratories in patients presenting in this way. In general there will be a clue from the circumstances in which the patient was discovered and from the previous history. Reliance is placed upon the assessment of metabolic and toxic metabolites in the blood and evidence should be sought for hepatic failure, renal failure, hyperglycaemia, hypoglycaemia, and disturbances of electrolytes or acidosis. Most commonly available drugs can now be assayed within blood, and serum enzymes should also be estimated. Problems inevitably arise when patients who are unconscious have been consuming alcohol and an assessment of the relevant importance of this in causing the unconsciousness may be difficult. Again the problem may be helped by the expedient of measuring blood alcohol levels.

Perhaps the most important single cause of unresponsiveness, which is directly treatable and correctable, is that of hypoglycaemia and this should have already been covered during the initial resuscitation of the patient. By this time in management the formal level of blood sugar will have been estimated and appropriate treatment for hypo- and hyperglycaemia may be instituted. The treatment of acid–base abnormalities will require not only routine biochemistry but arterial blood gas analysis to monitor progress. Usually a patient who has suffered from hypoxia or ischaemia will have been identified by the mode of presentation and by the normality of investigations thus far. The possibility of poisoning with carbon monoxide should be considered and excluded by the measurement of carboxyhaemoglobin. In general, patients who have suffered anoxic or ischaemic insult should be given 100% oxygen and the monitoring of PaO_2 will be important together with the maintenance of adequate circulation and oxygenation.

Patients who are in shock or hypertensive encephalopathy will be diagnosed by the level of blood pressure, and those with disturbed temperature regulation, by use of the thermometer, although a rectal thermometer may be required. These causes can then be corrected.

In patients with drug overdose the possibility of using specific antidotes should be considered: naloxone in patients in whom there is a high index of suspicion of opioid poisoning and benzodiazepine antagonists in self-poisoning with benzodiazepine. The use of analeptic agents in barbiturate poisoning cannot now be supported.[30] Consideration should also be given to clearing the ingested toxin from the stomach—the passage of a nasogastric tube should usually be considered and this is one indication for intubation of the trachea to prevent the risk of aspiration. The importance of the diagnosis of drug overdose coma is that such patients have a good prognosis provided that they are given adequate respiratory and circulatory support during their unconsciousness. They are, however, particularly liable to show sudden depression of brainstem responses and if the possibility of drug overdose is not considered their level of coma may be misinterpreted and their prognosis might be thought unduly pessimistic.

Prediction of outcome in coma

Having made an assessment of the cause of coma, established its severity, and introduced appropriate treatment, the physician should be able to identify the likely outcome to colleagues and to friends and relatives of the patient. Sedative drugs or alcohol overdose is not usually lethal and carries a good prognosis provided that circulation and respiration are protected. The physician can reasonably give a good prognosis in patients suffering from self-poisoning with sedative drugs provided that the complications of cardiac arrhythmia, aspiration pneumonia, and respiratory arrest are avoided or corrected. In non-traumatic coma other than that which is drug induced, those factors that determine the outcome have been defined[31] and include the cause of the coma, the depth of the coma, the duration of the coma, and certain clinical signs, among the most important of which are brainstem reflexes. Overall only 15% of patients in non-traumatic coma for more than six hours will make a good or moderate recovery; the other 85% will die, remain vegetative, or reach a state of severe disability in which they remain dependent.

Patients whose coma is due to metabolic reasons, including infection, organ failure, and biochemical disturbances, have a better prognosis. Thirty five per cent of patients will achieve moderate or good recovery; of those whose coma follows hypoxic ischaemic insult only 11% make such a recovery; of those in coma due to cerebrovascular disease only 7% can be expected to make such a recovery. Twenty per cent of patients in coma following hypoxic ischaemic injury will enter the vegetative state due to the likelihood of hypoxic ischaemia resulting in bihemispheric damage with relative sparing of the brainstem.

Apart from the diagnosis the depth of coma affects the individual prognosis. Those patients not showing eye opening after six hours of coma have only a 10% chance of making a good or moderate recovery whereas those whose eyes opened in response to painful stimuli have a 20% chance of making a good recovery. The longer the coma persists the less likely there is to be recovery; 15% of patients in coma for six hours make a good or moderate recovery compared with only 3% who remain unconscious for one week.[31]

The study of 500 patients reported by Levey *et al*[31] using prospective data from patients with clearly defined levels of coma, diagnoses, and outcomes showed that some clinical signs are significantly associated with a poor prognosis: in the total cohort of 500 patients, corneal reflexes were absent 24 hours after the onset of coma in 90 patients and this sign was incompatible with survival. In a more uniform group who suffered anoxic injury there were 210 patients: 52 of these had no pupillary reflex at 24 hours, all of whom died. By the third day 70 were left with a motor response poorer than withdrawal and all died. By the seventh day the absence of roving eye movements was seen in 16 patients all of whom died. The 95% confidence intervals for all of these criteria are given in table II.

At the opposite end of the scale more than 25% of patients who show roving conjugate eye movements within six hours of the

TABLE II—Clinical signs and prognosis

Time	Sign	Cohort	Patients with the sign	False positive survivors	95% confidence interval (%)
24 hours	Absent corneal response	500	90	0	0–5
24 hours	Absent pupillary response	210	52	0	0–5
3 days	Motor poorer than withdrawal	210	70	0	0–5
7 days	Absent roving eye movements	210	16	0	0–5

Summarised from Levy et al.[31]

onset of coma, or who show withdrawal responses to pain or eye opening to pain, will recover independence and make a moderate or good recovery. The use of combinations of clinical signs helps to improve the accuracy of prognosis: at 24 hours the absence of a corneal response, pupillary light reaction, or caloric or doll's eye response is not compatible with recovery to independence. Patients who are able to speak words within 24 hours or who show nystagmus on caloric testing are likely to make a good recovery (table III).[32]

The most accurate prediction of outcome in a patient in medical coma is still that which is obtained from the use of clinical signs and there is little to be added by more sophisticated testing other than in identifying the cause of the coma. It is possible to predict those patients who will not make a recovery and who will die in coma or who will enter a vegetative state within the first week of coma. It is rare for patients in medical coma who are in a vegetative state at one month to show any form of recovery.[33]

Continuation of care

The long term care of patients in coma may be undertaken in an intensive care unit, on a specialist ward, or later in a long stay hospital. It is important that those patients in whom prognosis is

23

TABLE III—Prediction of outcome of coma at 24 hours by a combination of clinical signs

		No. of patients	Percentage of patients with different outcomes		
			D/PVS	SD	MD/GR
500 patients					
Any two reacting: Pupils Corneals Oculovestibular	No	120	97	2	1
↓ Yes					
Motor better than flaccid	No	83	80	8	12
↓ Yes					
Motor withdrawal	No	135	69	14	17
↓ Yes					
Verbal moans	No	106	58	19	23
	Yes	56	46	13	41

Summarised from Levy et al.[31]
D/PVS = death or vegetative; SD = severe disability; MD/GR = moderate or good recovery.

hopeless should not be permanently exposed to the rigors of intensive care medicine, but should continue to receive basic care within routine hospital wards. So long as patients are considered to have a potential for recovery they should be looked after in intensive care units or on specialist wards. Their respiration, skin, circulation, and bladder and bowel function need attention, seizures controlled, and the level of consciousness regularly assessed and monitored. It is important that the mobility of joints and circulation to pressure areas are maintained during the long term care of the patient and the possibility of aspiration pneumonia, peptic ulceration, and other complications of long term intensive care be considered and avoided. In general, techniques such as mechanical ventilation and the use of steroid therapy are not to be used routinely in the management of the comatose patient since they do not improve prognosis and may specifically compromise recovery.[34]

Continuous vegetative state

The relative resilience of the brainstem allows it to survive injuries that may create irreversible damage to the cerebral hemispheres—then the patient will enter the state defined as vegetative. Retrospectively, after postmortem examination, it may be possible to identify massive neocortical damage which will indicate that the patient was permanently in the vegetative state,[35] although there are no laboratory means of confirming this before postmortem examination, the diagnosis of irreversibility can be established with a high degree of clinical certainty but is not absolute and is based on probability. It is suggested that the diagnosis may be considered when a patient has been in a continuing vegetative state following head injury for more than 12 months or following other causes of brain damage for more than 6 months.[36 37] Specialists in rehabilitation are concerned that physicians may take the attitude that there is no point in treating such patients, therefore creating a self fulfilling prophecy of poor prognosis, no treatment, and poor outcome.[38]

There is continuing debate as to the potential for recovery for patients who are vegetative. In patients who have suffered non-traumatic injury such as anoxia and ischaemia, the prognosis for recovery from the vegetative state is poor after the first few weeks. There are some reports of patients who have suffered coma as a result of head trauma in whom an improvement from the vegetative state has been recognised after months, but these anecdotal cases of recovery are difficult to validate and it seems possible that such patients were not truly vegetative, but rather in a state of profound disability with cognition, at the beginning of the observation.[39-41]

Investigations do not help to identify vegetative state because many types of EEG pattern have been recorded from near normality to a flat record and CT scans usually show considerable cortical atrophy with ventricular dilatation. Somatosensory evoked responses are said to show loss of the cortical component and positron emission tomography (PET) scans appear to show cortical metabolic underactivity. None is diagnostic in its results.[42]

Patients in a persisting vegetative state will often have received artificial ventilation at some time during their initial coma or resuscitation, but they are not truly respirator dependent and, as they are able to breathe, are only dependent upon carers for the

Management of medical coma

● The initial care for a patient in coma must be resuscitation by ensuring adequare oxygenation and circulation. A sample of blood should be withdrawn to estimate glucose and other parameters and, once stability is ensured, it is imperative to obtain an adequate history from those who brought the patient to the accident and emergency department or those who are responsible for the previous care.

● An assessment of the level of coma follows with an evaluation of those other features that may give clues as to aetiology, including temperature, heart rate, blood pressure, pattern of respiration, abnormalities in the skin, and focal signs in the chest, abdomen, or limbs. Neurological examination must include a search for evidence of trauma, tests for meningism, examination of the fundi, assessment of the brainstem reflexes, and the identification of any focal abnormality in face or limbs.

● The relevant investigations may then be considered, including biochemical and serological assessments, radiological imaging, and the possibility of EEG. Lumbar puncture will be indicated in certain circumstances and, with these investigations, the diagnosis of the aetiology of the coma should be established, corrective therapies instituted, and continuation of care and protection established.

● Most patients presenting to hospital in coma or lapsing into coma are ideally treated on an intensive care unit or a high dependency unit. The cause of the coma and the prognosis of the patient will determine their further follow up and the site of continuing care.

supply of liquid and nutrients, and the prevention of complications. The management of individual patients will depend upon circumstances, other aspects of the diagnosis, and consideration of prognosis.[43]

1 Bates D, Cartlidge NEF. The prognosis of medical coma. In: Tunbridge WMG, ed. *Advanced medicine*. London: Pittman Medical, 1981.
2 Plum F, Posner JB. *The diagnosis of stupor and coma*, 3rd ed. Philadelphia: Davis, 1980.
3 Brodal A. Neurological anatomy in relation to clinical medicine, 3rd ed. Oxford: Oxford University Press, 1981.
4 Jouvet M. The role of monoamines and acetyl choline containing neurones in the regulation of the sleep/wake cycle. *Rev Physiol* 1972;**64**:166–307.
5 Defeudis FV. Cholinergic roles in consciousness. In: Defeudis FV, ed. *Central cholinergic systems and behaviour*. London: Academic Press, 1974.

6 Tinuper P. Idiopathic recurring stupor; A case with possible involvement of the gamma aminobutyric acid(GABA)ergic system. *Ann Neurol* 1992;**31**:503–6.

7 Medical Research Council Brain Injuries Committee. A glossary of psychological terms commonly used in cases of head injury. MRC War Memorandum. London: HMSO, 1941.

8 Teasdale G, Jennett B. Assessment of coma and impaired consciousness: a practical scale. *Lancet* 1974;**2**:81–4.

9 Jennett B, Plum F. The persistent vegetative state: a syndrome in search of a name. *Lancet* 1972;**1**:734–7.

10 Cairns H. Disturbances of consciousness with lesions of the brain stem and diencephalon. *Brain* 1952;**75**:109–46.

11 Feldman MH. Physiological observations in a chronic case of locked in syndrome. *Neurol* 1971;**21**:459–78.

12 Harris JO, Berger JR. Clinical approach to stupor and coma. In: Bradley, Daroff, Fenichel, Marsden, eds. *Neurology in clinical practice*. London: Butterworth, 1991.

13 Fisher CM. The neurological examination of the comatosed patient. *Acta Neurol Scand* 1969;**45**(suppl 46):1–56.

14 De Jong RN. *The neurological examination*, 4th ed. Haggerstown: Harper and Rowe, 1979.

15 Crill WE. Horner's syndrome secondary to deep cerebral lesions. *Neurology* 1966;**16**:325–7.

16 Walsh FB, Hoyt WF. *Clinical neuro-ophthalmology*, 3rd ed. Baltimore: Williams and Wilkins, 1969.

17 Stewart JD, Kirkham TH, Mathieson G. Periodic alternating gaze. *Neurology* 1979;**29**:222–4.

18 Daroff RB, Hoyt FF. Supranuclear disorders of ocular control systems in man. In: Bach-y-Rita P, Collins C, Hyde G, eds. *The control of eye movements*. New York: Academic Press, 1971.

19 Fisher CM. Ocular bobbing. *Arch Neurol* 1964;**11**:543–6.

20 Leigh RJ, Shaw DA. Rapid regular breathing in unconscious patients. *Arch Neurol* 1976;**33**:356–61.

21 Jorgensen EO, Malchow-Moloer A. Natural history of global and critical brain ischaemia. *Resuscitation* 1981;**9**:133–91.

22 Synek VM. EEG abnormality grades and subdivisions of prognostic importance in traumatic and anoxic coma in adults. *Clin Electroencephalogr* 1988;**19**:160–6.

23 Engle J, Ludwig BI, Fetell M. Prolonged partial complex status epilepticus: EEG and behavioural observations. *Neurology* 1978;**28**:863–9.

24 Papanicolaou AC, Loring DW, Eisenberg HM, *et al.* Auditory brain stem evoked responses in comatosed head injured patients. *Neurosurgery* 1986;**18**:173–5.

25 Walser H, Emry M, Janzer R. Somatosensory evoked potentials in comatosed patients: correlation with outcome and neuropathological findings. *J Neurol* 1968;**233**:34–40.

26 Tasker RC, Matthew DJ, Kendall B. Computed tomography in the assessment of raised intracranial pressure in non-traumatic coma. *Neuropaediatrics* 1990;**21**:91–4.

27 Jaggi JL, Obrist WD, Jennarelli TA, Langfitt TW. Relationship of early cerebral blood flow and metabolism to outcome inacute head injury. *J Neurosurg* 1990;**72**:176–82.

28 Roine RO, Somer H, Caste M, *et al.* Neurological outcome after out of hospital cardiac arrest: prediction by cerebrospinal fluid enzyme analysis. *Arch Neurol* 1989;**46**:753–6.

29 Adams RD, Victor M. *Principles of neurology*, 4th ed. New York: McGraw Hill, 1989.

30 Schwartz GR. Emergency toxicology and general principles of medical management of the poisoned patient. In: Schwartz GR, Safar P, Stone N, *et al*, eds. *Principles and practice of emergency medicine*. London: WB Saunders, 1978.

31 Levy DE, Bates D, Caronna JJ, *et al.* Prognosis in non-traumatic coma. *Ann Intern Med* 1981;**94**:293–301.

32 Bates D. Coma. In: Swash M, Oxbury J, eds. *Clinical neurology*. Edinburgh: Churchill Livingstone, 1991.

33 Bates D. Defining prognosis in medical coma. *J Neurol Neurosurg Psychiatry* 1991;**54**:569–71.

34 Teasdale G. Prognosis of coma after head injury. In: Tunbridge WMG, ed. *Advanced medicine*. London: Pittman Medical, 1981.

35 Dogherty JH, Donald MD, Rawlinson DG, *et al.* Hypoxic-ischaemic brain injury in the vegetative state. *Neurol* 1981;**31**:991–7.

36 Andrews K. Managing the persistent vegetative state. *BMJ* 1992;**305**:486–7.

37 May PG, Kaelbling R. Coma of over a year's duration with favourable outcome. *Dis Nerv*

Syst 1968;**29**:837–40.

38 Rosenberg GA, Johnson SF, Brenner RP. Recovery of cognition after prolonged vegetative state. *Ann Neurol* 1977;**2**:167–8.

39 Snyder BD, Cranford RE, Rubens AB. Delayed recovery from postanoxic persistent vegetative state. *Ann Neurol* 1983;**14**:152–3.

40 Hansotia TI. Persistent vegetative state. *Arch Neurol* 1985;**42**:1048–52.

41 ANA Committee on Ethical Affairs. Persistent vegetative state: report of the American neurological association committee on ethical affairs. *Ann Neurol* 1993;**33**:386–90.

42 Multi-Society Task Force on PVS. Medical aspects of the persistent vegetative state (First Part). *N Eng J Med* 1994;**330**:1499–508.

43 Multi-Society Task Force on PVS. Medical aspects of the persistent vegetative state (Second part). *N Eng J Med* 1994;**330**:1572–9.

2 Head injury

J DOUGLAS MILLER

Head injury is one of the commonest disorders seen by doctors in hospital. It is therefore regrettable that in much of the United Kingdom today an unjustifiably pessimistic view about head injury continues to prevail. In fact, there have been major steps forward in understanding pathophysiology, facilitating diagnosis, and organising management of head injury. These have produced a 15–20% reduction in mortality following severe (coma producing) head injury with no increase in severe disability among survivors, and there is a strong indication that further improvements are possible. Determination of risk factors for secondary deterioration and a pre-emptive approach to management are important. Wider awareness of recent advances in thinking about traumatic brain injury is necessary so that resources can be appropriately allocated.

Epidemiology

Between 2000 and 3000 per million population are admitted to hospital each year because of head injury. For each patient admitted, three or four others have been seen in the accident and emergency department of the hospital or in the general practitioner's surgery and allowed home.[1 2]

Of those admitted to the hospital, approximately 5% or 100 per million per year, are suffering from severe head injury—in coma, scoring 8 or less on the Glasgow Coma Scale (GCS) with no eye opening, even to pain (table I). A further 5–10% are suffering from moderate traumatic brain injury, scoring between 9 and 12 on the Glasgow Coma Scale, while most (85–90%) are regarded

29

TABLE I—Glasgow Coma Scale for assessment of level of consciousness

Eye opening (E)

Spontaneous	4
To command	3
To pain	2
Nil	1

Best motor response (M)

Obeys commands	6
Localised pain	5
Normal flexion	4
Abnormal flexion	3
Extension	2
Nil	1

Verbal response (V)

Orientated speech	5
Disorientated speech	4
Words only	3
Sounds only	2
Nil	1

Severe head injury (coma) = E1, M5, V2 or less (GCS Sumscore 8 or less with no eye opening)

Moderate head injury	GCS Sumscore 9–12
Minor head injury	GCS Sumscore 13–15

as having suffered minor traumatic brain injury in terms of their level of consciousness on admission to hospital and score from GCS 13 to 15.[3-5] In fact, about a tenth of this group, although not obtunded significantly, are harbouring significant skull lesions which may include compound depressed skull fracture, linear skull fracture traversing an air sinus or dural venous sinus, or a small penetrating brain wound, each of which carries a potential risk of intracranial infection or haemorrhage.

In addition to the traumatic brain injury, many patients with head injury have extensive injuries elsewhere. In general, the more severe the traumatic brain injury, the greater the incidence of skull fracture and of multiple injury (table II).[6]

Pathophysiology of traumatic brain injury

It has been traditional to divide this into primary and secondary brain injuries. Primary brain injury was considered to be

TABLE II—Skull fractures, multiple injuries and severity of head injury (Edinburgh head injury admissions for 1981, 1986, and 1989)

	Severe GCS 3–8	Moderate GCS 9–12	Minor GCS 13–15	All head injuries
Number	302	492	3088	3882
Linear skull fracture	140 (46%)	152 (31%)	357 (12%)	649 (17%)
Depressed skull fracture	29 (10%)	9 (2%)	70 (2%)	108 (3%)
All skull fractures	169 (56%)	161 (33%)	427 (14%)	757 (20%)
Multiple injuries (% of number)	189 (63%)	183 (37%)	994 (32%)	1366 (35%)

Note that most patients with depressed skull fracture fall in the minor head injury group.

more or less complete at the time of impact and to be irreversible. The primary injuries include diffuse axonal injury consisting of scattered division of axons in the white matter of the brain signified within some days of injury by the development of retraction balls—swollen blobs of axoplasm. The distribution of these lesions is considered to be centripetal related to the force of injury so that extension of the lesions from the centrum semiovale down into the brainstem is a marker of an increasing degree of acceleration or deceleration associated with the injury.[7] The other form of primary brain injury is focal, caused by movement of the brain within the skull, and marked by subfrontal and temporal contusions and sometimes lacerations.[8] An additional form of focal brain injury is the cortical contusion and/or laceration that underlies the site of a direct blow on the skull, particularly if this is sufficiently severe to cause a depressed skull fracture.

The concept of primary diffuse axonal injury may now need to be modified in the light of recent evidence from experimental brain injuries. This suggests that while the brain movement associated with the injury may trigger off an axonal response, the subsequent events are progressive over a period of up to six hours, rather than being complete and final from the outset. These events consist of infolding of the axolemma and interruption of axoplasmic flow producing localised swelling of the axon at a stage when the axon still remains in continuity.[9 10] If the process continues, separation of the axon may follow with wallerian degeneration of the distal portion. It is possible therefore that, within the first few hours of head injury, at least, some of the diffuse axonal injury may be reversible. The process by which focal and polar brain contusions go on to produce brain necrosis is equally complex and is also prolonged over a period of hours. Cytotoxic processes include the release of free oxygen radicals, particularly the highly reactive hydroxyl radical, lipid peroxidation of cell membranes, opening of ion channels to influx of calcium, release of cytokines, and metabolism of free fatty acids into highly vasoreactive substances which may cause vasoconstriction and ischaemia.[11-14] Such processes may also be capable of interruption by mechanism-specific therapeutic agents such as lipid antioxidants, calcium channel blockers, and glutamate receptor antagonists. The search for secure evidence that new classes of drug based on these mechanisms reduce the morbidity and mortality of head injury will be one of the most important efforts of the 1990s.[15]

Secondary brain insults that may lead to ischaemic brain damage are extremely common after head injuries of all grades of severity, particularly if the head injury is associated with multiple injuries (box). Thus patients may suffer combinations of hypoxaemia, intracranial hypertension, arterial hypotension, pyrexia, and other adverse changes at recurrent intervals in the days following head injury.[16 17] These occur at a time when the normal regulatory mechanism by which the cerebrovascular resistance vessels can relax to maintain an adequate supply of oxygen and blood during such adverse events is impaired as a result of the original trauma.[18 19] In a recent detailed survey of 100 patients with severe, moderate, and minor head injury associated with other injuries, 92% of patients were found to have one or more

---

Box—Secondary insults to the injured brain

Systemic	*Intracranial*
Hypoxaemia	Haematoma (extradural,
Arterial hypotension	subdural, intracranial)
Hypercapnia	Brain swelling/oedema
Severe hypocapnia	Intracranial hypertension
Pyrexia	Cerebral vasospasm
Hyponatraemia	Intracranial infection
Anaemia	Epilepsy
Diffuse intravascular coagulopathy	

type of intracranial insult occurring for periods of five minutes or longer while being managed in a well staffed and well equipped intensive care unit (table III).[20 21]

Secondary brain damage is almost entirely ischaemic in type. It is extremely common and, as noted by Graham *et al*, continues to be found in more than 80% of fatal head injuries despite modern intensive management.[22 23] The ischaemic brain damage is, however, arrived at by a variety of intracranial or systemic mechanisms that are indicated in the box (page 31).

Another long held belief was that regeneration did not occur within the damaged CNS. It now appears that following traumatic brain injury there are vigorous attempts at regeneration within the brain, the proximal ends of severed axons produce multiple sprouts, and it is possible that some of the late improvements made by patients with severe diffuse axonal injury may represent successful regeneration. It seems sensible at this stage to at least admit the possibility of regeneration occurring, particularly in patients with diffuse axonal injury in whom there has been no major disruption of the cellular skeleton of brain tissue.[24]

In the light of current understanding of pathophysiology of traumatic brain injury, investigation and treatment of patients with head injury should be directed at early limitation of primary brain damage, prevention of secondary brain damage by early detection, and correction of adverse conditions in the form of

TABLE III—Frequency of secondary insults in 100 head injured patients during intensive care

Insult type	Number of patients monitored	Number in whom insult detected	Percentage of monitored patients
Raised intracranial pressure (>20 mm Hg)*	60	50	83
Reduced arterial pressure (<70 mm Hg)*	91	69	76
Reduced cerebral perfusion pressure (<60 mm Hg)*	58	45	78
Hypoxaemia (SaO$_2$ <90% or PaO$_2$ <8 kPa)*	90	39	43
Hypercapnia (PaCO$_2$ >6 kPa)*	57	17	30
Severe hypocapnia (PaCO$_2$ <3 kPa)*	57	21	35
Pyrexia (T >38° for more than 1 hour)	87	76	87

*For five minutes or more.

secondary insults, followed by maintenance of the patient in an optimal state of perfusion and brain nutrition to provide the most favourable milieu for any regeneration to take place.

Assessment and investigation

The goal of assessment is not only to discover how badly the patient has been injured, but also to determine the risk that further deterioration might supervene.

The assessment of the patient with head injury can begin at the roadside by the ambulance team who can report the obvious injuries, the level of blood pressure and heart rate, and score the patient on the Glasgow Coma Scale. Attention to the airway and circulation is of paramount importance during transportation of the patient to the hospital which should be an accident centre with the facilities implied by that term. Unfortunately, many injured patients arrive at the accident centre from the scene of the accident or from other hospitals in shock and/or hypoxic thereby considerably worsening the prognosis.[16 25]

Assessing and resuscitating the patient on arrival at the hospital should be done promptly and completely in the accident and emergency department. Security of the airway and stability of the circulation must be assured before the patient is moved anywhere in the hospital for any investigation or treatment, however urgent. All too often, the presence of a severe head injury leads to premature referral of the patient to the radiology department for CT before these basic conditions have been fulfilled, leading to predictably disastrous results if arterial hypotension occurs thereafter.

The neurological assessment of a patient with head injury is simplicity itself, consisting of scoring the patient on the Glasgow Coma Scale for the responses of eye opening, verbal response, and motor response to establish the level of consciousness, and noting any side to side difference in motor response so that hemiparesis may be detected. Painful stimuli must be applied above the neck as well as on the limbs, preferably supraorbital and mastoid process pressure, then heavy pressure on the nail beds of the little fingers and toes. This ensures that the lack of limb response due to high spinal cord injury is picked up. The only other essential element of the neurological examination at this stage is the pupillary response to light. Bilateral loss of pupillary light response is indicative of a lesion in the brainstem and is present in

20–25% of comatose patients with head injury.[26] Unilateral loss may be due to a lesion of the optic or oculomotor nerves and can be distinguished by comparing direct and consensual responses. Papilloedema is rare despite the fact that raised intracranial pressure is frequent.[27] Neurological examination is a valid index of brain damage only when blood pressure has been restored to a normal range and the patient is adequately oxygenated. Neurological assessment in the presence of ischaemia with or without hypoxia is unhelpful because it is unknown at that stage whether brain dysfunction is due to ischaemia or to injury.

In the patient with head injury it is crucial to discover all other injuries at this early stage of assessment. Pneumothorax or haemothorax needs to be detected and treated by chest drainage and, if there is any doubt about the possibility of intra-abdominal haemorrhage, then peritoneal lavage should be carried out. In a survey of 60 consecutive patients with severe head injury in whom concomitant trunk injury could not be excluded on history, peritoneal lavage revealed 10 positive cases with confirmation of a significant lesion in all 10 submitted to laparotomy. Only four of these patients were shocked on admission but it must be presumed that the remaining six would have become so had this injury remained undetected.[28]

Radiographs of the skull and a lateral radiograph of the cervical spine should be carried out in the accident and emergency department. The discovery of a fracture of the vault of the skull increases manyfold the risk that this patient, regardless of neurological status, will be harbouring an intracranial haematoma and is therefore an indication for recommending CT (table IV).[6 29 30] The discovery of a fluid level in the sphenoid sinus or intracranial air are indicative of basal skull fracture. These, and the presence of a depressed skull fracture or penetrating head wounds all signal an increased risk of intracranial infection.

CT has provided a major step forward in the management of head injuries in the last two decades. As CT becomes more widely available, the indications for CT after head injury are also widening and continue to yield positive findings. CT should be carried out on all patients with skull fracture, all patients who score below 15 on the Glasgow Coma Scale for 24 hours or more, and all patients with seizures or a focal neurological deficit.[29] Ideally every patient who has sustained a head injury and has been admitted to hospital should have CT.[31 32] In the head injured patient, CT may

TABLE IV—Intracranial haematoma (all types) versus skull fracture in different severities of head injury

Head injury	Haematoma (%)	No haematoma
Severe		
Fracture	74 (44)	94
No fracture	43 (32)†	91
Moderate		
Fracture	49 (29)	118
No fracture	25 (8)‡	299
Minor		
Fracture	42 (10)	391
No fracture	27 (1)§	2549

†$\chi^2 = 4\cdot49$; $p < 0\cdot05$.
‡$\chi^2 = 40\cdot26$; $p < 0\cdot001$.
§$\chi^2 = 123\cdot84$; $p < 0\cdot001$.

show an extracerebral haematoma—extradural or subdural; it will also show the amount of brain shift. Midline shift on CT greater than 10 mm and dilatation of the contralateral ventricle, or a loss of the image of the third ventricle and perimesencephalic cisterns indicate the presence or likelihood of high intracranial pressure.[33-35] CT may also show parenchymal lesions of increased density, indicating contusions, usually in the subfrontal and temporal area, deep intracerebral haematomas, and areas of lucency in the case of infarcts, although these become evident only after two or more days.

MRI is more sensitive in showing abnormal brain areas than CT and often yields positive findings in patients who have had what was considered to be only a minor head injury.[36] As most of these patients have returned to normality at six months, the significance of the MRI findings is uncertain.

Although seldom performed on head injured patients, there remains one important indication for angiography. This is for the patient who has an event leading to a head injury that is difficult to explain, where it may be suspected that a stroke or subarachnoid haemorrhage has occurred. Further indications for angiography may be the superimposition of suspected focal brain ischaemia due to traumatic vasospasm, an event that is seldom detected until the infarct has occurred.[37] Transcranial Doppler sonography may pick up some cases of post-traumatic cerebral vasospasm by documenting an abnormal increase in blood flow velocity in major intracranial vessels. However, such increases can be observed only if the cerebral perfusion pressure is normal.[38] Thus patients with raised intracranial pressure and vasospasm (a deadly combination) may fail to show increased velocity. Doppler sonography therefore requires to be accompanied by measurement of end tidal carbon dioxide and both arterial and intracranial pressure for correct interpretation of the findings.

Monitoring in patients with severe head injury

The normal brain requires a constant plentiful supply of blood, oxygen and glucose and, within limits, the resistance vessels of the cerebral circulation can respond by appropriate alterations of vascular calibre to alterations in perfusion pressure and the arterial tensions of oxygen and carbon dioxide. In the injured brain, these regulatory mechanisms are impaired.[18 19] A prime purpose of monitoring head injured patients is to measure continuously the arterial and intracranial pressure, the components of cerebral perfusion pressure ($CPP = BP - ICP$), and arterial oxygenation.[39] With this knowledge, levels can be adjusted to provide optimal perfusion and nutrition of the brain even when the normal regulatory mechanisms are impaired and cerebrovascular resistance is increased. Definition of these optimal levels is not straightforward, however, as these vary between patients and within individual patients over time. Another purpose of patient monitoring is to assess the effect of systemic events on brain function in a patient who is inaccessible to clinical evaluation.

In all patients with severe head injury, after a clear airway and adequate ventilation have been assured, arterial pressure should be monitored using an indwelling arterial cannula to provide a continuous record as well as convenient access for intermittent measurement of arterial blood gases. Arterial oxygen saturation should be monitored continuously using pulse oximetry. The issue of whether or not to monitor intracranial pressure is more controversial because current techniques are invasive and carry a risk of morbidity from intracranial infection (2–8%), intracranial haemorrhage (less than 1%), and epilepsy (less than 1%).[41] If it is accepted, however, that the cerebral perfusion pressure is important and that levels of arterial pressure are meaningless unless intracranial pressure is also known, then logic dictates that intracranial pressure should be monitored. Cerebral perfusion pressure is calculated from the difference between mean arterial and mean intracranial pressure using diastolic plus one third of pulse pressure or an electronically integrated mean pressure value. Recent studies indicate that a frequency of raised intracranial pressure of 80% or more is found in comatose head injured patients.[21][42] Although CT signs, such as loss of image of the third ventricle and perimesencephalic cisterns, are highly suggestive that intracranial pressure is, or will become, elevated, the absence of these findings is no guarantee of normal pressure. In eight severely head injured patients in whom admission CT showed no such indications of raised pressure, intracranial hypertension ensued in all but one case.[42a]

Intracranial pressure may be monitored by insertion of an intraventricular fluid filled catheter or by insertion of a solid state fibreoptic system into brain parenchyma, the lateral ventricle, or the subdural space.[43] Intracranial pressure should be monitored for three days after severe brain injury to cover the expected duration of formation of post-traumatic brain oedema and swelling. Monitoring can be continued for as long as episodes of intracranial hypertension occur and is normally discontinued after 48 hours of normal pressure recording.

In patients with severe head injury in whom raised intracranial pressure is anticipated, and particularly when treatment is required, much valuable information can be obtained from continuous monitoring of jugular venous oxygen saturation ($JvSO_2$).[40][44][45] This can now be measured continuously using an indwelling fibreoptic catheter system that requires to be precalibrated then calibrated in situ every 12 hours against measurements made by co-oximetry on withdrawn blood samples. $JvSO_2$ should lie in the range of 55–85%. Values above 85% are indicative of cerebral hyperaemia. Values below 55% indicate increasing cerebral oxygen extraction, and may occur when cerebral blood flow is reduced. Values below 45% indicate global cerebral ischaemia.

Continuous monitoring of brain electrical activity is valuable in the monitoring of the comatose head injured patient who is being artificially ventilated under the influence of muscle relaxant drugs. In such patients only the pupil light responses are available as an assessment of neurological function. Continuous measurements of EEG wave amplitude or frequency are helpful but need to be interpreted in the light of drug administration.

Velocity of blood flow in the intracranial arteries, notably the middle cerebral artery, can be measured intermittently or continuously for periods of several hours using transcranial Doppler sonography. With decreasing cerebral perfusion pressure, mean flow velocity decreases from the normal value of 55–65 cm/s but diastolic flow velocity decreases more than systolic flow velocity.[40 46] As a result, the pulsatility index, a dimensionless figure derived from the difference between systolic and diastolic flow velocity divided by mean flow velocity, increases from the normal value of around unity to three or more. Combined measurements of cerebral perfusion pressure, Doppler measurement of pulsatility index and JvSO$_2$ in patients with severe head injury have shown that below a threshold perfusion pressure level of 70 mm Hg, pulsatility index starts to increase and JvSO$_2$ starts to fall.[40] At perfusion pressures greater than 70 mm Hg there is no further increase in JvSO$_2$, suggesting that while a CPP level of 70 mm Hg is optimal for the head injured patient, the achievement of higher levels does not confer further advantage.

Doppler flow velocities may also be abnormally high (>100 cm/s) in the patient with head injury at perfusion pressure level of 70 mm Hg or above.[38] Such increased velocity may be due to a true increase in volume flow that would be signalled by an increase in JvSO$_2$ over 85%, or they may be caused by narrowing of the insonated vessels—cerebral vasospasm. In the latter case, JvSO$_2$ may be normal or low. While measurement of JvSO$_2$ can be used in this way to distinguish vasospasm from hyperaemia, it appears that inspection of the Doppler waveform can also provide this information, non-hyperaemic patients showing a dicrotic notch on the descending arm of the Doppler wave, whereas hyperaemic patients do not show such a notch.[47]

Management of patients with head injury

The goal of management of these patients is to prevent wherever possible the occurrence of secondary insults to the injured brain, both intracranial and systemic, and where this is not possible, to detect such insults as early as possible and reverse them. The injured brain is extremely vulnerable to such insults, for example, a single episode of arterial hypotension or raised intracranial pressure lasting only a few minutes may be sufficient to arrest the cerebral circulation which then fails to re-establish even when normal pressures have been regained and brain death ensues. Experimental data confirm this additive effect.[48] For this reason, a pre-emptive approach to head injury management is essential, aiming to identify patients and situations that carry a high risk of development of insults.

To ensure that the airway is clear and ventilation adequate, early endotracheal intubation and artificial ventilation is increasingly being employed to cover patients during transportation between hospitals and within the hospital, for example, between the accident and emergency department and CT imaging. It is crucial therefore that the level of consciousness of the patient be reliably assessed before the administration of sedative and/or relaxant drugs. In addition to assessing the severity of head injury, the earliest opportunity should be taken to assess the patient for any other injuries. Multiple injuries are present in more than 50% of patients with severe head injury and in a substantial proportion of patients with less severe injury. In a comatose patient it is important to exclude intra-abdominal bleeding, if necessary by peritoneal lavage, or mini-laparotomy, rather than await the onset of arterial hypotension. When arterial hypotension (systolic BP <90 mm Hg) is present it must be assumed that it is due to other injuries rather than to brain injury.

Patients with skull fracture with or without a depressed level of consciousness, abnormal neurological signs, or early seizures should all have CT as soon as possible, even if this means transfer from one hospital to another. More than 40% of comatose patients with head injury have intracranial haematomas and it is now clear that there are no clinical signs that allow the clinician to distinguish reliably between patients with intracranial haematomas and those with diffuse brain injury and swelling. Although it has been argued that transport of head injured patients from one hospital to another can be hazardous and time consuming, a recent study indicates that most delay occurs within the referring hospital because of slow recognition that the patient is at risk from intracranial bleeding.[49]

It cannot be emphasised enough that patients should be moved from the resuscitation area of the accident and emergency department only when the airway is secure and the circulation stable. If a stable circulation cannot be obtained, it must be assumed that the patient has occult intra-abdominal or other haemorrhage and steps must be taken to diagnose this by peritoneal lavage and correct it, whether by surgery or endovascular approaches. This takes precedence over the performance of CT and any intracranial surgery and in such cases CT should be deferred until the systemic emergency has been dealt with.

Aspects of surgical management

In cases where CT reveals an intracranial haematoma, the next decision is whether surgical evacuation is required. As a general rule, urgent evacuation of extracerebral haematomas that are associated with 5 mm or more of midline shift or are 25 ml or more in calculated volume, or both, should be carried out. The younger the patient the more ready the surgeon should be to evacuate a haematoma because of the less compliant nature of the craniospinal contents.

In cases where the extracerebral (extradural or subdural) haematoma is considered to be too small to warrant surgical evacuation, it is essential that CT be repeated after a few hours in all patients in whom the first CT scan has been carried out within six hours of injury. A significant number of such early diagnosed extradural haematomas will be found to have expanded considerably over the ensuing few hours, and it is in keeping with the pre-emptive approach to management that these haematomas be diagnosed before the patient manifests clinical signs of distress.[50]

The role of early operative treatment in the management of intracerebral haematomas and haemorrhagic contusions is more controversial.[26] Although some advocate early surgery in such cases, experience has shown that despite surgical treatment, postoperative intracranial hypertension continues to occur in virtually all patients, and a growing number of neurosurgeons prefer to manage such patients conservatively at first, relying upon continuous monitoring of arterial and intracranial pressure and repeat CT to pick up those cases in which a progressive increase in pressure and an increase in mass effect may warrant delayed operative evacuation of the haematoma.

In comatose patients in whom a sizeable extracerebral haematoma is disclosed, it is important that the brain be decompressed as soon as possible. A standard practice is to administer a large bolus dose of mannitol solution, 1 g/kg bodyweight, rapidly while the patient is still in the CT suite, then to transport the patient to operating theatre, and to proceed as quickly as possible to the point where the skull can be opened and haematoma evacuated from the extradural or subdural space. In this situation, minutes count but it is also important that decompression is effective and this usually demands more access than can be gained by a burr hole.

The other situation in which neurosurgical procedures may be required soon after injury is for complex head wounds such as a compound depressed skull fracture, particularly when dural tearing is involved as it is in 50% of cases.[51] While it is important that debridement of the wound, removal of haematoma or contaminating foreign matter, and sound wound closure be obtained quickly to avoid infection, there is not the same degree of urgency about these procedures as is necessary for evacuation of intracranial haematoma.[52] It is sensible for the team to take up to six hours if that is necessary to obtain the best possible operating conditions to minimise the extent of any brain swelling and possible extrusion of brain tissue of doubtful viability through the compound wound.

Non-operative management

In patients managed by artificial ventilation, arterial PCO_2 is kept in the range 3·5–4·5 kPa and SaO_2 should be kept as close to 100% as possible, employing where necessary an increase in the fractional concentration of inspired oxygen (FiO_2) and positive end expiratory pressure (PEEP). Arterial pressure should not be allowed to fall. The common causes of arterial hypotension are unsuspected hypovolaemia due to inadequate fluid replacement and the administration of sedative drugs such as barbiturates and propofol. The combination of hypovolaemia and sedative drug administration is particularly dangerous.[53 54]

Intracranial pressure should ideally be held below 20 mm Hg. Moderate increases to 25 mmHg or even 30 mm Hg may be tolerated provided arterial pressure is sufficient to yield a cerebral perfusion pressure of 70 mm Hg or more. When intracranial pressure rises above 25 mm Hg checks should be made for simple causes of intracranial hypertension such as excessive flexion or rotation of the neck, obstruction of the airway, loss of effect of relaxant drugs with the patient making respiratory efforts against the ventilator, elevations in arterial PCO_2 or body temperature, or occult epileptic seizures.[55] In patients receiving muscle relaxants seizures may be difficult to detect but may be signalled by bilateral pupillary dilatation and a small increase in arterial pressure accompanied by a larger increase in intracranial pressure. One of the advantages of continuous recording of brain electrical activity is that it becomes easier to detect such seizures.

Another important cause of intracranial hypertension is water overload causing dilutional hyponatraemia.[56 57] The most important surgical cause of intracranial hypertension is development of an intracranial mass lesion due to delayed haemorrhage or development of brain oedema and swelling. Surgical decompression may be required to reduce brain shift and distortion as well as reducing intracranial pressure.

When intracranial pressure rises above 25 mm Hg within the first 48 hours after injury, or 30 mm Hg thereafter and cerebral perfusion pressure is threatened, specific therapy may be required to reduce intracranial pressure if simple corrective measures have been applied and failed. Intracranial pressure therapy should ideally be directed at the cause of the increase in pressure, which may be divided simply into vascular and non-vascular causes. In the case of vascular intracranial hypertension there is vasodilatation with an increase in volume of blood in the capillary and venous beds, and the most appropriate therapy is one that will reduce the calibre of the cerebral resistance vessels. The simplest measure is hyperventilation with further reduction of arterial PCO_2 to 3·5 kPa with the aim of inducing some cerebral vasoconstriction. Although this is often a useful temporary measure the effect cannot be long lasting and there is a real risk that excessive cerebral vasoconstriction may result in ischaemia.[58] In this situation continuous monitoring of $JvSO_2$ is valuable. Excessive hyperventilation that produces cerebral ischaemia will be rapidly signalled by a fall in $JvSO_2$ to less than 45%. For a longer lasting effect, infusion of sedative or hypnotic drugs can be used— thiopentone sodium or propofol. These drugs are most effective if cerebrovascular carbon dioxide reactivity is preserved.[59] The use of these drugs must be very carefully monitored because of their effect on blood pressure. Again, continuous monitoring of $JvSO_2$ will provide an immediate indication if a moderate reduction in arterial blood pressure is sufficient to cause global cerebral ischaemia. This is a signal to reduce the infusion rate of the sedative drug, or even stop it altogether. Indomethacin infusion is under investigation as an alternative means of reducing raised intracranial pressure.[60]

In the case of intracranial hypertension of non-vascular origin, due to brain oedema, the most appropriate therapy is intravenous mannitol solution. When given for this purpose the lowest dose of mannitol should be used that is sufficient to lower intracranial pressure and improve cerebral perfusion pressure. As a rough guide a starting dose of 0·5 g/kg body weight should be used and subsequent doses adjusted upwards or downwards as determined by the response of intracranial pressure and cerebral perfusion pressure. The effect may be enhanced by administering frusemide while mannitol is being given and following the mannitol by albumin infusion.[61 62] Mannitol solution should not be administered if the serum osmolality is greater than 320 mmol/kg as it will not only be ineffective but carries a grave risk of producing renal failure. On occasion it may be necessary to support the arterial blood pressure with pressor agents to maintain an adequate level of cerebral perfusion pressure. At present there is no consensus on the best pressor agent to employ.

Drug therapy and head injury

There is no place for steroid therapy as a treatment for brain injury or for acute post-traumatic brain oedema. Numerous trials of steroids at various doses have produced either negative or inconclusive results and one study recorded an adverse effect of steroids in patients with severe head injury with raised intracranial pressure.[63 64]

At present, trials are under way on the effect of various neuroprotective drugs, calcium ion channel, or N-methyl-D-aspartate-type glutamate receptor blocking agents or antioxidants acting in the cell membrane. Although there is promising information from experimental studies, firm conclusions have not yet been reached on the value of neuroprotective agents in head injured patients.[15]

Prophylactic anticonvulsant drugs are no longer in vogue in the treatment of head injury following trials where no convincing preventative effect was shown. Post-traumatic epilepsy is, however, not uncommon. When it does occur later than one week from the time of injury then patients should be started on appropriate anticonvulsant drug therapy.

44

Similar controversy exists on the role of prophylactic antibiotic therapy in the case of patients with intracranial air, CSF rhinorrhoea, or otorrhoea and who are therefore at increased risk of developing meningitis after head injury. Opinions on the value of prophylactic antibiotics are sharply divided, with forceful opinions both for the need to provide adequate antibiotic prophylaxis and the opposing school which argues that such treatment only encourages the development of antibiotic resistant strains of bacteria.

Outcome from head injury

With increasing understanding of the pathophysiology of primary and secondary brain injury and the adoption of a preemptive approach to patient management based upon knowledge of risk factors for development of secondary brain damage, the mortality rate of severe head injury has fallen from 50% to between 30% and 40% over the past two decades.[26 65] The proportion of patients with severe head injury who remain severely disabled at six months or longer following head injury remains disappointingly at 10–20% while only a small number of patients survive in the persistent vegetative state. At six months or later only 1–3% of severely injured patients fall into this category. The remaining surviving patients divide more or less equally into those who make good recovery and return to the pre-injury level of function, even though there may be small residual deficits, and moderately disabled patients who, although independent for activities of daily living, do not ever return to their previous level of function. The challenge of the last years of this century will be to reduce the disability suffered by the survivors of severe and moderate head injury and thus improve the quality of life for these patients and their families.

One difficulty is that factors that predict increased mortality such as advancing age, low coma score, and signs of brainstem dysfunction are less effective in predicting disability in survivors.[66 67] There is a suggestion that secondary insults such as intracranial hypertension and low cerebral perfusion pressure are not only associated with higher mortality but also associated with an increase in severe disability.[26] It remains to be determined whether reduction in the burden of secondary insults suffered by patients with head injury will diminish disability in survivors.

45

Management of head injuries

● Assessment should begin at the scene of the accident at the same time as resuscitation with attention to airway and circulation which must be maintained throughout transfer and investigation.

● Neurological assessment includes scoring on the Glasgow Coma Scale, measurement of the pupil size and light response, and comparison of motor responses on the left and right side.

● Investigation includes a search for other injuries, plain radiographs of skull and cervical spine, imaging of the skull and brain by CT for all patients with impairment of consciousness or fracture of the skull, with radiographs of other areas and peritoneal lavage where indicated.

● In comatose patients and those with inadequate gas exchange, intubation and artificial ventilation are indicated.

● Extracerebral haematomas should be evacuated very urgently (within minutes) unless very small with no midline shift, in which case CT should be repeated. Mannitol (1 g/kg bodyweight) should be given while the patient is being prepared for surgery.

● In severe head injury (GCS 8 or less) monitoring of arterial and intracranial pressure, heart rate, body temperature, and arterial oxygen saturation should be done, and measurement of intracranial arterial blood flow velocity and jugular bulb oxygen saturation considered.

● Compound depressed fractures should be operated on urgently (within hours) to prevent infection. A dural tear is present in 50% of cases.

● Artificial ventilation and continuous monitoring should be continued until the patient is physiologically stable and, ideally, intracranial pressure has been normal for 48 hours.

● The use of prophylactic anticonvulsants and antibiotics is not currently recommended. Neuroprotective drugs are under investigation.

1 Kalsbeek WD, McLaurin RL, Harris BSH, Miller JD. The National Head and Spinal Cord Injury Surgery: Major findings. *J Neurosurg* 1980;**53** (Suppl):S19–31.
2 Jennett B, McMillan R. Epidemiology of head injury. *BMJ* 1981;**282**:101–4.
3 Teasdale G, Jennett B. Assessment of coma and impaired consciousness. *Lancet* 1974;**2**:81–4.

4 Miller JD, Jones PA. The work of a regional head injury service. *Lancet* 1985;**1**:1141–4.
5 Miller JD, Jones PA, Dearden NM, Tocher JL. Progress in the management of head injury. *Br J Surg* 1992;**79**:60–4.
6 Miller JD. Minor, moderate and severe head injury. *Neurosurg Rev* 1986;**9**:135–9.
7 Adams JH, Mitchell DE, Graham DI, Doyle D. Diffuse brain damage of immediate impact type. *Brain* 1977; **100**:489–502.
8 Adams JH. Head injury. In: Hume-Adams J, Corsellis JAN, Duchen LW, eds. *Greenfield's neuropathology*, 4th ed. London: Edward Arnold, 1984:85–124.
9 Yaghmai A, Povlishock J. Traumatically induced reactive change as visualised through the use of mono-clonal antibodies targeted to neurofilament subunits. *J Neuropathol Exp Neurol* 1992;**51**:158–76.
10 Povlishock JT. Traumatically induced axonal injury: pathogenesis and pathobiological implications. *Brain Pathol* 1992;**2**:1–12.
11 Kontos HA, Wei EP. Superoxide production in experimental brain injury. *J Neurosurg* 1986;**64**:803–7.
12 Ikeda Y, Long DM. The molecular basis of brain injury and brain edema: the role of oxygen free radicals. *Neurosurgery* 1990;**27**:1–11.
13 Hayes RL, Stonnington HW, Lyeth BG, Dixon CE, Yamamoto T. Metabolic and neurophysiologic sequelae of brain injury. A cholinergic hypothesis. *J Central Nervous System Trauma* 1986;**3**(2):163–73.
14 Wahl M, Unterberg A, Baethmann A, Schilling L. Mediators of blood-brain barrier dysfunction and formation of vasogenic brain edema. *J Cereb Blood Flow Metabol* 1988;**8**: 621–34.
15 Hall ED. The neuroprotective pharmacology of methyl prednisolone. *J Neurosurg* 1992; **76**:13–22.
16 Miller JD, Sweet RC, Narayan R, Becker DP. Early insults to the injured brain. *JAMA* 1978;**240**:4319–442.
17 Miller JD, Becker DP. Secondary insults to the injured brain. *J Roy Coll Surg Edin* 1982;**27**:292–8.
18 Lewelt W, Jenkins LW, Miller JD. Autoregulation of cerebral blood flow after experimental fluid percussion injury of the brain. *J Neurosurg* 1980;**53**:500–11.
19 Lewelt W, Jenkins LW, Miller JD. Effects of experimental fluid percussion injury of the brain on cerebrovascular reactivity to hypoxia and hypercapnia. *J Neurosurg* 1982;**56**:332–8.
20 Andrews PJD, Piper IR, Dearden NM, Miller JD. Secondary insults during intrahospital transport of head injured patients. *Lancet* 1990;**335**:327–30.
21 Jones PA, Andrews PJD, Midgley S, *et al.* Measuring the burden of secondary insults in head injured patients during intensive care. *J Anesth Neurosurg* 1994;**6**:4–14.
22 Graham DI, Adams JH, Doyle D. Ischaemic brain damage in fatal non-missile head injuries. *J Neurol Sci* 1978;**39**:213–34.
23 Graham DI, Ford I, Hume-Adams J, Doyle D, Teasdale GM, Lawrence AE, McLellan DR. Ischaemic brain damage is still common in fatal non-missile head injury. *J Neurol Neurosurg Psychiatry* 1989;**52**:346–50.
24 Povlishock JT, Erb DE, Astruc J. Axonal response to traumatic brain injury: reactive axonal change, deafferentation and neuroplasticity. *J Neurotrauma* 1992;**9**(Suppl 1):S189-200.
25 Gentleman D, Jennett B. Audit of transfer of unconscious head injured patients to a neurosurgical unit. *Lancet* 1990;**335**:330–4.
26 Miller JD, Butterworth JF, Gudeman SK, *et al.* Further experience in the management of severe head injury. *J Neurosurg* 1981;**54**:289–99.
27 Selhorst JB, Gudeman SK, Butterworth JF, Harbison JW, Miller JD, Becker DP. Papilledema after acute head injury. *Neurosurgery* 1985;**16**:357–63.
28 Butterworth JF, Maull KI, Miller JD, Becker DP. Detection of occult abdominal trauma in patients with severe head injuries. *Lancet* 1980;**2**:759–62.
29 Teasdale GM, Murray G, Anderson E, *et al.* Risks of acute traumatic intracranial haematoma in children and adults: implications for managing head injuries. *BMJ* 1990;**300**:363–7.
30 Chan KH, Mann KS, Yue CP, Fan YW, Cheung M. The significance of skull fracture in acute traumatic intracranial hematomas in adolescents: a prospective study. *J Neurosurg* 1990;**72**:189–94.
31 Bricolo AP, Pasut LM. Extradural haematoma: towards zero mortality. *Neurosurgery* 1984;**14**:8–12.

32 Servadei F, Piazza G, Seracchioli A, Acciarri N, Pozzati E, Gaist G. Extradural haematomas: an analysis of the changing characteristics of patients admitted from 1980 to 1986. Diagnostic and therapeutic implications in 158 cases. *Brain Injury* 1988;**2**:87–100.

33 Teasdale E, Cardoso E, Galbraith S, Teasdale G. CT scan in severe diffuse head injury: physiological and clinical consultations. *J Neurol Neurosurg Psychiatry* 1984;**47**:600–3.

34 Colquhoun IR, Burrows EH. The prognostic significance of the third ventricle and basal cisterns in severe closed head injury. *Clin Radiol* 1989;**40**:13–6.

35 Marshall LF, Marshall SB, Klauber MR, *et al*. A new classification of head injury based on computerised tomography. *J Neurosurg* 1991;**75**:S14-20.

36 Levin HS, Amparo E, Eisenberg HM, *et al*. Magnetic resonance imaging and computerised tomography in relation to the neurobehavioural sequelae of mild and moderate head injuries. *J Neurosurg* 1987;**66**:706–13.

37 Macpherson P, Graham DI. Correlation between angiographic findings and the ischaemia of head injury. *J Neurol Neurosurg Psychiatry* 1978;**41**:122–7.

38 Chan KH, Dearden NM, Miller JD. The significance of post-traumatic increase in cerebral blood flow velocity: a transcranial doppler ultrasound study. *Neurosurgery* 1992;**30**:697–700.

39 Miller JD, Stanek AE, Langfitt TW. Concepts of cerebral perfusion pressure and vascular compression during intracranial hypertension. In: Meyer JS, Schade JP, eds. *Progress in brain research, vol 35: cerebral blood flow*. Amsterdam: Elsevier, 1972:411–32.

40 Chan KH, Miller JD, Dearden NM, Andrews PJD, Midgley S. The effect of changes in cerebral perfusion pressure upon middle cerebral artery blood flow velocity and jugular venous oxygen saturation after severe brain injury. *J Neurosurg* 1992;**77**:55–61.

41 Lundberg N. Continuous recording and control of ventricular fluid pressure in neurosurgical practice. *Acta Psychiat Neurol Scand* 1960;**36**(Suppl 149):1–193.

42 Marmarou A, Anderson RL, Ward JD, *et al*. Impact of ICP instability and hypotension on outcome in patients with severe head trauma. *J Neurosurg* 1991;**75**:S59-66.

42a O'Sullivan MG, Statham PF, Jones PA, *et al*. Role of intracranial pressure monitoring in severely head injured patients without signs of intracranial hypertension on initial computerised tomography. *J Neurosurg* 1994;**86**:46–50.

43 Crutchfield JS, Narayan RK, Robertson CS, Michael LH. Evaluation of a fibreoptic intracranial pressure monitor. *J Neurosurg* 1990;**72**:482–7.

44 Dearden NM. Jugular bulb venous oxygen saturation in the management of severe head injury. *Curr Opin Anaesthesiol* 1991;**4**:279–86.

45 Sheinberg M, Kanter MJ, Robertson CS, Contant CF, Narayan RK, Grossman RG. Continuous monitoring of jugular venous oxygen saturation in head injured patients. *J Neurosurg* 1992;**76**:212–7.

46 Chan KH, Miller JD, Dearden NM. Intracranial blood flow velocity after head injury: relationship to severity of injury, time, neurological status and outcome. *J Neurol Neurosurg Psychiatry* 1992;**55**:787–91.

47 Chan KH, Dearden NM, Miller JD, Piper IR. Transcranial Doppler waveform differences in hyperaemic and non-hyperaemic patients after severe head injury. *Surg Neurol* 1992;**38**:433–6.

48 Jenkins LW, Moszynski K, Lyeth BG, *et al*. Increased vulnerability of the mildly traumatised rat brain to cerebral ischemia: the use of controlled secondary ischemia as a research tool to identify common or different mechanisms contributing to mechanical and ischemic brain injury. *Brain Res* 1989;**477**:211–24.

49 Marsh H, Maurice-Williams R, Hatfield R. Closed head injuries: where does delay occur in the process of transfer to neurosurgical care? *Br J Neurosurg* 1989;**3**:13–20.

50 Knuckey NW, Gelbard S, Epstein MH. The management of "asymptomatic" epidural hematomas. A prospective study. *J Neurosurg* 1989;**70**:392–6.

51 Miller JD, Jennett B. Complications of depressed skull fractures. *Lancet* 1968;**2**:991–5.

52 Sutcliffe JC, Miller JD, Whittle IR, Steers AJW. Gas gangrene occurring soon after compound depressed skull fracture. *Acta Neurochir* 1988;**95**:53–6.

53 Schwartz ML, Tator CH, Rowed DW, Reid SR, Megura K, Andrews DF. The University of Toronto Head Injury treatment study: a prospective randomised comparison of pentobarbital and mannitol. *Can J Neurol Sci* 1984;**11**:434–40.

54 Ward JD, Becker DP, Miller JD, *et al*. Failure of prophylactic barbiturate coma in the treatment of severe head injury. *J Neurosurg* 1985;**62**:383–8.

55 Miller JD, Dearden NM, Piper IR, Chan KH. Control of intracranial pressure in patients with severe head injury. *J Neurotrauma* 1992;**9**(Suppl 1):S317–26.

48

56 Arieff AI. Hyponatremia associated with permanent brain damage. *Adv Intern Med* 1987;**32**:325–44.
57 Bertrand YM, Herman A, Mahieu P, Roels J. Intracranial pressure changes in patients with head trauma during haemodialysis. *Intensive Care Med* 1983;**9**:321–3.
58 Muizelaar JP, Marmarou A, Ward JD, *et al.* Adverse effects of prolonged hyperventilation in patients with severe head injury: a randomised clinical trial. *J Neurosurg* 1991;**75**:731–9.
59 Nordstrom CH, Messeter K, Sundbarg G, Schalen W, Werner M, Ryding E. Cerebral blood flow, vasoreactivity and oxygen consumption during barbiturate therapy in severe traumatic brain lesions. *J Neurosurg* 1988;**68**:424–31.
60 Jensen K, Ohrstrom J, Cold JE, Astrup J. The effects of indomethacin on intracranial pressure, cerebral blood flow and cerebral metabolism in patients with severe head injury and intracranial hypertension. *Acta Neurochir* 1991;**108**:116–21.
61 Roberts PA, Pollay M, Engles C, Pendleton B, Reynolds E, Stevens FA. Effect on intracranial pressure of furosemide combined with varying doses and administration rates of mannitol. *J Neurosurg* 1987;**66**:440–6.
62 Albright AL, Latchaw RE, Robinson AG. Intracranial and systemic effects of osmotic and oncotic therapy in experimental cerebral edema. *J Neurosurg* 1984;**60**:481–9.
63 Braakman R, Schouten HJD, Van Dishoeck BM, Minderhoud JM. Megadose steroids in severe head injury results of a prospective double blind clinical trial. *J Neurosurg* 1983;**58**:326–30.
64 Dearden NM, Gibson JS, McDowall DG, Gibson RM, Cameron MM. Effect of high dose dexamethasone on outcome from severe head injury. *J Neurosurg* 1986;**64**:81–8.
65 Marshall LF, Gautille T, Klauber MR, *et al.* The outcome of severe closed head injury. *J Neurosurg* 1991;**75**:S28-36.
66 Jennett B, Teasdale G, Braakman R, Minderhoud J, Heiden J, Kurze T. Prognosis of patients with severe head injury. *Neurosurgery* 1979;**4**:283–9.
67 Braakman R, Gelpke GJ, Habbema JDF, Maas AIR, Minderhoud J. Systematic selection of prognostic features in patients with severe head injury. *Neurosurgery* 1980;**6**:362–70.

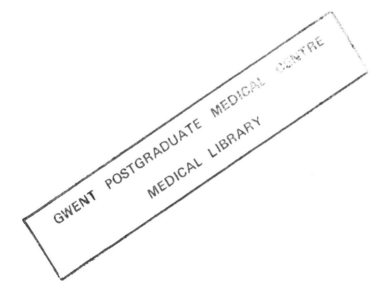

3 Ischaemic stroke

R S MARSHALL, J P MOHR

Epidemiological studies have quantified the seriousness of stroke. Its incidence averages 179 per 100 000 per year worldwide with a prevalence of 500–600 per 100 000. Eight to 20% of its victims die in the first 30 days.[1] Early recurrence adds to the neurological deficit and lengthens hospital stay. Late recurrence affects 4–14% per year and five year survival averages only 56% for men, 64% for women.[2] Overall, recurrence contributes to the $16 billion in health care costs and lost productivity seen annually in the United States alone.[3]

Once considered untreatable, ischaemic stroke has become subject to emerging therapies and is entering a new era, one that justifies a chapter focusing on treatment as well as the expected issues of diagnosis and delineation of risk factors. Increases in the understanding of the pathophysiology of stroke subtypes is steadily improving the outlook for more specific therapies for stroke analogous to the changes in outlook for myocardial infarction. Frustrated hopes for older therapies have given way to renewed confidence in newer lines of approach. Evidence from animal studies and preliminary clinical trials suggests that the ischaemic process may require several hours to develop, offering the possibility of preventing irreversible infarction. Uncontrolled intracellular influx of calcium is the current major culprit, although doubtless others will be as well documented in future. Antioxidants, free radical scavengers, and more exotic agents to block the developing necrosis after arterial occlusions are not yet well enough understood to predict their future in stroke therapy. Some of the older therapies such as anticoagulation are making a comeback while surgery for some indications has at last proved of value.

Hyperacute therapy for ischaemic stroke

Thrombolytic therapy

Increasing experience with thrombolytic agents, mainly recombinant tissue plasminogen activator (rTPA), has demonstrated instances of significant and sustained neurological improvement when thrombolytic treatment is initiated within the first few hours. Better outcomes are generally associated with documented recanalisation of the artery feeding the symptomatic region. What remains uncertain is whether the timing of therapy is more important than specific dose and whether delays increase the risk of complications, negating any benefits.

A multicentre, phase 1 trial evaluated the safety and efficacy of intravenous administration of rTPA in the treatment of acute ischaemic stroke.[4 5] Patients were stratified and evaluated separately for those treated within 90 minutes[4] and between 91 and 180[5] minutes of onset of stroke. An open-label, dose escalation study design was used. A total of 94 consecutive patients were treated with intravenous rTPA at one of seven doses, over 60 or 90 minutes. Subsequent use of anticoagulation was at the discretion of the investigators. Endpoints included intracerebral parenchymal haematoma (ICH), haemorrhagic transformation without ICH, systemic haemorrhagic complication, death, major neurological improvement at two and 24 hours, and neurological deterioration.

Of the 74 patients treated within 90 minutes, 32% had a decreased level of consciousness, 37% had gaze deviation, and 40% had hemiparesis. Major neurological improvement at two hours occurred in 30%, correlating with smaller infarct size, but not with patient age, race, gender, infarct location, severity of initial deficit, or presence of oedema. Improvement at 24 hours occurred in 46%. Neurological deterioration occurred in 11% (two with ICH) at 24 hours, and in 8% at 7–10 days. Six patients had died at 30 days and six more by three months. Asymptomatic bleeding occurred in 4% and was not dose related. Symptomatic bleeding correlated only with total dose. The three patients (4%) who developed ICH within 24 hours had all received doses greater than 0·85 mg/kg. Of the 20 patients treated at 91–180 minutes under the same study design, two had fatal ICH and three had major neurological improvement after 24 hours. Those who died had received higher doses (0·85 or 0·95 mg/kg).

Three other studies,[6-8] based on angiographic criteria for the diagnosis of arterial occlusion, used intravenous rTPA within six hours of onset of stroke. Recanalisation was demonstrated angiographically in 20–50%, asymptomatic haemorrhagic conversion in 30–40%, haemorrhage causing deterioration or death occurred in 10%, and good clinical outcome at 24 hours in 40%. Intraarterial thrombolysis with urokinase or streptokinase has also demonstrated some beneficial results in retrospective analyses.[9 10]

These encouraging findings have so far been in open-label studies and leave unresolved how well they compare with the natural history. In a recent study assessing 29 strokes within 12 hours of onset, 24% showed spontaneous improvement within the first hour after baseline examination, and 52% had improved by 18 hours after onset of stroke.[11] Spontaneous recanalisation has been documented in individual cases by angiogram or by Doppler sonography[12] in the same time frame as that from TPA, so eventually studies will have to involve a placebo group. At present, the main issues of safety are being studied in the hope that the justification for placebo studies will eventually be shown.

Neuronal rescue: calcium channel antagonists

Studies in vitro and animal models have indicated a pathological role of calcium entry in neuronal injury.[13-18] Ischaemia induces the release of excitatory amino acid neurotransmitters such as glutamate and glycine which promote calcium entry into neurons via such receptor-mediated membrane channels as the kainate, the a-amino-3-hydroxy-5-methyl-4-isoxazolepropionic acid (AMPA), and the N-methyl-D-aspartate (NMDA) channels. A variety of enzymatic reactions follow, including those mediated by calmodulin. Destruction of neurofilaments, disruption of cell membrane integrity and consequent cell death most likely result from the production of nitric oxide and the subsequent formation of other free radicals. The NMDA channel has at least six sites that may be susceptible to pharmacological blockade (table).[19] The glutamate recognition site has been blocked experimentally by the compound CGS-19755, the glycine site by HA-966, the "upper competitive site" by MK-801, NS-1102, and d-methorphan, the polyamine site by ifenprofil, and another competitive site by Mg^{2+}. At a sixth site—a site of phosphorylation—no antagonist has yet been identified. Enzymatic inhibition of nitric oxide synthetase by N-nitro-L-arginine also appears to protect against glutamate

TABLE Medical therapies for ischaemic stroke

Therapy	Agent	Comment
Protect brain metabolism		
Anaesthesia, hypothermia, barbiturates	Various	No proven value
Nitric oxide inhibitors	L-Arginine	In vitro studies[18]
Calcium channel antagonists		
Voltage dependent	Nicardipine	Slight benefit[20]
	Nimodipine	Benefit <12 h[22 23]
	PY 108–068	Inconclusive[120]
Receptor dependent	CGS-19755	In clinical trial[19]
(NMDA receptor)	HA-966	In vitro studies[19]
	Mg^{2+}	In vitro studies[19]
	MK-801	Trials cancelled[19]
	NS-1102	In vitro studies[19]
	d-Methorphan	In clinical trial[121]
	Ifenprofil	In vitro studies[19]
Lysis occluding clot		
Thrombolytic agents	rTPA	Phase I trials[4-8]
	Urokinase	Anecdotal benefit[9]
	Streptokinase	Anecdotal benefit[10]
Suppress systemic response to brain ischaemia	Naloxone	No proven value
Reduce sludging		
Haemodilution	Low molecular weight dextrans	No proven value
Red cell deformation	Pentoxifylline	No proven value
Anti-oedema agents	Steroids	No proven value
	Hyperosmolar agents	No proven value
Vasodilators	Nitroglycerin	No proven value
	Prostacycline	No proven value
Anticoagulants		
Intravenous	Heparin (pork, beef)	Conflicting results[24 25]
	Heparinoids (ORG 10172)	In clinical trial[27]
Oral	Warfarin	In trial *v* aspirin*
Platelet antiaggregants		
Cyclo-oxygenase pathway	Aspirin	In trial *v* warfarin*
cAMP phosphodiesterase pathway	Dipyridamole	No benefit alone[122]
	Sulphinpyrazone	No benefit alone[34]
Combined	Ticlopidine	Benefit *v* ASA in some[47 50]

*Warfarin-Aspirin Recurrent Stroke Study, funded by the National Institute of Neurologic Disease and Stroke, 17 July 1992. ASA = aspirin.

neurotoxicity.[17] Efficacy of these agents in humans awaits clinical trials.

Voltage-dependent calcium channel antagonists are the only agents that have reached the clinical trials stage. Verapamil, diltiazem, and nifedipine have poor brain penetration and have never been considered viable candidates for cerebral protection. Nicardipine was evaluated in a small phase I trial. Thirty five patients were randomised to receive 3–7 mg/kg per hour intravenously versus placebo.[20] All patients showed improvement, with a slight difference favouring nicardipine. No further studies were performed.

The greatest experience to date has been with nimodipine, which has less systemic effects than the other calcium channel blockers and penetrates the blood–brain barrier well. In a large multicentre trial of subarachnoid haemorrhage,[21] infarction was reduced by 34% and poor outcome by 40%. Early trials for ischaemic stroke using 120 mg/day showed decreased mortality when treatment was administered within 24 hours of stroke onset, but no significant difference in long term functional recovery. The largest trial, conducted by the Nimodipine Study Group,[22] enrolled 1064 patients for 21 days in doses of 60 mg, 120 mg, or 240 mg per day compared with placebo. Heparin was allowed in cases of suspected cardioembolic stroke. Exclusion criteria included intracranial haemorrhage and significant co-morbidity. Although no significant differences in mortality or neurological function were seen across the groups for the overall cohort treated within 48 hours of stroke, subgroup analysis of those patients treated with 120 mg/day within 18 hours of stroke onset showed significantly better outcome scores and a 30% reduction in frequency of deterioration. Benefit also correlated with negative initial brain CT.

Although this was the only trial among nine double-blind, placebo-controlled studies that showed such significant benefit, the numbers of those treated early in the other trials were too small for individual analysis. A meta-analysis of all nine trials, totalling 3714 patients, indicated a benefit for those receiving early therapy: the 616 patients treated within 12 hours showed a pooled odds ratio of 0·62 favouring nimodipine (95% CI, 0·44 to 0·87).[23] No effect on outcome was seen for age, sex, hypertension, diabetes, or cardiac disease. There was no drug effect for those treated within 13–24 hours, and a slightly worse outcome for those treated after 24 hours. Further studies appear to be in order, but, at the least, useful therapy seems to be in the offing. The human studies corroborate the animal models which emphasise the importance of early intervention.

Heparin

Unlike thrombolytic therapy, anticoagulation with intravenous heparin is not intended to dissolve thrombus, but to impair the thrombogenesis created by the "clotting cascade". Experience with warfarin and heparin dates back decades, and one might be forgiven for thinking that their usefulness has long been established; such is not the case. Brought early into clinical practice and never subjected to the kinds of trials demanded nowadays, warfarin anticoagulation has long been the standard treatment for patients with rheumatic mitral stenosis and prosthetic valves but is not likely to undergo any such trial in the near future. The debate on heparin use has continued unabated and only lately have major trials been mounted to establish its usefulness. Only two clinical trials in the CT era evaluated the effect of heparin anticoagulation in the treatment of acute stroke. One study treated patients with cardioembolic stroke and demonstrated probable benefit. The other study failed to show a treatment effect in non-cardioembolic stroke.

The first study[24] reported 45 patients randomised with presumed cardioembolic stroke to immediate anticoagulation with intravenous heparin versus delayed anticoagulation with warfarin after 14 days. The intravenous heparin group received a bolus of 5000–10 000 units of heparin within 48 hours of stroke onset, followed by a maintenance infusion to keep the partial thromboplastin time (PTT) at 1·5–2·5 times the patient's baseline. After at least 96 hours of heparin the study group was switched to long term anticoagulation with warfarin. Patients younger than 18 or older than 78 were excluded, as were those with persistent severe hypertension. Of the 24 patients randomised to early anticoagulation there were no recurrences and no haemorrhages during the two week study period. Of the 21 patients randomised to receive delayed anticoagulation, two had early recurrent embolism, one had a deep vein thrombosis, two had haemorrhagic conversions, and two died. The study was terminated early because of the strong trend towards benefit in the study group, despite the small sample size.

The second study[25] randomised 225 patients to receive either intravenous placebo or heparin within 48 hours of stroke onset, with a target PTT of 5–70 s. The study period was seven days and no long term anticoagulation was given. Patients were excluded from the study if they had a possible cardioembolic source, if their deficit was too severe or resolved before the start of therapy, if previous deficits existed, or if stroke progression was noted within one hour of study onset. No significant differences in stroke progression or death were seen at seven days. No difference in functional level was seen at one year. There were significantly more deaths in the heparin group at one year, although most of these deaths occurred 3–12 months after the initial stroke and "appeared to be unrelated to treatment".

Both studies suffered from a small sample size. They established that early recurrence was not so common as to make estimation of any therapeutic effect an easy task. Because the first study focused on cardioembolic stroke and the second excluded such patients, the conflicting conclusions cannot be directly compared. A subsequent meta-analysis[26] was unable to show a benefit of anticoagulation, although most trials surveyed were before CT. The findings were of sufficient interest that a multicentre trial is under way in the United States to compare a synthetic heparin with placebo in acute stroke.[27] No studies have so far determined whether differences for stroke exist according to the route of administration (intravenous or subcutaneous) or, if intravenous, whether continuous or bolus, or the exact dose and duration of therapy. The matter is not trivial as evidence favouring similar effects for intermittent subcutaneous heparin could easily allow treatment at home. Similarly, if continuous intravenous administration is needed, it could be given by subcutaneous pump, in either case sparing hospital expense in ambulatory patients.

Prevention of recurrence or first stroke

Whereas the treatment of stroke in the hyperacute phase is under intense study, better established but no less controversial is the initiation of prophylaxis for those at high risk and the long term management of stroke in the hope of preventing recurrence.

Long term oral anticoagulation

Large epidemiological studies, for which the Framingham

Study[28] is a model, have established a high risk for stroke in patients with cardiac disease. The highest risk was seen in patients with atrial fibrillation in combination with valvular disease. The overall risk of stroke in patients with chronic atrial fibrillation is 5% per year. With the decline in incidence of rheumatic heart disease and rising uncertainty of the best management for non-valvular atrial fibrillation, such patients have been considered suitable for such trials. Three large prospective, open-label trials indicate a benefit for long term anticoagulation and a low risk of serious complications.[29-32]

The three studies were the Copenhagen Atrial Fibrillation, Aspirin, Anticoagulation Study (AFASAK),[29] the Stroke Prevention in Atrial Fibrillation study (SPAF),[30 31] and the Boston Area Anticoagulation Trial for Atrial Fibrillation (BAATAF).[32] Overall, patients on warfarin had a 69% reduction in stroke risk in an "intention to treat" analysis and an 83% reduction in an "on-treatment" analysis.[33] Patients with strokes in the warfarin groups were no more likely to have haemorrhagic than ischaemic strokes. The rate of major bleeding was nearly identical for the warfarin and control groups at about 2%; minor bleeding was three times more likely in the warfarin group.

The design of the studies varied slightly. All three studies excluded highest risk cardiac patients; those with recent embolic events, recent myocardial infarction, and significant congestive heart failure or cardiomyopathy were not enrolled. SPAF excluded patients with lone atrial fibrillation, randomising them to aspirin (ASA) or placebo groups only because of a low stroke risk of less than 0·5% per year. AFASAK excluded patients with paroxysmal trial fibrillation for the same reason. The level of anticoagulation differed slightly. AFASAK used a prothrombin time of 1·5–2·0 times control, SPAF a prothrombin time of 1·3–1·8 times control, and BAATAF a prothrombin time of 1·2–1·5 times control. For the control groups AFASAK used ASA 75 mg/day or placebo, SPAF used 325 mg/day or placebo and BAATAF allowed ASA or no treatment to be used at the discretion of the investigators.

The AFASAK study randomised 1007 patients over a two year period. The unblinded warfarin group showed an incidence of transient ischaemic attack (TIA), stroke, or systemic thromboembolism of 2% per year compared with a 5·5% incidence in the ASA and placebo arms. Three of the five strokes in the warfarin group had strokes when they were off warfarin. Non-fatal bleeding occurred in 6% of the warfarin group (43% of these were found to have inflammatory or malignant disease) compared with 1% in the control groups. A drawback to this study was that 38% of patients in the warfarin group dropped out, mostly because of the inconvenience of frequent blood samples.

The SPAF study randomised 1330 patients and was terminated early at a mean follow up period of 1·3 years. The incidence of stroke or systemic embolism was 2·3% in the warfarin group, 3–6% in the ASA group, and 7·4% in the placebo group. In this study as well, four of six patients with ischaemic stroke in the warfarin group had strokes off therapy. Major bleeding complications were comparable in the warfarin, ASA, and placebo groups at 1·5%, 1·4%, and 1·6%, respectively.

Of the 420 patients randomised in the BAATAF study, followed for an average of 2·2 years, ischaemic stroke occurred in the warfarin group at a rate of 0·41% per year and in the control group at 2·98% per year for a risk reduction of 86%. The two strokes in the warfarin group occurred at prothrombin times of less than 1·2. Among the strokes in the control group, eight of 13 occurred in patients taking aspirin. The death rate in the warfarin group was 2·25% and, in the control group, 5·97%. Two fatal haemorrhages occurred, one presumed intracranial haemorrhage in the warfarin group and a pulmonary haemorrhage in the control group. Minor bleeding occurred in 38 patients in the warfarin group and in 21 patients in the control group.

Antiplatelet therapy

Aspirin therapy in primary and secondary stroke prevention has been widely employed because of its ease of administration, documented prophylactic effect in coronary artery disease, and because physicians and the public perceive it as a benign treatment. This last point is not entirely to its advantage: many patients (and some physicians) continue to think of it as adjunct therapy and often fail to mention its use when questioned about medications being taken. Other antiplatelet drugs such as sulphinpyrazone and dipyridamole used alone have not proved beneficial in clinical testing.[34]

More than 10 randomised, placebo-controlled trials of aspirin following TIA or minor stroke have been completed.[35-45] Most showed a significant risk reduction with aspirin. Given the decline in stroke incidence over the past decades, modern clinical trials of stroke prevention require approximately 1000 patients to be enrolled and followed for an average of five years to detect a 50% difference at a significance level of p < 0·05.[46] Smaller studies may suggest benefit when none exists or overlook a true benefit.

Of the four largest clinical trials—the United Kingdom trial,[35] the European,[36] the French,[37] and the Canadian[38]—all found some degree of benefit, ranging from 20% reduction in stroke and vascular death in the British trial to 50% reduction in stroke and stroke–death in the French trial. Two slightly smaller trials, the Danish[41] and the Swedish,[43] found no benefit. The Danish study used an ASA dose of 50–75 mg per day and the Swedish study entered only patients who had suffered major strokes. Differences from other studies are of uncertain significance. A lack of benefit in women, reported in the British and Canadian studies, may have been due to a lack of statistical power, as the risk of stroke and stroke recurrence is lower for women. The optimum dose of aspirin remains controversial. The Dutch trial for stroke prevention after TIA showed no difference between 30 mg/day and 283 mg/day.[45] The United Kingdom trial found no difference between 300 mg/day and 1300 mg/day but the meaning of the data has been disputed. The SPAF trial[31] in patients with atrial fibrillation found a benefit of ASA 325 mg/day, in a setting of atrial fibrillation, not TIA or prior stroke. Consequently, it remains unresolved whether ultra-low-dose aspirin or aspirin in doses as high as 1300 mg/day offer slight, wide, or no major differences in rates of first or recurrent stroke. The only source of agreement is that the higher doses produce more disagreeable gastrointestinal side effects.

Ticlopidine, a platelet antiaggregant newly available in North America, has been in use in Europe and the rest of the world for over 15 years. Its maximum antiplatelet action is at a dose of 500 mg/day, it reaches maximum effect at 3–5 days, and its effects last the lifetime of the platelets. Adverse side effects include gastrointestinal disturbance in 20% which may resolve with temporary dose reduction, rash in 10%, neutropenia in 2·4%, and severe neutropenia in 0·8% which is seen in the first few months and is reversible. Significant haemorrhage occurs in less than 1% and gastrointestinal bleeding is three times less common in patients taking 500 mg of ticlopidine than 1300 mg of ASA.[47] Two large clinical trials found a benefit over ASA and placebo.[47–49]

The Canadian–American Ticlopidine Study (CATS)[49] randomised 1053 patients with recent non-cardioembolic stroke to receive ticlopidine 250 mg twice daily or placebo. The study excluded patients who had significant co-morbidity and those with TIA alone. The incidence of primary endpoints (ischaemic stroke, myocardial infarction, and vascular death) was 10·8% in the ticlopidine group versus 15·3% in the placebo group for a relative risk reduction of 30·2% by "on-treatment" analysis. Intention-to-treat analysis concluded a 23% risk reduction for the treatment group. A total of 52% of patients in the ticlopidine group and 40% of those in the placebo group discontinued treatment. Relative reduction in stroke or stroke death was found on secondary analysis to be 33·5%. Ticlopidine proved equally effective in men and women.

The Ticlopidine–Aspirin Stroke Study (TASS)[47] randomised 3069 patients to ticlopidine 250 g twice daily or ASA 650 mg twice daily. They included patients with TIA, transient monocular blindness, or minor stroke. Average follow up period was 2·3 years. In their intention-to-treat analysis, they showed a 12% reduction of stroke or death. In a three year follow up, the incidence of fatal or non-fatal stroke was reduced by 21%. Twenty one per cent of the ticlopidine group and 14·5% of the ASA group discontinued the medicine.

For those who tolerate the medicine, ticlopidine appears to have a slight advantage over aspirin and a definite advantage over placebo in secondary stroke prevention. In a subsequent subgroup analysis of the two studies,[50] the patients who appeared to benefit more from ticlopidine than aspirin included women and those for whom aspirin therapy had failed. Patients with diabetes mellitus requiring treatment, those on antihypertensives, and those with elevated creatinine levels also showed greater treatment effects versus aspirin. It remains to be determined whether the slight improvement in stroke event rates, compared with aspirin, will offset the side effects and difficulties in monitoring to allow ticlopidine to become popular.

Modification of risk factors

A striking decline in age-specific stroke morbidity and mortality has been noted over the last 15 years in both women and men, with mortality rates falling in industrialised countries by

4·1–7·1%[51][52] Modification of diet and smoking behaviour, a decline in rheumatic heart disease, and improved treatment of hypertension and coronary artery disease have contributed.[51] Factors that influence stroke incidence include age greater than 65 and male gender.[53] Black men and women are twice as prone to stroke as white people and Hispanics,[54] even when controlling for a higher incidence of hypertension.[3] The difference for black patients has persisted throughout the period of overall declining mortality rates. Crucial to the management of stroke is an understanding of epidemiological predictors of stroke and stroke recurrence. Modification of risk factors has been shown to produce dramatic reductions in stroke risk.[55]

Among modifiable risk factors, hypertension overshadows the rest. From the Framingham Study, hypertension confers a relative risk of 4·0 for men and 4·4 for women. Borderline hypertension confers a relative risk of 2·0 and even isolated systolic hypertension, previously thought to be benign, carries a relative risk of 2·4.[1] One overview of 14 randomised drug trials showed a 40% reduction in stroke risk in patients able to lower their diastolic blood pressures an average of 6 mm Hg.[56]

The risk of smoking appears to be dose related: light smokers are twice as likely as the general population to develop stroke and heavy smokers (more than 25 cigarettes per day) four times as likely. Five years after cessation of smoking, the risk approaches that of the general population.[57][58] Diabetes mellitus confers a relative risk of 1·5–3·0, probably secondary to microvascular disease and a greater tendency to atherosclerosis.

Cardiac disease is a complex risk factor. Atrial fibrillation in the setting of rheumatic valvular disease confers a 17-fold risk and a fivefold risk exists for non-valvular atrial fibrillation.[28] A relative risk of 2·0 is seen for those with coronary artery disease, recent myocardial infarction, and congestive heart failure.[59][60] Left ventricular hypertrophy in the setting of advancing age and hypertension confers a relative risk of 4·0.[1] Increased risk may also be seen in patients with patent foramen ovale, mitral valve prolapse, atrial septal aneurysm, and aortic arch disease.[61]

A variety of laboratory abnormalities has been shown to correlate with higher stroke incidence. Elevated[62] and decreased[63] haematocrit may contribute, as well as protein C and S deficiencies, elevated fibrinogen,[3] and lupus anticoagulant/anticardiolipin antibodies[64–66] and antithrombin III levels.[67] Most

61

studies find a relationship between elevated lipids and athero-sclerosis in both coronary and carotid artery disease.[13]

Mild to moderate alcohol intake appears to confer a protective effect for ischaemic stroke with a relative risk of 0·3–0·5, where-as heavy drinking increases stroke risk, particularly for haemor-rhagic types.[68-70] Alcohol may be more associated with stroke recurrence.

Transient ischaemic attack may be considered both a manifes-tation and a risk factor for stroke. As a risk factor, TIA confers an independent relative risk of 3·9.[71] TIA precedes stroke in 10–14% of cases.

Because the rate of stroke recurrence is so high—ranging from 4% to 14% per year depending on the study—factors have been sought that independently influence stroke recurrence. In the Lehigh Valley study, the relative risk for recurrence was 41·4 for TIA, 8·0 for myocardial infarction or other coronary artery dis-ease, 5·6 for diabetes mellitus, and 4·5 for hypertension. Unlike initial stroke risk, age and sex did not influence recurrence.[53] The Stroke Data Bank found that hypertension, glucose level, and stroke subtype predicted 30 day recurrence, and only hyperten-sion predicted a two year recurrence.[72] The 30 day recurrence rate of stroke varied from 2·2% for lacunar syndromes to 7·9% for large artery atherosclerotic disease to up to 14% in the first two weeks for atrial fibrillation. A recent small case-control study identified potential cardioembolic aetiology as the single signifi-cant factor for 90 day recurrence.[73] Cardiac disease and hyperten-sion lower survival for recurrent stroke.[72]

In evaluating an individual patient's risk for stroke, the entire risk factor profile should be considered. Multiple risk factors are cumulative as in the case of hypertension which confers a relative risk of 4·0: adding coronary artery disease increases the relative risk to 8·4.[1]

Surgical intervention

Carotid endarterectomy was introduced in 1954.[74] At that time, even though its efficacy had not been proved, the operation grew in popularity from 15 000 in 1971 to 105 000 in 1985 in the United States.[75] Following the 1985 trial which suggested extracranial–intracranial bypass procedure to be an ineffective therapy,[76] a series of randomised clinical trials were initiated to assess the efficacy of endarterectomy. Three large, multicentre trials addressed the question of operating in the setting of symptomatic carotid artery disease.[77-79] Results from these trials demonstrate a 10–18% relative reduction in stroke risk for endarterectomy in high grade (>70%) stenosis. Mild to moderate disease as well as the question of asymptomatic carotid stenosis remain under investigation.

The North American Symptomatic Carotid Endarterectomy Trial (NASCET)[77] drew data from 50 centres in the United States and Canada, randomising patients to surgery and the best medical therapy (mostly ASA 1300 mg/day) or medical therapy alone. The patients were stratified to 30–69% stenosis or 70–99% stenosis documented by angiogram. After 659 patients had been randomised in the high-grade stenosis group—half the number projected to be needed to prove a 10% risk reduction—the study was terminated because of a dramatic therapeutic benefit favouring surgery. The cumulative risk of ipsilateral stroke at two years was found to be 9% in the surgical group and 26% in the medical group for a risk reduction of 17%. The cumulative risk of major or fatal ipsilateral stroke was 2·5% in the surgical and 13·1% in the medical group. The risk of all strokes was 12·6% versus 27·6%, and the risk of death or major stroke was 8% versus 18·1% for the surgical and medical group respectively. Average perioperative morbidity and mortality rate for all centres involved was 5·8%. Perioperative incidence of major stroke or death was 2·1%. The 30–69% stenosis group is still under investigation.

Another multicentre trial, the Veterans Administration study,[78] randomised 189 patients with greater than 50% internal carotid artery (ICA) stenosis to surgical plus medical therapy (ASA 325 mg) versus medical therapy alone, and found similar results. At a mean follow up of 11·9 months, crescendo TIAs and stroke were found in 7·7% of patients in the surgical group versus 19·4% in the medical group for a risk reduction of 11·7%. Patients with greater than 70% stenosis showed a risk reduction of 17·7%. Perioperative morbidity and mortality rate in this study was 5·5%.

The largest, longest running trial is the European Carotid Surgery Trial (ECST)[79] which also found a striking benefit of surgical intervention for high-grade carotid stenosis among the 2518 patients they recruited. Their comparison groups were surgery plus aspirin versus aspirin alone. The high-grade stenosis (>70%) portion was terminated for this trial as well after a 9·3% risk reduction was noted for stroke or death in less than 30 days and a

9·6% reduction in stroke or death at three years. Recruitment continues in this study also for patients with 30–69% stenosis.

What to do with asymptomatic carotid artery disease is less certain. Bruits are present in some 4–5% of the general population age 45 to 80. The reported risk of carotid stenosis without symptoms varies widely in the literature. Oft-quoted is a relatively small study which followed 50 patients with more than 50% stenosis, and found stroke in 4·5% and TIAs in 16.5%.[80] At the other extreme is a study following asymptomatic stenotic carotid arteries contralateral to operated symptomatic arteries which found no strokes in a 20 year follow up period.[81] Non-uniformity of definitions and follow up contributes to the problem in defining risk. In the Asymptomatic Carotid Artery Stenosis Study (ACAS),[82] a large multi-centre trial currently addressing the issue, 20% of patients have positive CT scans in the distribution of the "asymptomatic" ICA. Further, evidence of prior strokes may be found in up to 17% of all stroke patients presenting with their "first" acute stroke.[83]

Supplementary laboratory data may help assess the significance of a carotid stenosis. Positron emission tomography may identify areas of "misery perfusion" in the border-zone regions representing tissue at risk that could be better perfused after operation. Regional cerebral blood flow (rCBF) measurements may show low flow areas as well as areas of decreased vasoreactivity following carbon dioxide inhalation. The existence of adequate collaterals may be inferred by the re-establishment of low resistance flow in the common carotid artery on duplex Doppler sonography (ECA to ophthalmic to ICA collateral) or a reversal of flow in the anterior cerebral artery (ACA) on transcranial Doppler examination (collateral via the anterior communicating artery).

The one published multicentre trial of asymptomatic carotid stenosis (CASA-NOVA)[84] randomised 410 patients to surgery and medical therapy (ASA 330 mg, dipyridamole 75 mg) versus surgery alone. Those with more than 90% stenosis were excluded. Their endpoints were stroke or death. Patients were removed from the study and operated on if a TIA occurred in the ipsilateral territory, if more than 90% stenosis developed, or if there was bilateral disease of more than 50%. There was no difference between the two groups; however, the exclusion of patients with more severe arterial disease and the study's small size leave the issue unresolved. The ACAS trial may produce more data on the risk of asymptomatic disease at all degrees of stenosis.

Recommendations for management

From the outset of the encounter with an acute stroke patient, the conscientious clinician must accrue sufficient data to make informed and timely management decisions. Settling the diagnosis of stroke subtype is no longer a mere academic exercise but can help predict likely outcome and direct therapy (fig). From the history, TIAs, hypertension, increased blood glucose concentration, cardiac disease, and stroke subtype predict recurrence. Particular attention should be paid to indicators of cardioembolic source such as recent myocardial infarction, arrhythmias, or congestive heart failure. Headache suggests subarachnoid bleeding in the absence of focal signs. When severe headache coincides with focal signs, lobar haemorrhage is more common than ischaemic stroke.[85] Pain in the neck, side of face, teeth or jaw, or retro-orbital area may indicate vertebral or carotid artery dissection, even without a history of neck trauma.

The physical examination can give an impression of the size and a fair estimate of the location of the infarct, and thus guide the urgency of subsequent management steps. Hemiparesis and forced gaze deviation suggest a large hemisphere or critical brainstem lesion, particularly if accompanied by decreased level of consciousness, whereas hemiparesis involving the face, arm and leg in an alert patient suggests a small, deep lesion involving a confluence of motor fibres. When isolated, behavioural abnormalities such as aphasia or hemineglect without a gaze preference suggest smaller hemisphere lesions. General examination may reveal a carotid bruit, and physical examination and an electrocardiogram an arrhythmia, or signs of cardiomyopathy or congestive heart failure.

MRI should identify all but the smallest lesions and is superior to CT for brainstem and small, deep, so-called lacunar infarcts. CT is equal to MRI in documenting an infarct within the first hours[86] and is better for a diagnosis of acute haemorrhage or bony abnormalities. Either technology may miss an infarct within the first couple of hours of onset.

Data collected should suggest stroke aetiology. From 15% to 30% of strokes are embolic from a cardiac source such as atrial fibrillation or valvular disease. Although 5–6% of patients may have a fluctuating course, the classic clinical presentation of cardioembolic stroke is a sudden deficit, maximal at onset.[87 88]

65

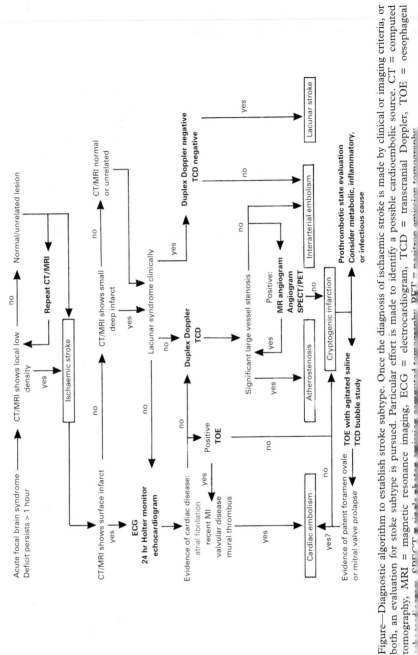

Figure—Diagnostic algorithm to establish stroke subtype. Once the diagnosis of ischaemic stroke is made by clinical or imaging criteria, or both, an evaluation for stoke subtype is pursued. Particular effort is made to identify a possible cardioembolic source. CT = computed tomography, MRI = magnetic resonance imaging, ECG = electrocardiogram, TCD = transcranial Doppler, TOE = oesophageal echocardiogram, SPECT = single photon emission computed tomography, PET = positron emission tomography.

Syndromes more likely to be embolic include hemianopia without hemiparesis, pure Wernicke's aphasia, and ideomotor apraxia.[89] CT and MRI which show a single cortical branch territory infarct are also consistent with an embolic source because atheroma rarely extends to the surface vessels, although the source of the inferred embolus may not be readily apparent even after full evaluation. Mainstem branch occlusions are also often embolic, but local atherostenosis is a possibility in such a setting as well. One difficult pitfall on initial CT is the deep-lying lucency involving the internal capsule and basal ganglia of some 2–3 cm in size, apparently sparing cortex, which can be labelled as a large lacune. Often such instances are also of embolic origin, involving several lenticulostriate branches of the middle cerebral artery from temporary occlusion of the middle cerebral stem, followed by rapid collateralisation from anterior or posterior cerebral branches or recanalisation of the occlusion with distal migration of the embolus. A right-to-left shunt, usually a patent cardiac foramen ovale, can be inferred when transcranial Doppler examination shows microbubbles in the intracranial vessels after injection of 10 ml of agitated saline in the antecubital vein[90] and contrast transoesophageal or standard transthoracic echocardiography usually can find the defect in the cardiac atrial wall or mitral valve prolapse.[61] Holter monitoring may infer a cardiac emboligenic source by documenting atrial fibrillation.

In 15% of cases, severe large vessel atherosclerosis is present and seems responsible for the stroke. It is best appreciated when there is severe, extracranial, internal carotid stenosis or occlusion and the "distal field" lesion is imaged on CT or MRI as an infarct high over the convexity, spreading caudally from the border-zone between arterial territories.[91 92]

The most common clinical profile of this type of infarct is fractional arm weakness (shoulder different from hand). Male gender, hypertension, and diabetes mellitus appear significantly more common in this group than in patients with cardioembolic stroke.[93] Although the standard angiogram most reliably demonstrates large vessel stenosis, when it is severe enough to be of haemodynamic significance, duplex Doppler sonography usually readily delineates the severity of the internal carotid stenosis and shows high velocity, turbulent flow. Intracranial internal carotid artery stenosis may produce detectable high resistance flow on Doppler examinations of the extracranial carotid. Transcranial

Doppler sonography often shows dampened pulsatility in the ipsilateral middle cerebral artery.[94-99] Duplex Doppler examination, in combination with magnetic resonance angiography, is rapidly becoming a reliable alternative to the more invasive traditional angiogram. Cerebral blood flow measurements with xenon CT, single photon emission CT (SPECT), and rCBF techniques are also being used to evaluate regional hypoperfusion.

In perhaps 15% of all strokes, large vessel atherosclerosis with less than haemodynamic stenosis (under 80% occluded or with an ulcerated plaque) occurs in the absence of a cardioembolic source and the cause is attributed to an artery to artery embolus. Embolic fragments may arise from atherosclerotic lesions in the ICA,[100-102] the basilar artery,[103] intracranial large vessels,[104 105] the proximal stump of an occluded carotid,[106] or the distal tail of a thrombus in an occluded ICA. Distinguishing interarterial embolism from possible cardioembolic aetiology may be difficult; however, interarterial embolism usually produces a smaller cortical infarct and cardioembolism is more often associated with a decreased level of consciousness and an abnormal initial CT.[93]

Small deep lesions in the subcortical white matter, the thalamus, the basal ganglia or the pons accompanied by an appropriate clinical syndrome suggest lacunar disease, accounting for 15–20% of all strokes.[107-109] Arteriolar wall lipohyalinosis, microatheroma, or even microemboli may produce the pathology.[110] Early studies described only a handful of classic syndromes, but case reports have expanded the number to more than 70.[111] Positive scans in the capsule, adjacent corona radiata, thalamus, or pons have been reported for clumsy hand-dysarthria, ataxic hemiparesis, and hemiballism; pure sensory syndromes have been associated with small thalamic lesions.[112] CT scans are positive in only half of lacunar strokes,[112 113] with MRI increasing the yield.[114] Larger lacunes are more often symptomatic. Hypertension is the risk factor most associated with lacunar infarction.

Despite efforts to arrive at a diagnosis, the cause of infarction in up to 40% of cases remains undetermined. This may result from an inability to perform appropriate laboratory studies because of the patient's advanced age or co-morbidity, or because of unwillingness on the part of the physician or patient. It may also result from improper timing of tests, such as an angiogram performed after an embolus has cleared, or a CT or MRI done before the infarction appears. In most of these cases, however, appropriate testing done at the proper time produces normal or ambiguous findings. Evaluation of patients classified as "infarct of undetermined cause" in the Stroke Data Bank revealed certain common features.[115] They tended not to have had previous TIAs, infarcts, carotid bruits, or cardiac risk factors. A total of 57% had clinically relevant CT images; surface infarcts were found in 40%. Hemispherical syndromes predominated in 66% and basilar syndromes occurred in 15%; 27% worsened in the hospital and 41% had moderate to severe weakness. Some of these cases may be explained by hypercoagulable states from protein C, free protein S, fibrinogen, lupus anticoagulant, or anticardiolipin antibody abnormalities.[116-118] Others may have had paradoxical emboli through a patent foramen ovale.[61 119] Migraine, meningitis, dissection, arteritis, or inherited metabolic abnormality may explain rare cases. Rather than force a classification into one of the four established categories, we recommend maintaining the classification of infarct of undetermined cause until a definite cause can be established.

Supported in part by TS32-NS-07-155-13S1 from the National Institute of Neurological Disorders and Stroke and by a gift from the Van Ingen Foundation.

Management of ischaemic stroke

● All patients with suspected stroke in which a deficit persists for more than one hour should undergo CT or MRI of the head. Subsequent investigation is directed towards identifying stroke aetiology.

● If the clinical picture, and CT or MRI appearances are consistent with a small or moderate-sized ischaemic stroke, heparin should be administered by intravenous infusion until the stroke subtype is determined, maintaining a partial thromboplastin time of 1·4–2 times control (but see pages viii and 55–56). This treatment may also be given if there is minor—but only minor—haemorrhagic infarction on brain imaging.

● If the stroke is large and disabling there is a greater risk of haemorrhagic transformation, and brain imaging should be repeated 48–72 hours after stroke onset. Anticoagulation treatment should be started only if haemorrhagic conversion has not occurred. If the clinical and imaging diagnosis is of intracranial haemorrhage, anticoagulants and antiplatelet agents should not be given.

● Investigation of stroke aetiology should focus first on cardioembolic sources and large vessel atherothrombosis. Transthoracic echocardiography, carotid duplex Doppler sonography, and transcranial Doppler examination should be performed in nearly all cases. MR angiography and transoesophageal echocardiography may deliver a diagnosis when the aforementioned studies are inconclusive.

● Patients with recent myocardial infarction, atrial fibrillation, valvular disease, or intracardiac thrombus should be given oral anticogulants for at least one year. The prothrombin time should be kept at 1·2–2·5 times control. If there is atrial fibrillation, warfarin should be continued indefinitely provided that reliable monitoring is available.

● If the stroke is small, the heart is normal, and a duplex Doppler sonogram shows significant carotid stenosis (greater than 70%) intravenous heparin should be continued until the exact degree of stenosis has been determined by digital subtraction angiography or MR angiography (if available). Prophylactic endarterectomy for patients with greater than 70% stenosis should be undertaken as soon as possible. For patients with lesser degrees of stenosis, Doppler monitoring should be undertaken at intervals of three, six, or 12 months to document those whose stenosis becomes more than than 70% and who then qualify for surgery.

● If no cardioembolic source or operable carotid stenosis is identified, and the patient is not considered at risk of haemorrhage, antiplatelet treatment with aspirin 325 mg daily should be given as chronic outpatient therapy. Ticlopidine may also be considered, particularly if the patient is female or has failed aspirin therapy. Close attention to the neutrophil count is essential when using ticlopidine.

1 Davis ND, Hachinski V. Epidemiology of cerebrovascular disease. In: Anderson D, ed. *Neuroepidemiology. A tribute to Bruce Schoenberg*. Boca Raton: CRC Press,1991:27-53.

2 Sacco RL, Wolf PA, Kannel WB, *et al*. Survival and recurrence: the Framingham Study. *Stroke* 1982;**13**:290-5.

3 Sacco RL. Frequency and determinants of stroke. In: Fisher, ed. *Stroke, diagnosis and treatment*. London: Gower Medical Publishing, 1994.

4 Brott TG, Haley EC, Levy DE, *et al*. Urgent therapy for stroke. Part I. Pilot study of tissue plasminogen activator administered within 90 minutes. *Stroke* 1992;**23**:632-9.

5 Haley EC, Levy DE, Brott TG, *et al*. Urgent therapy for stroke. Part II. Pilot study of tissue plasminogen activator administered 91-180 minutes from onset. *Stroke* 1992;**23**: 641-5.

6 Okada U, Sadoshima S, Nakane H. Early computerized tomographic findings for thrombolytic therapy in patients with acute brain embolism. *Stroke* 1992;**23**:20-3.

7 von Kummer R, Hacke W. Safety and efficacy of intravenous tissue plasminogen activator and heparin in acute middle cerebral artery stroke. *Stroke* 1992;**23**:646-52.

8 Del Zoppo GHL, Poeck K, Pessin MS, *et al*. Recombinant tissue plasminogen activator in acute thrombotic and embolic stroke. *Ann Neurol* 1992;**32**:78-86.

9 Mori E, Tabuchi M, Yoshida T, *et al*. Intracarotid urokinase with thromboembolic occlusion of the middle cerebral artery. *Stroke* 1988;**19**:802-12.

10 Hacke W Zeumer H, Ferbert A, *et al*. Intra-arterial thrombolytic therapy improves outcome in patients with acute vertebrobasilar occlusive disease. *Stroke* 1988;**19**:1216-22.

11 Biller J, Love BB, Marsh EE, *et al*. Spontaneous improvement after acute ischemic stroke: a pilot study. *Stroke* 1990;**21**:1008-12.

12 Mohr JP, Duterte DI, Oliveira VR, *et al*. Recanalization of acute middle cerebral artery occlusion. *Neurology* 1988;**38**:215.

13 Rothman SM, Olney JW. Glutamate and the pathophysiology of hypoxic ischaemic brain damage. *Ann Neurol* 1986;**19**:105-11.

14 Schlaepfer WW, Zimmerman UP. Mechanisms underlying the neuronal response to ischemic injury: calcium activated proteolysis of neurofilaments. *Prog Brain Res* 1985;**63**:185-96.

15 Simon RP, Swan JH, Griffiths T, *et al*. Blockade of N-methyl-D-aspartate receptors may protect against ischemic damage in the brain. *Science* 1984;**226**:850-2.

16 Choi DW Cerebral hypoxia: some new approaches and unanswered questions. *J Neurosci* 1990;**10**:2493-501.

17 Dawson VL, Dawson TM, London ED, *et al*. Nitric oxide mediates glutamate neurotoxicity in primary cortical culture. *Proc Natl Acad Sci USA* 1991;**88**:6368-71.

18 Dawson TM, Dawson VL, Snyder SH. A novel neuronal messenger molecule in brain: the free radical, nitric oxide. *Ann Neurol* 1992;**32**:297-311.

19 McCoulloch J. NMDA and non–NMDA receptor blockers. *Fourth international symposium on pharmacology of cerebral ischemia*. Marburg, Germany, July 1992.

20 Yatsu F. Nicardipine in acute stroke. In: Hartman A, Kuchinsky W, eds. *Cerebral ischemia and calcium*. Berlin: Springer-Verlag, 1989.

21 Teasdale G, PSokard J, Shaw D, *et al*. Treatment of subarachnoid hemorrhage with calcium-antagonist: a large randomized controlled trial. *International symposium on cerebral ischemia and calcium*. Chiemsee, West Germany, 12–15 June 1988, p9.

22 The American nimodipine study group. Clinical trial of nimodipine in acute ischemic stroke. *Stroke* 1992;**23**:3-9.

23 Mohr JP. Calcium antagonists in acute ischemic stroke. In: Krieglstein J, Oberpichler H, eds. *Pharmocology of cerebral ischemia*. Stuttgart: Wissenschaftliche Verlagsgesellschaft, 1992.

24 The cerebral embolism study group. Immediate anti–coagulation of embolic stroke: a randomized trial. *Stroke* 1983;**14**:668-76.

25 Duke RJ, Bloch RF, Turpie AGC, *et al*. Intravenous heparin for the prevention of stroke progression in acute partial stable stroke: a randomized controlled trial. *Ann Intern Med* 1986;**105**:825-8.

26 Jonas S. Anticoagulant therapy in cerebrovascular disease: review and meta-analysis. *Stroke* 1988;**19**:1043-8.

27 Gordon-D-L, Linhardt R, Adams HP Jr. Low–molecular–weight heparins and heparinoids and their use in acute or progressing ischemic stroke. *Clin-Neuropharmacol* 1990;**13**: 522-43.

28 Wolf PA, Dawber TR, Thomas HE, *et al*. Epidemiologic assessment of chronic atrial fibrillation and risk of stroke: the Framingham study. *Neurology* 1978;**28**:973-7.

71

29 Petersen P, Godtfredsen J, Boysen C, *et al.* Placebo-controlled, randomized trial of warfarin and aspirin for prevention of thromboembolic complications in chronic atrial fibrillation: The Copenhagen AFASAK study. *Lancet* 1989;1:175–9.

30 The Stroke Prevention in Atrial Fibrillation Investigators. Preliminary report of the stroke
prevention in atrial fibrillation study. *N Engl J Med* 1990;322:863–8.

31 The Stroke Prevention in Atrial Fibrillation Investigators. The stroke prevention in atrial
fibrillation study: final results. *Circulation* 1991;84:527–39.

32 The Boston Area Anticoagulation Trial for Atrial Fibrillation Investigators. The effect of
low-dose warfarin on the risk of stroke in patients with non-rheumatic atrial fibrillation.
N Engl J Med 1990;323:1505–11.

33 Albers GW, Sherman DG, Gress DR, *et al.* Stroke prevention in nonvalvular atrial fibrillation: a review of prospective randomized trials. *Ann Neurol* 1991;30:511–8.

34 Barnett HJM. Aspirin in stroke prevention: an overview. *Stroke* 1990;21(suppl IV):
40–3.

35 UK-TIA Study Group: United Kingdom transient ischemic attack (UK-TIA) Aspirin
trial: interim results. *BMJ* 1988;296:316–20.

36 The ESPS Group. The European Stroke Prevention Study. *Stroke* 1990;21:1122–30.

37 Guiraud-Chaumeil B, Rascol AD, Boneu B, *et al.* Prevention des recidives des accidents
vasculaires cerebraux ischemiques par les anti-agregants plaquettaires. *Rev Neurol* 1982;
5:367–5.

38 The Canadian Cooperative Study Group: a randomized trial of aspirin and sulfinpyra-
zone in threatened stroke. *N Engl J Med* 1978;299:53–9.

39 Fields WS, Lemak NA, Frankowske RF, *et al.* Controlled trials of aspirin in cerebral
ischaemia. *Stroke* 1977;8:301–14.

40 Reuther R, Domdorf W, Loew D. Behandlung transitorischischamischer Attacehn mit
Acetylsalicylsaure. *Münch Med Wochenschr* 1980;122:795–8.

41 Boysen G, Sorensen PS, Juhler M, *et al.* Danish very-low-dose aspirin after carotid
endarterectomy trial. *Stroke* 1988;19:1211–5.

42 Sorensen PS, Pedersen H, Marquardsen, *et al.* Acetylsalicylic acid in the prevention of
stroke in patients with reversible cerebral ischemic attacks: a Danish cooperative study.
Stroke 1983;14:15–22.

43 Britton M, Helmers C, Samuelsson K. High-dose acetylsalicylic acid after cerebral
infarction—a Swedish cooperative study. *Stroke* 1987;18:325–34.

44 Bousser MG, Eschwege E, Hagenau M, *et al.* "AICLA" controlled trial of aspirin and
dipyridamole in the secondary prevention of athero-thrombotic cerebral ischaemia. *Stroke*
1983;14:5–14.

45 The Dutch TIA trial study group. A comparison of two doses of aspirin (30 mg vs. 283
mg a day) in patients after a transient ischemic attack or minor ischemic stroke. *N Engl J
Med* 1991;325:126–6.

46 Taylor DW, Sacken DI, Haynes RB. Sample size for randomized trials in stroke prevention: how many patients do we need? *Stroke* 1984;15:968–71.

47 Hass WK, Easton HD, Adams HP, *et al*, for the Ticlopidine Aspirin Stroke Study Group.
A randomized trial comparing ticlopidine hydrochlorine with aspirin for the prevention of
stroke in high-risk patients. *N Engl J Med* 1989;321:501–7.

48 Albers GW. Role of ticlopidine for prevention of stroke. *Stroke* 1992;23:912–6.

49 Gent M, Blakely JA, Easton JD, *et al.* The Canadian American Ticlopidine Study
(CATS) in thromboembolic stroke. *Lancet* 1989;1:1215–20.

50 Grotta JC, Norris JW, Kamm B, *et al.* Prevention of stroke with ticlopidine: Who benefits
most? *Neurology* 1992;42:111–5.

51 Barnett HJM. 35 years of stroke prevention: challenges, disappointments and successes.
Cerebrovasc Dis 1992;1:61–70.

52 Schoenberg BS, Schulte BPM. Cerebrovascular disease: epidemiology and geopathology.
In: Vinken PJ, Bruyn GW, Klawasn HL, eds. *Handbook of clinical neurology.* New York:
Elsevier Publishers, 1988.

53 Meehan EF, Sobel E, Alter M, *et al.* The Lehigh Valley Stroke Program: establishing a
communitywide, hospital-based stroke register. *Am J Prev Med* 1986;2:97–102.

54 Sacco RI, Hauser WA, Mohr JP. Hospitalized stroke in blacks and hispanics in northern
Manhattan. *Stroke* 1991;22:1491–6.

55 Dunbabin DW, Sandercock PAG. Preventing stroke by the modification of risk factors.
Stroke 1990;21 (suppl):IV36–9.

56 Collins R, Peto R, MacMahon S, *et al.* Blood pressure, stroke and coronary heart disease:

Part II. Effects of short-term reductions in blood pressure and overview of the unconfounded randomised drug trials in an epidemiological context. *Lancet* 1990;**335**:827–38.

57 Wolf PA, D'Agostino B, Kannel WB, *et al.* Cigarette smoking as a risk factor for stroke: the Framingham Study. *JAMA* 1988;**259**:1025.

58 Abbott RD, Yin Y, Reed DM, *et al.* Risk of stroke in male cigarette smokers. *N Engl J Med* 1986;**315**:717–20.

59 Gillum RF, Fabsitz RR, Feinleib M, *et al.* Community surveillance for cerebrovascular disease: the Framingham cardiovascular disease survey. *Public Health Rep* 1978;**93**: 438–42.

60 Davis PH, Dambrosia JM, Schoenberg BS, *et al.* Risk factors for ischemic stroke: a prospective study in Rochester, Minnesota. *Ann Neurol* 1987;**22**:319–27.

61 DiTullio M, Sacco RL, Gopal A, *et al.* Prevalence of patent foramen ovale in older cryptogenic stroke patients assessed by contrast echocardiography. *J Am Soc Echocardiogr* 1991;**4**:294.

62 Wolf PA, Kannel WB, McGee DL. Prevention of ischemic stroke: risk factors. In: Barnett HJM, Mohr JP, Stein BM, Yatsu FM, eds. *Stroke: pathophysiology, diagnosis and management.* New York: Churchill Livingstone, 1986.

63 Kiyohara Y, Ueda K, Hasuo Y, *et al.* Hematocrit as a risk factor of cerebral infarction: long-term prospective population survey in a Japanese rural community. *Stroke* 1986;**17**:687.

64 Briley DP, Coull BM, Goodnight SH. Neurological disease associated with antiphospholipid antibodies. *Ann Neurol* 1989;**25**:221–7.

65 Nencini P, Baruffi MC, Abbate R, *et al.* Lupus anticoagulant and anticardiolipin antibodies in young adults with cerebral ischaemia. *Stroke* 1992;**23**:189–93.

66 Hess DC, Krauss, J, Adams RJ, *et al.* Anticardiolipin antibodies: a study of frequency in TIA and stroke. *Neurology* 1991;**41**:1181–9.

67 Takano K, Yamaguchi T, Uchida K. Markers of a hypercoagulable state following acute ischemic stroke. *Stroke* 1992;**23**:194-8.

68 Wolf PA, D'Agostino RB, Odell P, *et al.* Alcohol consumption as a risk factor for stroke: the Framingham Study. *Ann Neurol* 1988;**24**:177.

69 Gill GS, Zezulka AV, Shipley MJ, *et al.* Stroke and alcohol consumption. *N Engl J Med* 1986;**315**:1041–6.

70 Stampfer NJ, Colditz GA, Willett WC, *et al.* A prospective study of moderate alcohol consumption and the risk of coronary disease and stroke in women. *N Engl J Med* 1988;**319**:267–73.

71 Matsumoto N, Whisnant JP, Kurland LT, *et al.* Natural history of stroke in Rochester, Minnesota, 1955 through 1969: an extension of a previous study. *Stroke* 1973;**4**:20–9.

72 Sacco RL, Foulkes MA, Mohr JP, *et al.* Determinants of early recurrence of cerebral infarction: Stroke Data Bank. *Ann Neurol* 1989;**25**:382–90.

73 Goldstein LB, Perry A. Early recurrent ischemic stroke: a case-control study. *Stroke* 1992;**23**:1010–3.

74 Eastcott HHG, Pickering GW, Rob CG. Reconstuction of internal carotid artery in a patient with intermittent attacks of hemiplegia. *Lancet* 1954;**2**:994–6.

75 Polcras R, Dyken ML. Dramatic changes in the performance of endarterectomy for diseases of the extracranial arteries of the head. *Stroke* 1988;**19**:1289–90.

76 EC-IC Bypass Study Group: Failure of extracranial-intracranial arterial bypass to reduce the risk of ischemic stroke: results of an international randomized trial. *N Engl J Med* 1985;**313**:1191–1200.

77 North American Symptomatic Carotid Endarterectomy Trial Collaborators. Beneficial effect of carotid endarterectomy in symptomatic patients with high-grade carotid stenosis. *N Engl J Med* 1991;**325**:452.

78 Mayberg MR, Wilson SE, Yatsu F, *et al.* Carotid endarterectomy and prevention of cerebral ischaemia in symptomatic carotid stenosis. *JAMA* 1991;**266**:3289–94.

79 European Carotid Surgery Trialists' Collaborative Group. MRC European Carotid Surgery Trial: interim results for symptomatic patients with severe (70–99%) or with mild (0–29%) carotid stenosis. *Lancet* 1991;**337**:1235–43.

80 Podore PC, DeWeese JA, May AG, Rob CG. Asymptomatic contralateral carotid artery stenosis: a five year follow-up study following carotid endarterectomy. *Surgery* 1980;**88**:748–52.

81 Levin SM, Sondheimer FK, Levin JM. The contralateral diseased but asymptomatic carotid artery: to operate or not? An update. *Am J Surg* 1980;**140**:203–5.

73

82 The Asymptomatic Carotid Atherosclerosis Study Group: Study design for randomized prospective trial of carotid endarterectomy for asymptomatic atherosclerosis. *Stroke* 1989;**20**:844–9.
83 Chodosh EH, Foulkes MA, Kase CS, *et al.* Silent stroke in the NINCDS Stroke Data Bank. *Neurology* 1988;**38**:1674–9.
84 The CASANOVA Study Group. Carotid surgery versus medical spy in asymptomatic carotid stenosis. *Stroke* 1991;**22**:1229–35.
85 Massaro AR, Sacco RL, Timsit SG, *et al.* Early clinical discriminators between cerebral infarction and hemorrhagic stroke. *Ann Neurol* 1990;**30**:246–7.
86 Mohr JP, Biller J, Hilal SK, *et al.* MR vs CT imaging in Acute Stroke. *Stroke* 1992;**23**:142.
87 Fisher CM, Pearlman A. The non-sudden onset of cerebral embolism. *Neurology* 1967;**17**:1025–32.
88 Mohr JP, Caplan LR, Melske JW, *et al.* The Harvard cooperative stroke registry; a prospective registry of cases hospitalized with stroke. *Neurology* 1978;**28**:754–62.
89 Bogousslavsky J, Cachin C, Regli F, *et al.* Cardiac sources of embolism and cerebral infarction-clinical consequences and vascular concommitants: the Lausanne Stroke Registry. *Neurology* 1991;**41**:855–9.
90 Massaro AR, Hoffman M, Sacco RL, *et al.* Detection of paradoxical cerebral embolism using transcranial Doppler in a patient with infarct of undetermined cause. *Cerebrovasc Dis* 1993;**3**:116–9.
91 Carpenter DA, Grubb RL, Jr, Powers WJ. Borderzone hemodynamics in cerebrovascular disease. *Neurology* 1990;**40**:1587–92.
92 Powers WJ. Cerebral hemodynamics in ischemic cerebrovascular disease. *Ann Neurol* 1991;**23**:231–40.
93 Timsit S, Sacco RL, Mohr JP, *et al.* Early clinical differentiation of atherosclerotic and cardioembolic infarction: Stroke Data Bank. *J Neurol* 1990;**237**:140.
94 Caplan LR, Brass LM, Dewitt ID, *et al.* Transcranial doppler ultrasound: present status. *Neurology* 1990;**40**:696–700.
95 Tatemichi TK, Chamorro A, Petty CW, *et al.* Hemodynamic role of ophthalmic artery collateral in internal carotid artery occlusion. *Neurology* 1990;**40**:461–4.
96 Zanette EM, Fieschi C, Bozzao L, *et al.* Comparison of cerebral angiography and transcranial Doppler sonography in acute stroke. *Stroke* 1989;**20**:899–903.
97 DeWitt LD, Wechsler LR. Transcranial Doppler. *Stroke* 1988;**19**:915–21.
98 Grolimund P, Seller RW, Aaslid R, *et al.* Evaluation of cerebrovascular disease by combined extracranial and transcranial Doppler sonography. Experience in 1039 patients. *Stroke* 1987;**18**:1018–24.
99 Zierler RE, Kohler TR, Strandness DE Jr. Duplex scanning of normal or minimally diseased carotid arteries: correlation with arteriography and clinical outcome. *J Vasc Surg* 1990;**12**:447–54.
100 Beal MF, Williams RS, Richardson EP, *et al.* Cholesterol embolism as a cause of transient ischemic attacks and cerebral infarction. *Neurology* 1981;**31**:860–5.
101 David NJ, Gordon KK, Friedberg SJ, *et al.* Fatal atheromatous cerebral embolism associated with bright plaques in the retinal arterioles. *Neurology* 1963;**13**:708–13.
102 Zatz LM, Iannone AM, Eckman PB, *et al.* Observations concerning intracerebral basilar occlusion. *Neurology* 1965;**15**:390–401.
103 Castaigne P, Lhermitte F, Cautier JC, *et al.* Arterial occlusions in the vertebro-basilar system—a study of forty four patients with post-mortem data. *Brain* 1973;**96**:133–54.
104 Adams HP, Gross CE. Embolism distal to stenosis of the middle cerebral artery. *Stroke* 1981;**12**:228–9.
105 Masuda J, Ogata J, Yutani C, *et al.* Artery to artery embolism from a thrombus formed in stenotic middle cerebral artery. Report of an autopsy case. *Stroke* 1987;**18**:680–4.
106 Barnett HJM, Peerless SJ, Kaufmann JCE. "Stump" of internal carotid artery—a source for further cerebral embolic ischaemia. *Stroke* 1978;**9**:448–56.
107 Bogousslavsky JK, Van Melle G, Regle F. The Lausanne Stroke Registry: analysis of 1000 consecutive patients with first stroke. *Stroke* 1988;**19**:1083–92.
108 Foulkes MA, Wolf PA, Price TR, *et al.* The Stroke Data Bank: design, methods, and baseline characteristics. *Stroke* 1988;**19**:547–51.
109 Bamford J, Sandercock P, Jones L. The natural history of lacunar infarction: the Oxfordshire Community Stroke Project. *Stroke* 1987;**18**:545–51.
110 Fisher CM. Lacunes: Small deep cerebral infarcts. *Neurology* 1965;**15**:774–84.
111 Fisher CM. Lacunar infarcts—a review. *Cerebrovasc Dis* 1991;**1**:311–20.

112 Chamorro AM, Sacco RI, Mohr JP, *et al*. Lacunar infarction: Clinical–CT correlations in the Stroke Data Bank. *Stroke* 1991;**22**:175–81.

113 Rascol A, Clanet M, Manelfe C. Pure motor hemiplegia: CT study of 30 cases. *Stroke* 1982;**13**:11–7.

114 Hommel M, Besson G, Le Bas JF, *et al*. Prospective study of lacunar infarction using magnetic resonance imaging. *Stroke* 1990;**21**:546–54.

115 Sacco RL, Ellenberg JA, Mohr JP, *et al*. Infarction of undetermined cause: the NINCDS Stroke Data Bank. *Ann Neurol* 1989;**25**:382–90.

116 Hart RG, Kanter MC. Hematologic disorders and ischemic stroke. A selective review. *Stroke* 1990;**21**:1111–21.

117 Sacco RL, Owen J, Mohr JP *et al*. Free protein S deficiency: a possible association with intracranial vascular occlusion. *Stroke* 1989;**20**:1657–61.

118 Levine SR, Kim S, Deegan MJ, *et al*. Ischemic stroke associated with anticardiolipin antibodies. *Stroke* 1987;**18**:1101–6.

119 Lechat P, Mas JL, Lascault G, *et al*. Prevalence of patent foramen ovale in patients with stroke. *N Engl J Med* 1988;**318**:1148–52.

120 Wiernsperger N, Gygax P, Hofmann A. Calcium antagonist PY 108-068: demonstration of its efficacy in various types of experimental brain ischaemia. *Stroke* 1984;**15**:679–85.

121 Steinberg CK, Panahian N. "Therapeutic window" for NMDA antagonist protection against focal cerebral ischaemia may be narrow. *Fourth international symposium on pharmacology of cerebral ischaemia*. Marburg, Germany, July 1992.

122 Acheson J, Danta G, Hutchinson EC. Controlled trial of dipyridamole in recent cerebral vascular disease. *BMJ* 1969;**1**:614–5.

4 Delirium

DAVID TAYLOR, SHÔN LEWIS

The concept of delirium has been with us for over two thousand years. Greek physicians, such as Hippocrates, described its essential features[1] and the Roman writer Celsus distinguished it from mania and depression.[2] Galen differentiated between primary (idiopathic) and secondary (symptomatic) forms of the disorder.[3]

Delirium is common in the hospital setting.[4] It often goes undiagnosed in its early stages[5] and may therefore present as a neurological emergency. If untreated, it is associated with a high mortality.[6] This chapter will therefore pay close attention to the diagnosis of the condition and its proper management. In addition, we will review its epidemiology, aetiology, and pathogenesis.

Terminology

A general problem in psychiatry has been the complex etymology of clinical terms. This problem has been largely rectified as a result of the move towards operational definitions in both the ICD–10 *International classification of mental and behavioural disorders* (box 1)[7] and the American *Diagnostic and statistical manual of mental disorders*, 4th edition, revised (DSMIV) (box 2).[8] "Delirium" is now the accepted term for acute, transient, global, organic disorders of higher nervous system function involving impaired consciousness and attention. It is synonymous with the "acute confusional state" of ICD–9,[9] which term it replaced, and is also referred to as "acute organic reaction" and "acute brain syndrome".

Box 1—ICD–10 diagnostic criteria for delirium

For a definite diagnosis, symptoms, mild or severe, should be present in each one of the following areas:
(a) impairment of consciousness and attention (on a continuum from clouding to coma; reduced ability to direct, focus, sustain, and shift attention);
(b) global disturbance of cognition (perceptual distortions, illusions, and hallucinations—most often visual; impairment of abstract thinking and comprehension, with or without transient delusions, but typically with some degree of incoherence; impairment of immediate recall and of recent memory but with relatively intact remote memory; disorientation for time as well as, in more severe cases, for place and person);
(c) psychomotor disturbances (hypo- or hyperactivity and unpredictable shifts from one to the other; increased reaction time; increased or decreased flow of speech; enhanced startle reaction);
(d) disturbance of the sleep–wake cycle (insomnia or, in more severe cases, total sleep loss or reversal of the sleep–wake cycle; daytime drowsiness; nocturnal worsening of symptoms; disturbing dreams or nightmares, which may continue as hallucinations after awakening);
(e) emotional disturbances, for example, depression, anxiety or fear, irritability, euphoria, apathy, or wondering perplexity.

The onset is usually rapid, the course diurnally fluctuating, and the total duration of the condition less than six months. The above clinical picture is so characteristic that a fairly confident diagnosis of delirium can be made even if the underlying cause is not firmly established. In addition to a history of an underlying physical or brain disease, evidence of cerebral dysfunction (such as, an abnormal EEG, usually but not invariably showing a slowing of the background activity) may be required if the diagnosis is in doubt.

The problem remains of a lack of consensus as to what constitutes the definition of some particular symptoms or signs in psychiatry. Neither ICD–10[7] nor DSMIV[8] contains glossary definitions for all the clinical features of delirium. In this chapter, symptoms and signs will be defined with regard to their clinical utility in diagnosing delirium. It should be borne in mind, however, that many terms such as "consciousness"[10] and "memory"[11] are

Box 2—DSMIV diagnostic criteria for delirium

(a) Disturbance of consciousness (i.e., reduced clarity of awareness of the environment) with reduced ability to focus, sustain, or shift attention.

(b) A change in cognition (such as memory deficit, disorientation, language disturbance) or the development of a perceptual disturbance that is not better accounted for by a preexisting, established, or evolving dementia.

(c) The disturbance develops over a short period of time (usually hours to days) and tends to fluctuate during the course of the day.

(d) There is evidence from the history, physical examination, or laboratory findings that the disturbance is caused by the direct physiological consequences of a general medical condition.

Coding note: If delirium is superimposed on a preexisting Dementia of the Alzheimer's Type or Vascular Dementia, indicate the delirium by coding the appropriate subtype of the dementia, e.g., 290.3 Dementia of the Alzheimer's Type, With Late Onset, With Delirium.

Coding note: Include the name of the general medical condition on Axis I, e.g., 293.0 Delirium Due to Hepatic Encephalopathy; also code the general medical condition on Axis III (see Appendix G for codes).

used differently by different groups, even within medicine. The terms "confusion", "clouding", and "sensorium" in particular should be avoided on account of their lack of standard definitions.

Epidemiology

Sophisticated epidemiological data are now available for most psychiatric disorders. Accurate data on incidence, prevalence, and mortality in delirium, however, are difficult to come by. The comparison of estimates across studies is hampered by methodological differences. Methods of case finding and diagnosis will influence rates obtained, as will the patient population and the setting (community, general medical, surgical, or geriatric in-patient) in which the disorder is diagnosed.[12] Most incidence and prevalence studies of delirium have been conducted in inpatient settings. One notable exception is the Eastern Baltimore Mental Survey, a large community based survey forming part of the Epidemiologic Catchment Area (ECA) programme.[13] This study aimed to look at the prevalence of delirium in the general adult population aged between 18 and 64 years. A total of 810 individuals were subjected to psychiatric evaluation, and a point prevalence rate of 0·4% was calculated, rising to 1·1% for those aged 55 years and over.

Several other risk factors could be identified. When compared with dementia sufferers and to individuals of the same age who did not suffer from a psychiatric disorder, delirium sufferers were found to have more medical conditions, take more medication, and have higher levels of physical disability.

Whereas prevalence rates in the community are low, in hospital settings they are high. It has been estimated that 10% of all medical and surgical inpatients meet criteria for delirium at some point during their stay.[4] Delirium may therefore represent the mental disorder with the single highest incidence.[14]

As with community subjects, advanced age is a potent risk factor for delirium in inpatient surveys. Among elderly general medical inpatients, rates of 30%[15] or even 50%[16] have been reported, although a more conservative estimate of 17%[17] is probably more realistic. Rates of delirium in elderly surgical patients are broadly similar, although following operation for hip fracture the rate may be as high as 50%.[18]

A pre-existing dementia seems also to be a risk factor, independent of age. A large Finnish study[19] found that, in 2000 patients aged 55 and over admitted to medical wards, delirium was present in over 40% of those patients with evidence for an established dementia, compared with 15% on admission for the group as a whole.

The diagnosis of delirium carries a significant mortality rate,[6] particularly in the elderly.[20] Development of delirium doubles the risk of the patient dying[21] over a period of hours to weeks, depending on the underlying condition. Of equal importance, however, is the fact that successful treatment of the condition eliminates much of this excess mortality. Even so, death occurs in

25% of elderly patients with delirium in hospital.[13] This under-
lines the importance of early detection and urgent treatment.

Aetiology

Delirium is a consequence either of a primary brain lesion or of
cerebral involvement secondary to systemic illness, including
those cases caused by substances such as drugs and toxins. A wide
variety of causes act by way of a common pathway of electrical or
chemical disturbance to produce the clinical syndrome.[22]

Some causes of delirium are given in box 3. Almost any sufficiently severe acute medical or surgical condition may, under the
right circumstances, cause the syndrome. Although most cases of
the clinical syndrome present little difficulty in determining a

---

Box 3—Causes of delirium

(a) Primary central nervous system causes
     Head injury
     Cerebrovascular: stroke, transient ischaemic attack,
       subarachnoid haemorrhage, subdural haematoma,
       extradural haematoma
     Raised intracranial pressure
     Intracranial infection: encephalitis, meningitis.
     Epilepsy: ictal, post-ictal

(b) Secondary to systemic illness
     Infections: chest, urinary tract, septicaemia, malaria, HIV
     Cardiovascular: infarction, cardiac failure, arrhythmia
     Metabolic: hypo/hyperglycaemia, uraemia, hepatic failure,
       electrolyte disturbances
     Endocrine: addisonian crisis, disturbance of thyroid,
       parathyroid
     Alcohol: Wernicke's encephalopathy, delirium tremens
     Toxins, e.g. carbon monoxide
     Illicit drugs, e.g. amphetamine, cocaine
     Prescribed drugs: psychotropic drugs, steroids, digoxin,
       cimetidine, anticonvulsants, anticholinergics, overdosage

(c) Rare causes
     Systemic lupus erythematosus, porphyria, vitamin B-12 or
       folate deficiency, pellagra, heavy metal poisoning,
       hypothermia, Wilson's disease, remote effect of
       carcinoma, hypertensive encephalopathy

---

cause, a substantial minority of patients (as high as 5–20% of the elderly delirious)[20] never receive an aetiological diagnosis. In this situation, it may be necessary to reconsider the diagnosis, but cases remain where the clinical diagnosis is not in doubt, and the aetiological agent simply remains unidentified. It must also be remembered that more than one aetiological factor may be contributing to the patient's delirium, particularly in the elderly.[23]

The commonest causes of delirium include alcohol abuse and withdrawal, stroke, diabetes, ischaemic heart disease, pneumonia, and urinary tract infections.[24] Almost any medically prescribed drug can cause delirium if taken in sufficient overdose, but anticholinergic and hypnotic agents in particular are known for their propensity to provoke the disorder, especially in the elderly.[25]

Pathology and pathogenesis

The neuropathology associated with delirium is obviously determined by the cause of the underlying disorder, but it is important to note that brains of patients dying with delirium often reveal no obvious macroscopic or microscopic pathological changes,[26] reflecting the fact that many cases are related to systemic disturbance resulting in global higher nervous system dysfunction at a cellular or molecular level. This consideration limits enquiry into which sites are critical in mediating the psychological disturbance in delirium. The frontal lobes are known to subserve psychological functions considered to be of primary importance in delirium, such as attention.[27] Localised lesions elsewhere in the brain may also cause the condition.[28] This observation has three possible explanations: a widely distributed substrate for consciousness and attention (which appears to be the case, including the prefrontal, cingulate, and parietal cortices, the reticular activating system, and thalamic projections),[22] functional diaschisis,[29] or increased intracranial pressure.[30] Any or all of these three explanations may be relevant in an individual patient. Likewise, although it has been argued that lesions of the right cerebral hemisphere are more prone to result in delirium,[28] as a result of attentional processes possibly being dominant on the right side,[31] left sided lesions may also give rise to the condition.[32]

Although it is often assumed that delirium is associated with impaired cerebral oxidative metabolism, there is little direct evidence either to support or refute this claim. Normal cerebral function relies almost entirely on the oxidative metabolism of glucose.[33] In the normal subject there is usually a close correlation between neural activity, regional cerebral metabolism, and cerebral blood flow.[34] Studies of cerebral metabolic rate in delirium are rare and lack consistency in their results. In one study, a correlation was demonstrated between cerebral metabolic rate and level of consciousness:[33] cerebral oxygen consumption decreased as the subjects passed from normal consciousness through "confusion" to coma. Delirium, however, can occur in the absence of, or precede, failure of cerebral metabolism[35] and additional mechanisms must therefore play a part.

Studies on delirious patients measuring regional cerebral blood flow are equally sparse and contradictory. In the conscious state, the frontal lobes are activated relative to post-frontal regions of the brain. A case of delirium has been reported showing an absence of this normal physiological "hyperfrontality" on measurement of cerebral blood flow.[36] Another study reported no correlation between cerebral blood flow and psychological impairment in delirium tremens.[37]

In the delirious patient, the deviation of electrical activity on the EEG from that of the normal waking state correlates well with the clinical condition:[38] in most cases, the greater the slowing of the EEG trace, the more clinically impaired the patient.[38] Delirium associated with withdrawal states such as delirium tremens does not follow this general rule and tends to be associated with fast wave activity superimposed on generalised slowing of the trace, suggesting additional pathogenic mechanisms.[39] The rate of change of frequency is important: single EEG recordings may occasionally give a false impression in delirious patients with unusually high or low premorbid baseline frequencies,[40] implying the desirability of serial EEG recordings in the diagnosis of delirium. These changes are reversible and mirrored in the patient's clinical recovery.[39 41]

EEG recordings made during the day in delirious patients reveal disorder of the circadian rhythm, with traces characteristic of wakefulness, somnolence, and sleep emerging in a disorganised manner. Night traces likewise display breakdown of the normal rhythm of sleep stage progression as well as reduction in the overall sleep time.[42]

The exact nature of the neurochemical correlates of delirium are poorly understood. Claims have been made for the primacy of acetylcholine in this context on both clinical[43] and experimental[44] grounds. In the past, similar claims were made in Alzheimer's dementia research which proved to be unfounded, and caution is therefore essential in ascribing a primary role for acetylcholine in the pathogenesis of delirium. Nonetheless, hypoxia occurring with decreased cerebral oxidative metabolism results in a generalised decrease in neurotransmitter synthesis, preferentially affecting acetylcholine.[45] Blockade of central cholinergic projections certainly can result in delirium[44] and it is of some interest that anticholinergic agents reduce cerebral perfusion in the frontal cortex.[46] Cerebral structures and pathways implicated in higher CNS processes such as consciousness and attention are legion[47 48] and the primary neurochemical abnormality in delirium has yet to be clarified.

Clinical features

As noted by Lishman,[49] one of the most intriguing aspects of delirium is the constancy of the clinical picture despite the wide variety of different causes.

Traditionally, impaired *consciousness* is the cardinal feature of delirium. The main problem here is that consciousness is a complex, ill-defined concept. A number of different aspects of consciousness have been described including awareness (of the external environment), alertness, and wakefulness.[22] Awareness is always impaired in delirium. DSMIV[8] requires the presence of a disturbance of consciousness in the form of reduced clarity of awareness of the environment. Alertness to environmental stimuli may be abnormally elevated or lowered. If hyperalert, the patient responds to stimuli without discrimination, with the clinical result that he or she is distracted by irrelevant events at the expense of the more relevant. It is characteristic of delirium tremens and may be accompanied by overactivity. If hypoalert, there is an overall reduction in response to environmental stimuli; for example, the patient may remain mute as the physician attempts to take a history. This is characteristically seen in metabolic encephalopathies and may be associated with underactivity. Any one individual delirious patient, however, may alternate between hyper- and hypoalertness, as well as exhibiting relatively lucid periods.

The sleep–wake cycle is disrupted in delirium: the patient may exhibit excessive drowsiness by day with or without insomnia at night. In severe cases there may be total insomnia or reversal of the cycle. Sleep may be accompanied by nightmares which may then merge into frank hallucinations on wakening.

Impaired ability to focus, sustain, or shift *attention* is seen in delirium.[8] Thus questions may need to be repeated because the patient's attention wanders, or the patient may perseverate in the answer to a previous question rather than appropriately shift attention. The patient may have difficulty with such basic bedside tasks as serial sevens (subtraction of seven from 100, then seven from 93 and so on), and digit span (immediate verbal recall of a string of digits). It is, however, essential to appreciate that impairment on any basic test of attention is not an absolute indication of dysfunction: possible confounding factors include the patient's age, level of educational attainment, and coexisting anxiety. It has been claimed that serial sevens and digit span do not even allow differentiation of organic from "functional" disorders, let alone delirium from dementia.[50 51] If doubt remains about the presence of attentional deficit, one means of helping to decide the matter is to give increasingly simple tasks, such as requesting the months of the year or days of the week in reverse, serial threes or serial ones (asking the patient to subtract one from 20, then one from 19 and so on).

These impairments of attention are essentially impairments of immediate memory. A number of forms of *memory* impairment may be seen in delirium. Immediate ("working") memory relates to the ability to hold information for very short periods of only a few seconds. In contrast, recent memory refers to information recalled after a delay of minutes. Remote memory refers to the recall of events that occurred days, weeks, months, or years previously.[52]

In delirium, disordered immediate memory is primary. Secondary, anterograde recent memory deficits result, and remote memory deficits may also be present,[39] although generally there is relative preservation of remote memory except in the most severe cases. Thus the amnestic deficit, although primarily anterograde, may as a result contain retrograde elements.

Recent memory deficit may be elicited by the patient's inability to recall completely after five minutes a seven-unit name and address or even three nouns (for example, apple, book, coat) after correct registration and subsequent distraction (e.g. with another cognitive task. Registration (the immediate repetition of the units) is obviously contingent on adequate attentional processes and it therefore follows that, if those processes are impaired to such an extent that the patient cannot correctly register the units, then formal testing of recent memory will result in impaired performance.

Disorientation for time, place, and person reflects abnormalities in immediate, recent, and remote memory.[53] It does not refer to the parietal lobe phenomenon of "topographical disorientation". Disorientation for the exact time of day is considered a sensitive indicator of delirium.[54] As the disorder progresses and becomes more established the patient characteristically loses the ability to correctly identify the day of the week, the month of the year, or even the year itself. In relatively mild cases of the disorder the patient may be fully orientated for place and person but disorientated for time.

Disorientation for place refers to the patient's inability to identify correctly where he or she is physically located at the time of interview. Some consideration must be given to the context in which the interview occurs when assessing this. For example, a patient at home may be able to identify this correctly, yet become disorientated for place when admitted to hospital.[55][56] Presumably in such cases a relatively unimpaired access to the remote memory store compensates for the underlying functional deficit.

Misidentification of persons often occurs and usually involves mistaking unfamiliar persons for familiar.[57] Here again context is important. For example, a patient's inability to identify his or her recently acquired hospital doctor would not give as much cause for concern as being unable to recognise a spouse. Global misidentification of persons is common in delirium and must be differentiated from prosopagnosia which is a selective inability to recognise an individual by facial characteristics; this occurs as a result of damage to the non-dominant occipitotemporal gyrus.

Thought content in delirium has often been noted to have an oneroid (dream-like) quality.[58][59] Delusions, when they occur, are typically transitory and fragmentary, and usually of a persecutory nature. Different studies put their prevalence at between 40% and 100%.[60-62]

Patients often experience abnormal perceptions. These have been shown to be related to impairments of perceptual processing.[63] The percept may be distorted, and happens most often in the visual modality. Examples include metamorphopsia (distortions in the perceived size of objects including macropsia and micropsia), dysmorphopsia (alterations in shape), and polyopsia (a single object perceived as multiples). In addition, the patient may have difficulty in distinguishing between internal mental events and external percepts. Perceptual misidentifications (illusions) are also common, as in delirium tremens where, for example, an innocuous wallpaper pattern may be perceived by the patient as a host of unpleasant scurrying animals. Less commonly, the abnormal percepts have absolutely no basis in external reality (hallucinations). They occur in between 40% and 75% of all cases of delirium[60-62 64] and are more common in younger patients. Again, they are most often visual.[60] They vary in complexity from simple geometric shapes and colours to the highly detailed, such as people, animals, or the physical environment. They are most frequently associated with hyperalert states of delirium such as occur commonly with withdrawal states associated with alcohol, hypnotics, and anxiolytics, and intoxication states associated, for example, with anticholinergic drugs.

Mood disturbance is frequent, in particular irritability, agitation, aggression, anxiety, depression, apathy, perplexity, or suspiciousness.[60 61] Euphoria may also occur, but is less common.[22] The mood and its behavioural consequences shift frequently and rapidly from one state to another, giving a characteristic lability of mood. Anxiety or fear is often seen in hyperalert states and will be accompanied by overactivity of the autonomic nervous system. Mood disturbances can be marked and present an urgent management problem: undertreated agitation may result in injury to the patient or others.

The abnormalities in mentation present in delirium result in directly observable abnormalities of behaviour, including speech. The patient may be either underactive or overactive or may irregularly alternate between the two. The level of activity tends to correlate with the level of conscious alertness exhibited by the patient at the time. In general, hyperalertness is associated with general motor overactivity which is at best semi-purposeful, such as repeatedly getting out of bed in an attempt to leave the hospital. On other occasions the behaviour is essentially purposeless, for example, picking at the bedclothes (carphology) and purposeless tossing and turning in the bed (sactitation). Speech may be increased in quantity, rate, and volume; in some cases it may be frankly incoherent. There may be associated defects such as alexia[65] and agraphia.[66] In contrast, hypoactivity is associated with general underactivity, prolongation of the reaction time, and speech which is reduced in quantity, slow, monotonous, and low in volume. In severe cases the patient may be stuporous and mute. It is important to emphasise that these two dimensions of the clinical syndrome are not distinct subtypes of delirium, as both may occur in irregular alternation during any one illness. It is equally important to bear in mind that the popular medical conception of delirium corresponds to hyperactivity; it follows that in hypoactive patients a diagnosis of delirium may be missed.[39]

Clinical information on both recent and remote memory can sometimes be inferred from the patient's spontaneous behaviour and speech. For example, he may insist that he is seeing his wife for the first time that day even though she had been talking with him at his bedside just a few minutes earlier (impaired recent memory). He may believe, despite being in hospital, that he is living at a location he left many years earlier and may talk of going out to work at what was his occupation there at that time (impairment of recent memory with inappropriate accessing of remote memory). If severely ill, he may claim never to have met his wife and children before (impairment of remote memory). Confabulation is the term for the giving of false past personal information in the context of a recent memory deficit, and is presumed to be an attempt by the patient to obscure the memory deficit.

The *clinical course* of an episode of delirium is influenced by individual patient variables such as age and general physical condition, the cause of the disturbance, and the speed and efficacy of management interventions. Certain statements, however, apply to delirium in general. Onset is typically sudden, developing over hours or days, and often begins at night. In those cases with a relatively gradual onset, there may be a prodromal period in which the patient complains of various non-specific symptoms such as malaise, irritability, sleep disruption, nightmares, and difficulty in concentrating. Once established, the clinical picture tends to fluctuate in intensity. Lucid intervals occur most commonly during the day, and the usual pattern is nocturnal worsening, when levels of conscious awareness and attention are lowered, with abnormally raised or lowered levels of conscious alertness. If the underlying disease is severe and progressive, the patient may lapse into an increasingly pronounced stupor, followed by coma and death. This downward spiral is sometimes preceded by a period of

5 Acute behaviour disturbances

G G LLOYD

Psychiatric disorders are commonly encountered in neurological practice and most neurologists accept the need to assess and manage behavioural problems. The more complicated cases require expert psychiatric intervention and, for optimum care, it is essential that there is close collaboration between neurologist and psychiatrist.

Many neurological conditions, particularly those with cerebral involvement, increase the risk of developing a psychiatric disorder. Furthermore psychiatric disorders can be associated with symptoms such as headache, dizziness, and weakness which suggest neurological disease but for which no organic explanation can be found. This phenomenon, known as somatisation, is being increasingly recognised and accounts for a substantial proportion of patients who are referred to neurological departments.

Schiffer[1] evaluated a consecutive series of 241 patients attending an American neurology service and found that 101 (41·9%) had symptoms sufficient to warrant a psychiatric diagnosis according to DSM–III criteria. Of 57 inpatients, 10 were considered to have a primary psychiatric disorder and five of these had no neurological illness. Among 184 outpatients, 32 had a primary psychiatric disorder and 30 of these had no neurological illness. Kirk and Saunders[2] had previously described a retrospective survey from a neurological clinic in northeast England and reported that, during a four year period, 358 (13·2%) of 2716 patients had a psychiatric disorder with no evidence of neurological illness.

102

with
inje
sed
spe
a d
mai
of
exp
not
foll
viev
inte
and
ulai
mei
of i
dur

So

T
rep
mec
unli
at ti
mec

Ac

P
and
and
nial
bod
mu
eith
the
and
deli
D

response include natu
or terrorist activity, a1
disorder has been esti
tain multiple injuries a
  There is a delay be
symptoms which rang
The typical symptoms
event ("flashbacks"),
emotional blunting, av
original trauma, depre

Management of an:
therapy, involving rela
tating situation, is of
panic disorder when t
chologist should asse
behaviour or cognitive
elzine is a useful adju
Drug treatment is more
phenelzine and imipran
  There has been con
ment of people who h
and who are at risk of
psychiatric disorders.[3]
tant.[36] Various techn
therapy and cognitive
allow the patient to r
tional response in a ca
ment of avoidance
established, either tric
inhibitors can provide

Dissociative (conv

  This group of diso
The term "hysteria" i
different ways; as a re:
and ICD–10 but it is
clinical practice.
  Dissociative disord
suggest lesions in the

prot
sele
moc
  A
effec
a sp
ther
ticul
stup
inta
Hea
to t1
ond
Act
dep1
  T
treat
of th
tinu
whic

Ma1
  T
of c
enh:
pres
loss
irrit

If the psychiatric disorder underlying the neurological symptoms is not recognised, patients can be subjected to unnecessary and expensive investigations.[3] They may receive symptomatic treatment which fails to alleviate their condition and they will become dissatisfied with the result of their treatment and try to consult other specialists in the hope of finding a more effective remedy.

Some of the psychological symptoms and behavioural disturbances which the neurologist encounters are of sudden onset and require urgent attention. This review describes the clinical features and management of those disorders that are most likely to give rise to acute behavioural problems in neurological practice.

Affective disorders

The fundamental disturbance is a change of mood (or affect), either depression or elation. Mood disturbance is not necessarily the most prominent symptom, however, and it may be masked by a wide range of other abnormalities which at first sight suggest the presence of organic disease. Affective disorders have a tendency to recur. When the recurrences always take the same form, the condition is referred to as unipolar affective disorder; when the mood change varies between depression or elation it is described as bipolar affective disorder.

Depressive disorder

Depression not associated with organic disease usually presents to the neurologist with symptoms such as headache, dizziness, disturbance of higher mental function, and facial or bodily pain.[4] Psychological symptoms, emotional conflicts, and life stresses may not be volunteered and are only elicited by tactful, direct questioning on the part of the examining doctor. Fitzpatrick and Hopkins[5] assessed a series of patients referred to a neurologist with headaches not due to structural disease and found that 37% had an affective disorder of at least mild severity. The preoccupation with pain may dominate the clinical picture to such an extent that the patient does not appear depressed and does not readily admit to feeling depressed. This has been described in relation to facial pain;[6] the cognitive features of depression such as self reproach, suicidal thinking, and psychomotor retardation were uncommon but, in addition to pain, the patients complained of insomnia, fatigue, irritability, and agitation.

103

Phobic anxiet

A phobia
situation wh:
precipitates
tered clinica
are particula:
centration, d
sis comes fro
situations wh
phobia the c
supermarket:

Panic disordei

The char:
whelming an
particular si
palpitations,
dominate the
ety, often in
attack or brai
ation which
bodies which
ings and are
may be mist:
disease, or i
neurological
ential diagr
hypoglycaem

A typical
Patients bec
learn to avoi
embarrassing
there is no e;
ciated with a

Post-traumati

This synd
stressful expe
is quite outs
likely to cau
danger of de
sustained m:

severe head injury reported that the prevalence of personality change increased with time; at five years after the injury, 74% of patients were described by their relatives as having undergone a personality change. Threats or gestures of violence had occurred in 54% while there had been an actual assault on a relative in 20% of cases. Other problems which had occurred included trouble with the law (31%), childishness (38%), and being upset by minor changes in routine (38%).[53]

Brain injury can produce an exaggeration of premorbid personality traits so that a person with an obsessional personality becomes even more meticulous and preoccupied with detail, whereas someone with a psychopathic personality becomes more impulsive and irresponsible. Among a group of patients with Wilson's disease, psychopathic personality traits were significantly related to the severity of neurological symptoms, particularly dysarthria, bradykinesia, and rigidity.[54] If the damage is localised to particular parts of the brain, the personality changes tend to be more specific.[55 56] Frontal lobe damage is associated with apathy, lack of initiative, tactlessness, irritability, euphoria, and disinhibition. Although the patient's demeanour is predominantly listless there may be unpredictable outbursts of aggression or sexually disinhibited behaviour. Social skills tend to be lost with a failure to consider the feelings of other people and the impact of tactless remarks. The ability to plan ahead is impaired with the result that irresponsible decisions may be taken with little concern about their outcome.

Irritability and aggressive outbursts are especially associated with temporal lobe pathology. Herpes simplex encephalitis has an affinity for the temporal lobes, so behavioural manifestations are common during the acute stages of the illness and after recovery if there is residual brain damage. Patients who survive temporal lobe damage may manifest the features of the Kluver–Bucy syndrome which include hypersexuality, aggressive outbursts, excessive oral behaviour, and visual agnosia.

Management of aggressive behaviour—Box 4 summarises the conditions in which unpredictable outbursts of aggression may occur.

Patients who are potentially violent should not be interviewed in an isolated room; when the risk is particularly high the doctor should not be alone with such patients. Adequate staff should be available nearby. The immediate aims are to control the risk of

---

Box 4—Neurological and psychiatric disorders associated with aggression

- Acute delirium
- Brain damage—especially to frontal and temporal lobes
- Epilepsy
- Functional psychoses—schizophrenia, bipolar affective disorder
- Alcohol abuse—intoxication, withdrawal
- Drug abuse—intoxication, withdrawal, threatening behaviour to obtain drugs
- Personality disorder

---

violence, to diagnose the underlying disorder, and to administer specific treatment. A detailed history and full physical and mental state assessment are rarely possible; immediate treatment has to be arranged before complete information is available.

Every effort should be made to calm patients by sympathetic understanding and reassurance. Violence is often a response to paranoid experiences and patients can be pacified if they believe that the doctor appreciates the reasons for their behaviour. If this can be achieved medication may be accepted voluntarily; otherwise compulsory treatment becomes unavoidable if patients are endangering themselves or others. Physical restraint should be applied with the assistance of security staff; the safety of all involved is best ensured by having more than a sufficient number of staff available. At least one person should restrain each limb while another administers medication.[57][58] Haloperidol 10–20 mg intramuscularly or droperidol 5–15 mg intravenously are the preferred drugs, except for cases of alcohol or drug misuse or patients with serious physical illness. Benzodiazepines should then be given instead—for example, diazepam 10 mg by slow intravenous injection or lorazepam 2 mg intramuscularly. Once the risk of aggression has been controlled it is nearly always necessary to arrange admission to an appropriate inpatient unit to begin a diagnostic evaluation and specific treatment for the underlying condition when the diagnosis has been clarified.

119

Management of acute behaviour disturbances

● Acute behaviour disturbances are commonly encountered in neurological practice. Psychiatric disorders may accompany neurological disease or may present with somatic symptoms that suggest neurological lesions but for which no organic pathology can be detected.

● Evidence of intellectual impairment, particularly reduced level of consciousness, disorientation, and memory deficits, enables conditions such as delirium, which are due to overt physical disease, to be distinguished from affective, anxiety, and acute psychotic disorders. The psychotic disorders are not usually associated with overt physical disease although in a few patients they may be the presenting manifestations of an occult lesion in the central nervous system or elsewhere. The likelihood of this increases with advancing age and if there is no previous personal or family history of psychiatric illness or no apparent psychosocial precipitating factor.

● Successful management requires close collaboration between neurologists and psychiatrists. It is essential to be familiar with the psychotropic drugs that are most appropriately used for patients with neurological disorders. Tricyclic antidepressants and selective serotonin re-uptake inhibitors are both used for treating depression but the latter group of drugs may prove more acceptable because of their lower incidence of side effects.

● Acute psychotic disorders require treatment with neuroleptic drugs, the main groups being the phenothiazines and butyrophenones. Rapid control of acute psychosis is essential when it is associated with aggressive behaviour and it is important that clinicians are familiar with regimens of parenteral neuroleptic administration and indications for compulsory treatment.

1 Schiffer RB. Psychiatric aspects of clinical neurology. *Am J Psychiatry* 1983;**140**:205–7.
2 Kirk C, Saunders M. Primary psychiatric illness in a neurological outpatient department in north-east England. *J Psychosom Res* 1977;**21**:1–5.
3 Lloyd G. Somatization: a psychiatrist's perspective. *J Psychosom Res* 1989;**33**:665–9.
4 Kirk C, Saunders M. Primary psychiatric illness in a neurological outpatient department in North East England: an assessment of symptomatology. *Acta Psychiatr Scand* 1977:**56**:294–302.
5 Fitzpatrick R, Hopkins A. Referrals to neurologists for headaches not due to structural disease. *J Neurol Neurosurg Psychiatry* 1981;**44**:1061–7.

6 Lascelles RG. Atypical facial pain and depression. *Br J Psychiatry* 1966;**112**:651–9.
7 Fullerton DT, Harvey RF, Klein MH, Howell T. Psychiatric disorders in patients with spinal cord injuries. *Arch Gen Psychiatry* 1981;**38**:1369–71.
8 Judd FK, Stone J, Weber JE, Brown DJ, Burrows GD. Depression following spinal cord injury: a prospective inpatient study. *Br J Psychiatry* 1989;**154**:668–71.
9 World Health Organization. The ICD-10 classification of mental and behavioural disorders: clinical descriptions and diagnostic guidelines. Geneva: WHO, 1992.
10 Lloyd GG. Psychiatry in general medicine. In: Kendell RE, Zealley AK, eds. *Companion to psychiatric studies*, 5th ed. Edinburgh: Churchill Livingstone, 1993:779–92.
11 Whitlock FA. *Symptomatic affective disorders*. London: Academic Press, 1982.
12 Ron MA. Psychiatric manifestations of frontal lobe tumours. *Br J Psychiatry* 1989;**155**:735–8.
13 Ron MA, Logsdail SJ. Psychiatric morbidity in multiple sclerosis: a clinical and MRI study. *Psychol Med* 1989;**19**:887–95.
14 Berrios GE, Quemada JI. Depressive illness in multiple sclerosis: clinical and theoretical aspects of the association. *Br J Psychiatry* 1990;**156**:10–16.
15 Kearney TR. Parkinson's disease presenting as a depressive illness. *J Irish Med Assoc* 1964;**54**:117–19.
16 Mindham RHS. Psychiatric symptoms in Parkinsonism. *J Neurol Neurosurg Psychiatry* 1970;**33**:188–91.
17 Lyon RL. Huntington's chorea in the Moray Firth area. *BMJ* 1962;**1**:1301–6.
18 Folstein SE, Abbott MH, Chase GA, Jenson BA, Folstein MF. The association of affective disorder with Huntington's disease in a case series and in families. *Psychol Med* 1983;**13**:537–42.
19 Eastwood MR, Rifat SL, Nobbs H, Ruderman J. Mood disorder following cerebrovascular accident. *Br J Psychiatry* 1989;**154**:195–200.
20 Robinson RG, Starr LB, Kubos KL, *et al.* A two-year longitudinal study of post-stroke mood disorder: findings during the initial evaluation. *Stroke* 1983;**14**:736–41.
21 Starkstein SE, Robinson·RG. Affective disorders and cerebrovascular disease. *Br J Psychiatry* 1989;**154**:170–82.
22 House A, Dennis M, Mogridge L, Warlow C, Hawton K, Jones L. Mood disorders in the first year after stroke. *Br J Psychiatry* 1992;**158**:83–92.
23 House A, Dennis M, Molyneux A, Warlow C, Hawton K. Emotionalism after stroke. *BMJ* 1989;**298**:991–4.
24 Stenager EN, Stenager E. Suicide and patients with neurologic diseases: methodological problems. *Arch Neurol* 1992;**49**:1296–303.
25 Stenager EN, Stenager E, Koch-Henderson N, *et al.* Suicide and multiple sclerosis: an epidemiological investigation. *J Neurol Neurosurg Psychiatry* 1992;**55**:542–5.
26 Nordentoft M, Breum L, Munck LK, Nordestgaartd AG, Hunding A, Bjaeldager PAL. High mortality by natural and unnatural causes: a 10 year follow up study of patients admitted to a poisoning treatment centre after suicide attempts. *BMJ* 1993;**306**:1637–41.
27 Hawton K, Fagg J, Platt S, Hawkins M. Factors associated with suicide after parasuicide in young people. *BMJ* 1993;**306**:1641–4.
28 Kreitman N. Suicide and parasuicide. In: Kendell RE, Zealley AK, eds. *Companion to psychiatric studies*, 5th ed. Edinburgh: Churchill Livingstone, 1993:743–60.
29 Lishman WA. *Organic psychiatry: the psychological consequences of cerebral disorder*, 2nd ed. Oxford: Blackwell, 1987.
30 Joyston-Bechal MP. Clinical features and outcome of stupor. *Br J Psychiatry* 1966;**112**: 967–81.
31 Johnson J. Stupor: a review of 25 cases. *Acta Psychiat Scand* 1984;**70**:370–7.
32 Starkstein SE, Pearson GD, Boston J, Robinson RG. Mania after brain injury: a controlled study of causative factors. *Arch Neurol* 1988;**44**:1069–73.
33 Jorge RE, Robbinson RG, Starkstein SE, Arndt SV, Forrester AW, Geisler FH. Secondary mania following traumatic brain injury. *Am J Psychiatry* 1993;**150**:916–21.
34 Mayou R. Psychiatric aspects of road traffic accidents. *Int Rev Psychiatry* 1992;**4**:45–54.
35 Rosser R, Dewer S. Therapeutic flexibility in post disaster response. *J R Soc Med* 1991;**84**: 2–3.
36 Ramsay R. Post traumatic stress disorder: a new clinical entity? *J Psychosom Res* 1990;**34**: 355–65.
37 Davidson J. Drug therapy of post traumatic stress disorder. *Br J Psychiatry* 1992;**160**: 309–14.

38 Marsden CD. Hysteria: a neurologist's view. *Psychol Med* 1986;**16**:277–88.
39 Lloyd GG. Hysteria: a case for conservation? *BMJ* 1986;**294**:1255–6.
40 Trimble MR. *Neuropsychiatry*. Chichester: John Wiley & Sons, 1981.
41 Ljunberg L. Hysteria: a clinical prognostic and genetic study. *Acta Psychiat Scand* 1957;**32**:Suppl 112.
42 Pincus J. Hysteria presenting to the neurologist. In: Roy A, ed. *Hysteria*. Chichester: John Wiley & Sons, 1982.
43 Fenton GW. Epilepsy and hysteria. *Br J Psychiatry* 1986;**149**:28–37.
44 Roy A. Hysterical fits previously diagnosed as epilepsy. *Psychol Med* 1977;**7**:271–3.
45 Kopelman MD. Amnesia: organic and psychogenic. *Br J Psychiatry* 1987;**150**:428–42.
46 Keane JR. Hysterical gait disorders: 60 cases. *Neurology* 1989;**39**:586–9.
47 Perry JC, Jacobs D. Clinical applications of the amytal interview in psychiatric emergency settings. *Am J Psychiatry* 1982;**139**:552–9.
48 Taylor D, Lewis S. Delirium. *J Neurol Neurosurg Psychiatry* 1993;**56**:742–51.
49 Friedman JH. The management of levodopa psychoses. *Clin Neuropharmacol* 1991;**14**:283–95.
50 Feinstein A, Ron MA. Psychosis associated with demonstrable brain diseases. *Psychol Med* 1990;**20**:793–803.
51 Kellam AMP. The neuroleptic malignant syndrome, so-called: a review of the world literature. *Br J Psychiatry* 1987;**150**:752–9.
52 Kellam AMP. The (frequently) neuroleptic (potentially) malignant syndrome. *Br J Psychiatry* 1990;**157**:169–73.
53 Brooks N, Campsie L, Symington C, Beatty A, McKinlay W. The five year outcome of severe blunt head injury: a relative's view. *J Neurol Neurosurg Psychiatry* 1986;**49**:764–70.
54 Dening TR, Berrios GE. Wilson's disease: a prospective study of psychopathology in 31 cases. *Br J Psychiatry* 1989;**155**:206–13.
55 McClelland RJ. Psychosocial sequelae of head injury: anatomy of a relationship. *Br J Psychiatry* 1988;**153**:141–6.
56 Trimble MR. Behaviour and personality disturbances. In: Bradley WG, Daroff RB, Fenichel GM, Marsden CD, eds. *Neurology in clinical practice*, vol. 1. London: Butterworth-Heinemann, 1991:81–100.
57 Sheard MH. Clinical pharmacology of aggressive behaviour. *Clin Neuropharmacol* 1988;**11**:483–92.
58 Goldberg RJ, Dubin WR, Fogel BS. Behavioural emergencies: assessment and psychopharmacologic management. *Clin Neuropharmacol* 1989;**12**:233–48.

122

6 Tonic–clonic status epilepticus

SIMON SHORVON

Tonic–clonic status epilepticus can be defined as a condition in which prolonged or recurrent tonic–clonic seizures persist for 30 minutes or more. From indirect studies, the annual incidence of tonic–clonic status has been estimated to be approximately 18–28 cases per 100 000 persons (9000–14 000 new cases each year in the United Kingdom, or 45 000–70 000 cases in the United States).[1,2] It is most frequent in children, the mentally handicapped, and in those with structural cerebral pathology (especially in the frontal areas). In established epilepsy, status may be precipitated by drug withdrawal, intercurrent illness or metabolic disturbance, or the progression of the underlying disease, and is more common in symptomatic than in idiopathic epilepsy. About 5% of all epileptic adult clinic patients will have at least one episode of status in the course of their epilepsy,[1,2] and in children the proportion is higher (10–25%).[1-3] Most status episodes, however, do not develop in known epileptic patients, and in such cases are almost always due to acute cerebral disturbances; common causes are cerebral infection, trauma, cerebrovascular disease, cerebral tumour, acute toxic or metabolic disturbance, or febrile illness (in children). Recent studies have shown status to account for about 4% of admissions to neurological intensive care,[4] and 5% of all visits to a university hospital casualty department.[5] The mortality of tonic–clonic status is about 5–10%, most patients dying of the underlying condition, rather than the status itself or its treatment.[1,2] Permanent neurological and mental deterioration may result from status, particularly in young children, the risks of morbidity being greatly increased the longer the duration of the status episode.[36] Tonic–clonic status is only one of the forms of status epilepticus (see box 1), and indeed is not the most common. Nevertheless, unlike other types, it is a medical emergency. Treatment is urgent because the longer seizures continue, the worse the outcome and the more hazardous is therapy. Successful management is a balance between the conflicting requirements of controlling seizure activity as quickly as possible, and minimising physiological changes and medical complications.

Pathophysiology of tonic–clonic status epilepticus

The pattern of seizures in tonic–clonic status evolves over time. There is often a premonitory stage of minutes or hours, during

---

Box 1—Classification of status epilepticus (derived from Shorvon[2])

Confined to the neonatal period
Neonatal status
Status in neonatal epilepsy syndromes

Confined to infancy and childhood
Infantile spasm (West's syndrome)
Febrile status epilepticus
Status in childhood myoclonic syndromes
Status in benign childhood partial epilepsy syndromes
Electrical status during slow wave sleep (ESES)
Syndrome of acquired epileptic aphasia

Occurring in childhood and adult life
Tonic–clonic status
Absence status
Epilepsia partialis continua (EPC)
Myoclonic status in coma
Specific forms of status in mental handicap
Myoclonic status in other epilepsy syndromes
Non-convulsive simple partial non-convulsive status
Complex partial status
Boundary syndromes

Confined to adult life
De novo absence status of late onset

---

which epileptic activity increases in frequency or severity from its habitual level. This clinical deterioration is an augury, often stereotypical, of impending status, and urgent therapy may well prevent its full development. At the onset of status, the attacks typically take the form of discrete grand mal seizures. As time passes, however, the convulsive motor activity often evolves, first to become continuous, and then clonic jerking becomes less pronounced and less severe, and finally ceases altogether. This is the stage of "subtle status epilepticus",[7 8] by which time the patient will be deeply unconscious, and the prognosis is poor. In parallel to this clinical evolution, there is also sometimes a progressive change in the EEG,[9] although how consistently such a progressive clinical and EEG pattern occurs is not known. Autonomic changes in status can be profound, and dominate the clinical picture. These include hyperpyrexia, tachycardia, cardiac arrhythmia, blood pressure changes, apnoea, sweating, hypersecretion, and massive noradrenaline and adrenaline release. Other profound endocrine changes also occur.

The physiological changes in status are often divided into two phases, the transition from phase 1 to 2 occurring after about 30–60 minutes of continuous seizures.[2 10–12] Although this is a generally useful concept, it must be recognised that there is great variation. Both the rate and extent of physiological change are dependent on many other factors, including the anatomical site of the epileptic focus, the severity of the seizures, the underlying aetiology, and the treatment employed. Nevertheless, this staging of changes is helpful in devising a rational plan for therapy.

Phase 1

From the onset of status, seizure activity greatly increases cerebral metabolism. Physiological mechanisms are initially sufficient largely to compensate for this pertubation. Cerebral blood flow is increased, and initially the delivery of glucose to the active cerebral tissue is maintained. Later systemic and cerebral lactate levels rise, and a profound lactic acidosis may develop.[13] There are massive cardiovascular and autonomic changes. Blood pressure rises, as does cardiac output and rate. The autonomic changes result in sweating, hyperpyrexia, bronchial secretion, salivation and vomiting, and adrenaline and noradrenaline release. Endocrine and autonomic changes also cause an early rise in sugar levels.

125

Phase 2

As the seizure activity progresses, the compensatory physiological mechanisms begin to fail. Cerebral autoregulation breaks down progressively, and thus cerebral blood flow becomes increasingly dependent on systemic blood pressure.[10-12] Hypotension develops due to seizure-related autonomic and cardiorespiratory changes and drug treatment, and in terminal stages may be severe. The falling blood pressure results in falling cerebral blood flow and cerebral metabolism. The high metabolic demands of the epileptic cerebral tissue cannot be met and ischaemic or metabolic damage may ensue.[14-16] The tendency to hypotension can be greatly exacerbated by intravenous antiepileptic drug therapy, especially if infusion rates are too fast. Pressor agents are often necessary in prolonged therapy.

Systemic and cerebral hypoxia are common in status, due to: central respiratory failure (greatly exacerbated by drug medication); the increased oxygen requirements of convulsions; and later pulmonary artery hypertension and pulmonary oedema.[2 11] Because of this, assisted ventilation is often required early in the course of status.

Intracranial pressure may rise precipitously in status. The combined effects of systemic hypotension and intracranial hypertension can result in a compromised cerebral circulation and cerebral oedema, particularly in children.[12] Intracranial pressure monitoring is advisable in prolonged severe status, especially in children, when raised intracranial pressure is suspected; the need for active medical or surgical therapy is, however, largely determined by underlying pathology.

Cardiovascular changes in late status can also be serious. Pulmonary hypertension and oedema are frequent, even in the presence of systemic hypotension. Pulmonary artery pressures can rise to dangerous levels, well in excess of the osmotic pressure of blood, causing oedema and stretch injuries to lung capillaries.[17] Cardiac arrhythmias in status are the result of direct seizure-related autonomic activation, catecholamine release, hypoglycaemia, lactic acidosis, electrolyte disturbance, or cardiotoxic therapy. The autonomic effects are sometimes caused by simultaneous discharges in sympathetic and parasympathetic pathways. Intravenous sedatives depress cardiac function, and the drug effects can be potentiated by pre-existing compromise of cardiac function. In spite of the greatly increased demand, cardiac output can fall due to decreasing left ventricular contractility and stroke volume,[18] causing cardiac failure. The prodigious noradrenaline and adrenaline release also contributes to the cardiac dysfunction, arrhythmia, and tachycardia. Measures to control cardiac failure and arrhythmia are often needed.

Spectacular hyperpyrexia can also develop in status,[7] [13] and may also require specific treatment.

There are many metabolic and endocrine disturbances in status, the commonest and most important being: acidosis (including lactic acidosis), hypoglycaemia, hypo/hyperkalaemia, and hyponatraemia. Lactic acidosis is almost invariable in major status epilepticus,[13] from its onset, due to neuronal and muscle activity, the acceleration of glycolysis, tissue hypoxia, impaired respiration, and catecholamine release. Acute tubular necrosis due to myoglobinuria or dehydration, and occasionally fulminant renal failure, may occur. Hepatic failure is a not uncommon terminal event in status, due to other physiological disturbances, drug treatment, or underlying disease. Rhabdomyolysis, resulting from persistent convulsive movements, can develop early in status and precipitate renal failure if severe, and can be prevented by artificial ventilation and paralysing drugs. Disseminated intravascular coagulation is another rare but serious development in status which will require urgent therapy. Other medical complications in status are listed in box 2, and are usually due to the autonomic activity, seizures, or drug treatment.

Antiepileptic drug pharmacology

As fast drug absorption is essential in status, all drugs are administered parenterally. Midazolam and paraldehyde can be given intramuscularly, diazepam, midazolam, and paraldehyde by the rectal route, but all others must be given by intravenous injection. It is desirable in status for drugs to have a rapid onset and a prolonged duration of action. Unfortunately, rapidly acting drugs are usually highly lipid-soluble (for example, diazepam, midazolam, chlormethiazole, propofol), tending to redistribute quickly from cerebral tissue to accumulate in the larger peripheral lipid compartments (fat stores). Because of this, after a single intravenous injection, there is a rapid fall in cerebral drug levels; the initial injection therefore has a short-lived effect. Repeated dosing of such lipid-soluble drugs results in progressive drug

Box 2—Medical complications in tonic–clonic status epilepticus (derived from Shorvon[2])

Cerebral
Hypoxic/metabolic cerebral damage
Seizure-induced cerebral damage
Cerebral oedema and raised intracranial pressure
Cerebral venous thrombosis
Cerebral haemorrhage and infarction

Cardiovascular, respiratory, and autonomic
Hypotension
Hypertension
Cardiac failure, tachy- and bradyarrhythmia, arrest
Cardiogenic shock
Respiratory failure
Disturbances of respiratory rate and rhythm, apnoea
Pulmonary oedema, hypertension, embolism
Pneumonia, aspiration
Hyperpyrexia
Sweating, hypersecretion, tracheobronchial obstruction
Peripheral ischaemia

Metabolic
Dehydration
Electrolyte disturbance (especially hyponatraemia, hyperkalaemia, hypoglycaemia)
Acute renal failure (especially acute tubular necrosis)
Acute hepatic failure
Acute pancreatitis

Other
Disseminated intravascular coagulopathy/multiorgan failure
Rhabdomyolysis
Fractures
Infections (especially pulmonary, skin, urinary)
Thrombophlebitis, dermal injury

accumulation in the fat stores. The clinical effect of subsequent doses will therefore differ greatly from that of the first injection, as redistribution to the already drug-rich fat stores will not readily occur. In this situation, new drug administration can cause very high cerebral levels which persist for long periods of time. These high levels may precipitate hypotension, sedation, or cardiorespiratory failure; a serious risk with the repeated administration of diazepam, midazolam, chlormethiazole, clonazepam, pentobarbitone, or thiopentone. Less lipid-soluble drugs are relatively slower to act, but have a much longer lasting effect without a high risk of accumulation (for example, phenytoin, lorazepam, phenobarbitone). For lipid-soluble drugs, the rate of injection must also be carefully monitored, as too rapid a rate of administration will cause very high cerebral levels, and the risk of sudden cardiorespiratory arrest or hypotension. For less lipid-soluble drugs (such as lorazepam), the rate of injection is not critical. An ideal antiepileptic drug: should have no active metabolites (diazepam, midazolam, lignocaine, and thiopentone have active metabolites); should not interact with other medication; should not have saturable metabolism (both phenytoin and thiopentone have saturable pharmacokinetics at therapeutic levels); should not be unduly affected by hepatic or renal blood flow or disease (chlormethiazole is an example of a drug whose metabolism is greatly effected by both hepatic disease and changes in hepatic blood flow); should show no tendency to autoinduction (thiopentone, phenobarbitone, and phenytoin are all subject to strong autoinduction); should have strong antiepileptic action (the non-barbiturate anaesthetics have little or no intrinsic antiepileptic action, a conundrum for their use in status which has not been fully explored); and should be stable in solution and unreactive with giving sets (a problem with paraldehyde, diazepam, and thiopentone).

General measures

For the new patient presenting as an emergency in status, it is helpful to plan therapy in a series of progressive phases (box 3).

First stage (0–10 minutes)

Oxygen and cardiorespiratory resuscitation—It is first essential to assess cardiorespiratory function, to secure the airway, and to resuscitate where necessary. Oxygen should always be administered, as hypoxia is often unexpectedly severe.

Second stage (1–60 minutes)

Monitoring—Regular neurological observations and measurements of pulse, blood pressure, ECG, and temperature should be initiated. Metabolic abnormalities may cause status, or develop

---

Box 3—General measures (derived from Shorvon[2])

1   (0–10 minutes)
    Assess cardiorespiratory function
    Secure airway and resuscitate
    Administer oxygen

2   (0–60 minutes)
    Institute regular monitoring (see text)
    Emergency antiepileptic drug therapy (see text)
    Set up intravenous lines
    Emergency investigations (see text)
    Administer glucose (50 ml of 50% solution) and/or
        intravenous thiamine (250 mg) as high potency intra-
        venous Parentrovite) where appropriate
    Treat acidosis if severe

3   (0–60/90 minutes)
    Establish aetiology
    Identify and treat medical complications
    Pressor therapy where appropriate

4   (30–90 minutes)
    Transfer to intensive care
    Establish intensive care and EEG monitoring (see text)
    Initiate seizure and EEG monitoring
    Initiate intracranial pressure monitoring where appro-
        priate
    Initiate long term, maintenance, antiepileptic therapy

These four stages should be followed chronologically; the first
and second within 10 minutes, and stage 4 (transfer to intensive
care unit) in most settings within 60–90 minutes of
presentation.

---

during its course, and biochemical, blood gas, pH, clotting, and
haematological measures should be monitored.

Emergency anticonvulsant therapy—This should be started (see
below).

Intravenous lines—These should be set up for fluid replacement
and drug administration (preferably with 0·9% sodium chloride
(normal or physiological saline) rather than 5% glucose solutions). Drugs should not be mixed and, if two antiepileptic drugs

are needed (for example, phenytoin and diazepam), two intravenous lines should be sited. The lines should be in large veins, as many antiepileptic drugs cause phlebitis and thrombosis at the site of infusion. Arterial lines must *never* be used for drug administration.

Emergency investigations—Blood should be drawn for the emergency measurement of blood gases, sugar, renal and liver function, calcium and magnesium levels, full haematological screen (including platelets), blood clotting measures, and anticonvulsant levels. Fifty millilitres of serum should also be saved for future analysis especially if the cause of the status is uncertain. Other investigations depend on the clinical circumstances.

Intravenous glucose and thiamine—Fifty millilitres of a 50% glucose solution should be given immediately by intravenous injection if hypoglycaemia is suspected. If there is a history of alcoholism, or other compromised nutritional states, 250 mg of thiamine (for example, as the high potency intravenous formulation of Parentrovite, 10 ml of which contains 250 mg) should also be given intravenously. This is particularly important if glucose has been administered, as a glucose infusion increases the risk of Wernicke's encephalopathy in susceptible patients. Intravenous high dosage thiamine should be given slowly (for example, 10 ml of high potency Parentrovite over 10 minutes), with facilities for treating the anaphylaxis which is a potentially serious side effect of Parentrovite infusions. Routine glucose administration in non-hypoglycaemic patients should be avoided as there is some evidence that this can aggravate neuronal damage.

Acidosis—If acidosis is severe, the administration of bicarbonate has been advocated in the hope of preventing shock, and mitigating the effects of hypotension and low cerebral blood flow. In most cases, however, this is unnecessary and more effective is the rapid control of respiration and abolition of motor seizure activity.

Third stage (0–60/90 minutes)

Establish aetiology—The ranges of causes of status depend primarily on age and the presence or absence of established epilepsy. The investigations required depend on clinical circumstances. CT and CSF examination are often necessary—the latter should be

131

carried out only with facilities for resuscitation available as intracranial pressure is often elevated in status.

If the status has been precipitated by drug withdrawal, the immediate restitution of the withdrawn drug, even at lower doses, will usually rapidly terminate the status.

Physiological changes and medical complications—The physiological changes of uncompensated status, listed above, may require specific therapy. Active treatment is most commonly required for: hypoxia, hypotension, raised intracranial pressure, pulmonary oedema and hypertension, cardiac arrythmias, cardiac failure, lactic acidosis, hyperpyrexia, hypoglycaemia, electrolyte disturbance, acute hepatic or renal failure, rhabdomyolysis, or disseminated intravascular coagulation.

Pressor therapy—Dopamine is the most commonly used pressor agent, given by continuous intravenous infusion. The dose should be titrated to the desired haemodynamic and renal responses (usually initially between 2 and 5 μg/kg per minute, but this can be increased to over 20 μg/kg per minute in severe hypotension). Dopamine should be given into a large vein as extravasation causes tissue necrosis. ECG monitoring is required, as conduction defects may occur, and particular care is needed in dosing in the presence of cardiac failure.

Fourth stage (30–90 minutes)

Intensive care—If seizures are continuing in spite of the measures taken above, the patient must be transferred to an intensive care environment, and the usual intensive care measures instituted.

Intensive care monitoring—In severe established status, intensive monitoring may be required, including: intra-arterial blood pressure, capnography, oximetry, central venous pressure, and Swan–Ganz monitoring.

Seizure and EEG monitoring—In prolonged status, or in comatose ventilated patients, motor activity can be barely visible. In this situation, continuous EEG monitoring using a full EEG or a cerebral function monitor is necessary. The latter must be calibrated individually, and then can register both burst suppression and seizure activity. Burst suppression provides an arbitrary physiological target for the titration of barbiturate or anaesthetic therapy. Drug dosing is commonly set at a level that will produce burst suppression with interburst intervals of between 2 and 30 seconds.

Intracranial pressure monitoring and cerebral oedema—Continuous intracranial pressure monitoring is advisable, especially in children in the presence of persisting, severe, or progressive elevated intracranial pressure. The need for active therapy is usually determined by the underlying cause rather than the status. Intermittent positive pressure ventilation, high-dose corticosteroid therapy (4 mg dexamethasone every 6 hours), or mannitol infusion may be used (the latter is usually reserved for temporary respite for patients in danger of tentorial coning). Neurosurgical decompression is occasionally required.

Long term anticonvulsant therapy—Long term, maintenance, anticonvulsant therapy must be given in tandem with emergency treatment. The choice of drug depends on previous therapy, the type of epilepsy, and the clinical setting. If phenytoin or phenobarbitone has been used in emergency treatment, maintenance doses can be continued orally (through a nasogastric tube) guided by serum level monitoring. Other maintenance antiepileptics can be started also, giving oral loading doses.

Stages in emergency drug treatment

The drug treatment of tonic–clonic status epilepticus can also be usefully divided into stages[2] (table I). A suggested regime for a typical new case presenting as an emergency is given in box 4.

Premonitory stage

In patients with established epilepsy, tonic–clonic status seldom develops without warning. Usually, a prodromal phase (the premonitory stage) presages status, during which seizures become increasingly frequent or severe. Urgent drug treatment will usually prevent the evolution into true status. One of three drugs is used (diazepam, midazolam, or paraldehyde), and each is highly effective.

The earlier treatment is given the better. It is easier to prevent the evolution of epilepsy to status epilepticus than to treat the established condition. If the patient is at home, antiepileptic drugs

TABLE I—Antiepileptic drugs used in status epilepticus (derived from Shorvon[2])

Stage	Method of administration
1 *Premonitory stage*	
Diazepam	IV bolus or rectal solution
Midazolam	IM, IV bolus, rectal solution
Paraldehyde	Rectal solution, IM
2 *Early status*	
First line	
Lorazepam	IV bolus (repeated if necessary)
Diazepam	IV bolus (repeated if necessary)
Second line	
Lignocaine	IV bolus and short infusion
Clonazepam	IV bolus
Paraldehyde	Rectal solution, IM
Phenytoin	IV bolus
3 *Established status*	
First line	
Phenobarbitone	IV loading and then repeated IV/oral boluses
Phenytoin (± diazepam)	IV loading and then repeated IV/oral boluses
Second line	
Clonazepam	IV bolus or short infusion
Chlormethiazole	IV bolus and continuous infusion
Paraldehyde	IV infusion
Diazepam	Short IV infusion
Midazolam	Short IV infusion
4 *Refractory status*	
First line	
Thiopentone	IV bolus and infusion
Propofol	IV bolus and infusion
Second line	
Pentobarbitone	IV bolus and infusion
Isoflurane	Inhalation
Etomidate	IV bolus and infusion

IV = intravenous; IM = intramuscular; rectal = rectal administration

should be administered before transfer to hospital, or in the casualty department before transfer to the ward. The acute administration of either diazepam or midazolam will cause drowsiness or sleep, and occasionally cardiorespiratory collapse, and should be carefully supervised.

Stage of early status epilepticus (0–30 minutes)

Once status epilepticus has developed, treatment should be carried out in hospital, under close supervision. For the first 30–60

Box 4—Emergency antiepileptic drug regimen for status in newly presenting adult patients (derived from Shorvon[2])

Premonitory stage	Diazepam 10–20 mg given IV or rectally, repeated once 15 minutes later if status continues to threaten. IV injection at a rate not exceeding 2–5 mg/minute *If seizures continue, treat as below.*
Early status	Lorazepam (IV) 0·07 mg/kg (usually a 4 mg bolus, repeated once after 10–20 minutes; rate not critical) *If seizures continue 30 minutes after first injection, treat as below.*
Established status	Phenobarbitone bolus of 10 mg/kg at a rate of 100 mg/minute (usually 700 mg over seven minutes in an adult) *and/or* Phenytoin infusion at a dose of 15–18 mg/kg at a rate of 50 mg/minute (eg, 1000 mg in 20 minutes; with diazepam if not already given—IV 10–20 mg) *If seizures continue for 30/60 minutes or longer, treat as below.*
Refractory status	General anaesthesia, with either propofol or thiopentone. Anaesthetic continued for 12–24 hours after the last clinical or electrographic seizure, then dose tapered

In the above scheme, the refractory stage (general anaesthesia) is reached 60/90 minutes after the initial therapy. This scheme is suitable for usual clinical hospital settings. In some situations, general anaesthesia should be initiated earlier and, occasionally, should be delayed.

minutes or so of continuous seizures, physiological mechanisms compensate for the greatly enhanced metabolic activity. This is the stage of *early status,* and it is usual to administer a fast-acting benzodiazepine drug.

In most clinical settings, intravenous lorazepam or diazepam (but not both together) is the drug of choice. Rectal or intramuscular paraldehyde is a useful alternative to the benzodiazepine drugs in early status, where facilities for intravenous injection or for resuscitation are not freely available (for instance in nursing homes, where it can be administered by nursing staff). In patients in respiratory failure, intravenous lignocaine may be preferable. Intravenous phenytoin is sometimes given with diazepam at this stage, although this is usually unnecessary.

In most patients, therapy will be highly effective. Continuous inpatient observation should follow. In previously non-epileptic patients, chronic antiepileptic therapy should be introduced, and in those already on maintenance antiepileptic therapy this should be reviewed.

Stage of established status epilepticus (30–60/90 minutes)

The *stage of established status* can be operationally defined as status which has continued for 30 minutes in spite of early stage treatment. The time period is chosen because physiological decompensation will usually have begun. Intensive care facilities are desirable. There are two alternative first-line treatment options, both with significant drawbacks, and status at this stage carries an appreciable morbidity. These are subanaesthetic doses of phenobarbitone, or phenytoin, both given by intravenous loading followed by repeated oral or intravenous supplementation. Diazepam is often given with phenytoin (either at this or the early stage of status), combining the fast-acting but short-lasting effect of diazepam with the slow-onset but long-lasting effect of phenytoin.

Numerous second-line treatment options exist, including chlormethiazole given by intravenous bolus and continuous infusion, and continuous intravenous infusions of clonazepam, diazepam, paraldehyde or midazolam, at various doses. Although once popular, continuous benzodiazepine infusions are hazardous and now not generally recommended. Lorazepam and lignocaine are essentially short term therapies, and so should not be employed at this stage.

Stage of refractory status epilepticus (after 60/90 minutes)

If seizures continue for 60–90 minutes after the initiation of therapy, the stage of *refractory status* is reached and full anaesthesia required. This applies to an average case, and in many emergency situations (for example, postoperative status, severe or complicated convulsive status, patients already in intensive care), anaesthesia can and should be introduced earlier. Prognosis will now be much poorer, and there is a high mortality and morbidity.

Anaesthesia can be induced by barbiturate or non-barbiturate drugs. A number of anaesthetics have been administered, although few have been subjected to formal evaluation and all have drawbacks. The most commonly used anaesthetics are the intravenous barbiturate thiopentone or the intravenous non-barbiturate propofol. Other drugs in current use include the infusional anaesthetic isoflurane, and the intravenous anaesthetics pentobarbitone (not available in the UK) and etomidate.

Patients require the full range of intensive care facilities, including EEG monitoring, and care should be shared between anaesthetist and neurologist. Experience with long term administration (hours or days) of the newer anaesthetic drugs is very limited. The non-barbiturate anaesthetics have little intrinsic antiepileptic activity (indeed some are proconvulsant), but it is not clear to what extent (if any) this is a disadvantage. The modern anaesthetics, on the other hand, have important pharmacokinetic advantages over the more traditional barbiturates.

Antiepileptic drugs

Diazepam

Diazepam[19-23] has a time honoured place as a drug of first choice in premonitory or early stages of status. Its pharmacology and clinical effects have been extensively studied in adults, children, and the newborn, and it has been shown to be highly effective in a wide range of status types. Diazepam can be given by intravenous bolus injections or by the rectal route in the premonitory stage, and has a rapid onset of action. Sufficient cerebral levels are reached within one minute of a standard intravenous injection, and rectal administration produces peak levels at about 20 minutes. The drug is rapidly redistributed, and has a relatively short duration of action after a single intravenous injection. After repeated dosing, as drug concentrations in the peripheral compartments (lipid stores) increase, this redistribution does not occur. Thus repeated bolus injections produce high peak levels which persist, carrying an attendant risk of sudden and unexpected CNS depression and cardiorespiratory collapse.

137

Diazepam is metabolised by hepatic microsomal enzymes. Respiratory depression, hypotension, and sedation are the principal side effects. Sudden apnoea can occur, especially after repeated injections or if the injection is administered at too fast a rate.

Bolus intravenous doses of diazepam should be given in an undiluted form at a rate not exceeding 2–5 mg/minute, using the Diazemuls formulation. Diazepam may be given rectally, either in its intravenous preparation infused from a syringe via a plastic catheter, or as the ready made, proprietary, rectal tube preparation Stesolid which is a convenient and easy method. Diazepam suppositories should not be used, as absorption is too slow. The adult bolus intravenous or rectal dose in status is 10–20 mg, and additional 10 mg doses can be given at 15 minute intervals, to a maximum of 40 mg. In children, the equivalent bolus dose is 0·2–0·3 mg/kg. A continuous infusion of benzodiazepine has also been used, but there is now little place for this mode of administration. The solution should be freshly prepared, and no drugs should be admixed.

The usual intravenous formulation is as an emulsion (Diazemuls) in a 1 ml ampoule containing 5 mg/ml or as a solution in 2 ml ampoules containing 5 mg/ml. Stesolid is the usual rectal formulation—a 2·5 ml rectal tube containing 5 mg or 10 mg diazepam. The intravenous solution can also be instilled rectally.

Midazolam

Midazolam[24-27] has only recently been introduced in status, and clinical experience is limited. Unique among the drugs in status, it can be given by intramuscular injection, as well as by the rectal or intravenous routes. Bioavailability after intramuscular injection is about 80–100%, and peak levels are reached after about 25 minutes although there is marked individual variation. Its elimination kinetics are dependent on hepatic blood flow. The lipid solubility of the drug, and hence its cerebral action, is reduced as pH falls. Action is short lived, and there is a strong tendency to relapse following a single bolus injection. It is cleared from the body faster than diazepam, and there is thus less tendency to accumulate. Midazolam exhibits the same toxic effects as other benzodiazepines, including sedation, hypotension, and cardiorespiratory depression. Respiratory arrest may occur occasionally even after intramuscular injection so careful monitoring is imperative.

Intramuscular use in premonitory status, where immediate facilities for intravenous injection are often not available, is a great advantage. This is the main current role for midazolam in status, but further experience may widen its indications.

Midazolam is usually given intramuscularly or rectally in premonitory status, at a dose of 5–10 mg (in children 0·15–0·3 mg/kg), which can be repeated once after 15 minutes or so. A 5–10 mg intravenous bolus injection can also be given (repeated to a maximum of 0·3 mg/kg in adults), and there is limited experience of an intravenous infusion. Midazolam is available in 5 ml ampoules containing 2 mg/ml or 2 ml ampoules containing 5 mg/ml.

Paraldehyde

Paraldehyde[28-30] is a thoroughly old fashioned medication, but is still widely used in the treatment of status epilepticus. Its main indication is as an alternative or sequel to the administration of diazepam in the stage of premonitory or early status. It is especially useful in situations where intravenous administration is difficult, or where conventional antiepileptic drugs are contra-indicated or have proved ineffective. The drug is usually given rectally (or less often intramuscularly), and absorption by both routes is fast and complete. The onset of action is rapid and paraldehyde is effective for many hours. Seizures tend to recur less after control is achieved than with the shorter acting benzodiazepines, anaesthetic drugs, or chlormethiazole. Paraldehyde has no strong tendency to accumulate, and the risks of hypotension or cardiorespiratory depression are low. Toxicity is unusual providing: the correct dose is not exceeded; the solution is freshly made; the paraldehyde is not decomposed; and it is diluted satisfactorily. Inappropriately diluted or decomposed paraldehyde is highly toxic by any route of administration. The intramuscular injection must be into deep (usually gluteal) muscle, well away from the sciatic nerve. In established status, paraldehyde can be given by intravenous infusion, but this is a complicated and fraught procedure, and one which is now very rarely recommended. The drug also reacts with rubber and plastic, and so, if infused, must be given via glass giving sets and syringes. An injection using a plastic syringe, however, is acceptable if given rapidly after drawing the solution up.

In early status, paraldehyde can be given at a dose of 10–20 ml of 50% solution rectally or intramuscularly (children 0·07–0·35 ml/kg), which can be repeated once after 15–30 minutes.

In established status in adults, it can be given by continuous infusion, as a solution of 15 ml ampoules in 500 ml of 5% dextrose freshly made up every three hours, given at a dose of 15–30 ml every three hours (that is, approximately 100–200 mg/kg per hour). There is now no place for the bolus injection of undiluted paraldehyde even into a fast running drip. In neonatal status, an infusion of 200 mg/kg per hour can be given for at least three hours, or an initial infusion of 200 mg/kg followed by 16 mg/kg for 12 hours.

Paraldehyde is supplied in 10 ml ampoules (approximately 10 g) in darkened glass to prevent decomposition. For rectal or intramuscular administration, it is diluted in equal measure with 0·9% sodium chloride (normal saline) or arachis oil. For intravenous administration, it should be given as a 5% infusion in 5% dextrose, freshly made up every three hours.

Chlormethiazole

Chlormethiazole[31–34] is widely used at the stage of established status, by continuous intravenous infusion. Distribution is very rapid, and there is a large volume of distribution. A single intravenous injection has a very rapid effect, which is very short lived. Chlormethiazole is thus best given as a continuous infusion, and the dose can be titrated according to effect on a moment to moment basis, without inducing deep anaesthesia. This ability to titrate the dose is very useful, and unique among the drugs used in status. On longer term therapy, however, as the drug concentrations in peripheral lipid compartments approach saturation levels, this property is lost. Sudden accumulation may cause persistingly high blood levels, resulting in sudden cardiorespiratory collapse, cardiac arrhythmia, hypotension, or deep sedation. In view of this risk, prolonged use of the drug should be avoided where possible. If a long term infusion (>12 hours) is judged necessary, it is wise to reduce the dose every few hours to minimise accumulation. There is a tendency for seizures to recur as chlormethiazole is weaned, and longer term oral replacement therapy is sometimes required. On prolonged therapy there is a danger of fluid overload, and electrolyte supplementation may be required as the infusion fluid is electrolyte deficient. The elimination of chlormethiazole is markedly affected by changes in hepatic blood flow and by hepatic disease. The drug is absorbed by PVC on prolonged contact. Although its pharmacokinetics are well studied, there have been no formal clinical trials of chlormethiazole in status, and published experience of its use, especially in the long term and in children or the newborn, is very limited.

In status, an initial intravenous infusion of 40–100 ml of the 0·8% solution is given (that is, 320–800 mg) at a rate of 5–15 ml/minute. The infusion is continued at a minimum dose which will control seizures (commonly 0·5–4 ml/minute, maximum 20 ml/minute in adults). When seizures are controlled (for 12 hours in a case of adult status), the rate of infusion should be slowly reduced. It is not uncommon for seizures to recur on chlormethiazole withdrawal, in which case the minimum effective dose should again be determined and continued. Sometimes, switching from the intravenous to oral form (1–3 capsules of 192 mg chlormethiazole base a day, or 1–3 tablets of 500 mg chlormethiazole edisylate, or 5–15 ml of chlormethiazole edisylate syrup) is necessary as status resolves. An infusion rate of 0·01 ml/kg per minute (0·08 mg/kg per minute) in children has been recommended, increasing every 2–4 hours until seizures are abolished or drowsiness intervenes. The drug is usually supplied in 500 ml bottles of a 0·8% solution of chlormethiazole edisylate (8 mg/ml) in dextrose and sodium hydroxide.

Lorazepam

Lorazepam[23 35-39] is indicated in the early stage of status only, where its lack of accumulation in lipid stores, its strong cerebral binding, and long duration of action are very significant advantages over diazepam. The pharmacology and clinical effects of lorazepam have been well characterised in adults, in children, and in the newborn, and the drug has been the subject of large scale clinical trials. Lorazepam is remarkably effective in controlling seizures in the early stage of status. Its main disadvantage is the rapid development of tolerance. Initial injections of lorazepam are effective for about 12 hours (longer than with diazepam), but repeated doses are much less effective, and the drug has no place as long term therapy. Lorazepam has sedative effects shared by all the benzodiazepine drugs used in status, but sudden hypotension or respiratory collapse is less likely because of its relative lipid insolubility and the lack of accumulation after single bolus injections.

Lorazepam is administered by intravenous bolus injection. As distribution is slow, the rate of injection is not critical. In adults, a bolus dose of 0·07 mg/kg (to a maximum of 4 mg) is given, and this can be repeated once after 20 minutes if no effect has been observed. In children under 10 years, bolus doses of 0·1 mg/kg are recommended. Long term infusion of lorazepam should not be used. It is usually available as a 1 ml ampoule containing 4 mg of lorazepam.

Phenytoin

Phenytoin[40-43] is a drug of first choice in established status. Its pharmacology and clinical effects are well documented, and there is extensive experience in status in adults, children, and the newborn. It is a highly effective anticonvulsant, with the particular advantage of a long duration of action. It can also be continued as chronic therapy. Phenytoin causes relatively little respiratory or cerebral depression, although hypotension is more common. The initial infusion of phenytoin takes 20–30 minutes in an adult, and the onset of action is slow. It is therefore often administered in conjunction with a short-acting drug with a rapid onset of action, such as diazepam. The notorious saturable pharmacokinetics of phenytoin cause less problems in the emergency setting than in chronic therapy, but careful serum level monitoring is essential. The usual phenytoin solutions have a pH of 12, and if added to bags containing large volumes of fluid at lower than physiological pH (for example, 5% glucose) precipitation may occur in the bag or tubing; use in a solution of 0·9% sodium chloride (normal saline) (5–20 mg/ml) is safer. There is also a serious risk of precipitation if other drugs are added to the infusion solution. Administration via a side arm, or directly using an infusion pump, is preferable. Phenytoin should not be given by either rectal or intramuscular injection. ECG monitoring is advisable while administering phenytoin.

The rate of infusion of phenytoin solution should not exceed 50 mg/minute, and it is prudent to reduce this to 20–30 mg/minute in the elderly. The adult dose is 15-18 mg/kg; usually about 1000 mg, therefore taking at least 20 minutes to administer. Regrettably, a lower dose is too often given, which results in suboptimal cerebral levels. This is a common and potentially serious mistake. Phenytoin therapy can be continued after intravenous loading by oral or further intravenous daily dosages of 5–6 mg/kg, guided by blood level measurements. For older children, the dose of phenytoin is as for adults. For the newborn a dose of 15–20 mg/kg, injected at a rate not exceeding 1 mg/kg per minute, should be given. Phenytoin is usually available as 5 ml ampoules containing phenytoin sodium 250 mg.

Phenobarbitone

Phenobarbitone[43-46] is a drug of choice for the treatment of established status. It is highly effective, has a rapid onset of action, and prolonged anticonvulsant effects. It has stable and non-reactive physical properties, and convenient pharmacokinetics. Wide experience has been gained of its use in adults and in children, and few drugs are as well tried in the newborn. It has stronger anticonvulsant properties than most other barbiturates, and may be preferentially concentrated in metabolically active epileptic foci. As well as excellent anticonvulsant properties, it may also have cerebral-protective action. Acute tolerance to the antiepileptic effect is unusual, in contrast to the benzodiazepines and, once controlled, seizures do not tend to recur. The main disadvantages of phenobarbitone are its potential to cause sedation, respiratory depression, and hypotension; although in practice these effects seem slight except at high levels or with rapidly rising levels, its safety at even high doses is well established. The well known chronic side effects of phenobarbitone in long term therapy are of no relevance in the emergency situation of status. The drug is eliminated slowly and, although this is of no importance on initial phenobarbitone loading, on prolonged therapy there is a danger of accumulation and blood level monitoring is essential. In the newborn period dosing is more difficult than in adults, as the pharmacokinetics change rapidly during the first weeks and months of life. The drug has a strong tendency to autoinduction. Phenobarbitone is a stable preparation which does not easily decompose, and the drug is not absorbed by plastic. It should not be used in a solution containing other drugs (for example, phenytoin), as this may result in precipitation.

The usual recommended adult intravenous loading dose is 10 mg/kg, given at a rate of 100 mg/minute (that is, a total of about 700 mg in seven minutes). This should be followed by daily maintenance doses of 1–4 mg/kg. The initial maximum adult dose should not exceed 1000 mg as the drug is not very lipid soluble and, in obese patients, the guide (in mg/kg) may be unreliable. In neonates, initial phenobarbitone loading doses of between 12 and

20 mg/kg have been recommended to produce therapeutic levels, with subsequent supplementation of 3–4 mg/kg per day, to a maximum dose of 40 mg/kg. In older children, loading doses of between 5 and 20 mg/kg are recommended and maintenance doses of 1–4 mg/kg, although much higher doses have been safely given. After loading, maintenance doses can be given by the oral, intravenous, or intramuscular route. Phenobarbitone is usually presented in 1 ml ampoules containing 200 mg of phenobarbitone sodium.

Thiopentone

Thiopentone[47–50] is the compound traditionally used for barbiturate anaesthesia in status epilepticus, at least in Europe. It is an effective antiepileptic drug, and may have additional cerebral-protective effects. In the doses used in status it has an anaesthetic action, and all patients require intubation and most artificial ventilation. The most troublesome side effect is persisting hypotension and many patients require pressor therapy. Thiopentone has saturable pharmacokinetics, and a strong tendency to accumulate. Thus if large doses are given, blood levels may remain very high for protracted periods, and days may pass before consciousness is recovered after drug administration is discontinued. Blood level monitoring, both of the thiopentone and its active metabolite pentobarbitone, is therefore essential on prolonged therapy. Other toxic effects on prolonged therapy include pancreatitis and hepatic disturbance, and thiopentone may cause acute hypersensitivity. It should be administered cautiously in the elderly, and in those with cardiac, hepatic, or renal disease. Although it has been in use since the 1960s in status, formal clinical trials of its safety and effectiveness in either adults and children are few. A full range of intensive care facilities are required during thiopentone infusions. Central venous pressure should be monitored, and blood pressure monitored via an arterial line. Swan–Ganz monitoring is sometimes advisable, and EEG or cerebral function monitoring is essential if thiopentone infusions are prolonged. A concomitant dopamine infusion is frequently needed to maintain blood pressure. Thiopentone can react with polyvinyl infusion bags or giving sets. The continuous infusion should be made up in 0·9% sodium chloride (normal saline). The intravenous solution has a pH of 10·2–11·2, is incompatible with a large number of acidic or oxidising substances, and no drugs should be added. The aqueous solution is unstable if exposed to air.

The dose regimen commonly used is as follows: thiopentone is given as a 100–250 mg bolus over 20 seconds, with further 50 mg boluses every 2–3 minutes until seizures are controlled, with intubation and artificial ventilation. The intravenous infusion is then continued at the minimum dose required to control seizure activity (burst suppression on the EEG), usually between 3 and 5 mg/kg per hour, and at thiopentone blood levels of about 40 mg/l. After 24 hours, the dose should be controlled by blood level monitoring. At this point, metabolism may be near saturation, and daily or twice daily blood level estimations should be made to ensure that levels do not rise excessively. The dose should be lowered if systolic blood pressure falls below 90 mm Hg, or if vital functions are impaired. Thiopentone should be continued for no less than 12 hours after seizure activity has ceased, and then slowly discontinued. The usual preparation is as a 2·5 g vial with 100 ml of diluent to produce a 2·5% solution.

Propofol

In recent times, there has been a vogue for the use of non-barbiturate anaesthesia in status; of the currently available compounds, propofol[51-54] is probably the drug of choice. Published experience, however, is very limited of its use in status, or indeed of its long term administration in any clinical situation. Propofol is a highly effective and non-toxic anaesthetic. Although, in experimental models, it has intrinsic anticonvulsant properties, it has caused seizures in anaesthetic practice. Propofol is extremely soluble in lipid and has a high volume of distribution. It thus acts extremely rapidly in status. Its effects are maintained while the infusion is continued, and recovery following discontinuation of the drug is also very quick—in marked contrast to thiopentone. Theoretically, there is a danger of accumulation on very long term therapy, but this has not been reported in practice. Propofol administration causes profound respiratory and cerebral depression, requiring the use of assisted respiration, the full panoply of intensive care, and monitoring, but only mild hypotension, and has few cardiovascular side effects. Long term administration causes marked lipaemia and may result in acidosis. It may cause involuntary movements which should not be mistaken for seizures. Although propofol has been the subject of only a few case reports, it is widely used in status, and warrants further formal study. Its safety in young children has not been established.

145

TONIC-CLONIC STATUS EPILEPTICUS

In status, the following regimen can be used: initially a 2 mg/kg bolus dose is given, which can be repeated if seizures continue, succeeded by an infusion of 5–10 mg/kg per hour guided by EEG. The dose should be gradually reduced, and the infusion tapered 12 hours after seizure activity is halted. In the elderly, doses should be lower. It is available as 20 ml ampoules containing 10 mg/ml as an emulsion.

Other drugs

A wide variety of other drugs have been used in status, including clonazepam, lignocaine, pentobarbitone, etomidate, magnesium sulphate, clorazepate, corticosteroids, valproate, and lamotrigine. Few of these (or indeed the first line) drugs have received adequate formal clinical study in status, and their relative merits are largely uncertain. An exciting area of future research is the use of cerebral protective agents, to prevent status-induced cerebral damage. A more detailed discussion of the drugs used in status can be found in larger reviews.[2 16 55]

Box 5—Common reasons for the failure of emergency drug therapy to control seizures in status epilepticus

- Inadequate emergency antiepileptic drug therapy (especially the administration of drugs at too low a dose)

- Failure to initiate maintenance antiepileptic drug therapy (seizures will recur as the effect of emergency drug treatment wears off)

- Hypoxia, hypotension, cardiorespiratory failure, metabolic disturbance

- Failure to identify the underlying cause

- Failure to identify other medical complications (including hyperthermia, disseminated intravascular coagulation, hepatic failure)

- Misdiagnosis (pseudostatus is more common than epileptic status at least in specialist neurological practice)

Management of tonic–clonic status epilepticus

● The annual incidence of tonic–clonic status is about 18–28 cases per 100 000 persons. It occurs most frequently in children, the mentally handicapped, and in those with structural cerebral disorders. It can develop de novo usually due to an acute cerebral insult, or in patients with established epilepsy where drug withdrawal is often the immediate cause. Mortality rate is about 5–10%, with most patients dying of the underlying condition rather than the status itself.

● Experimental work suggests that compensatory physiological mechanisms protect homoeostasis for the first 30–60 minutes of continuing seizures. If seizures persist for longer periods, however, a series of physiological changes occur, resulting in the breakdown of cerebral autoregulation and a fall in cerebral blood flow. The failure to meet the high metabolic demands of cerebral tissue can result in permanent cerebral damage.

● Other complications include hyperpyrexia, massive autonomic activation, pulmonary hypertension and oedema, intracranial hypertension, cardiac arrhythmia and failure, hypoglycaemia, acidosis, rhabdomyolysis, disseminated intravascular coagulation, and cardiac, respiratory, renal, or hepatic failure.

● General treatment measures should proceed in stages: firstly, cardiorespiratory function should be secured; secondly, regular, monitoring and emergency drug therapy should be commenced, and investigations initiated; thirdly, aetiology should be established, and hypotension and medical complications treated. If seizures are continuing, the patient should be transferred to intensive care, and seizure, EEG, and sometimes intracranial pressure monitoring applied.

● A suggested regimen for emergency antiepileptic drug therapy is as follows: (1) *premonitory stage*: diazepam 0·2–0·3 mg/kg (usual adult dose 10–20 mg) can be given by intravenous or rectal administration. (2) *Early status*: lorazepam 0·07 mg/kg (usual adult dose 4 mg), which can be repeated after 10 minutes. (3) *Established status*: phenobarbitone 10 mg/kg given intravenously at an infusion rate of 100 mg/minute (usual adult dose is 700 mg given over seven minutes), or phenytoin at a dose of 15–18 mg/kg at a rate of 50 mg/minute (usual adult dose is 1000 mg given over 20 minutes). (4) *Refractory status*: general anaesthesia with either thiopentone initially with a 100–250 mg bolus injection, followed by further 50 mg boluses, and then a continuous infusion (usual dose 3–5 mg/kg per hour), or propofol initially with a 2 mg/kg bolus dose, repeated if necessary, and then a continuous infusion of 5–10 mg/kg per hour. Maintenance antiepileptic drug therapy should be given concurrently.

Failure of antiepileptic treatment

The antiepileptic drugs used in status are highly effective. If seizures continue despite emergency therapy, it is important to reassess the clinical circumstances, as there are often complicating remediable factors influencing the response to treatment. The most common of these are listed in box 5.

1 Hauser WA. Status epilepticus: epidemiological considerations. *Neurology* 1990;**40**(suppl 2):9–12.
2 Shorvon SD. *Status epilepticus: its clinical features and treatment in children and adults.* Cambridge: Cambridge University Press, 1994.
3 Aicardi J, Chevrie JJ. Convulsive status epilepticus in infants and children. A study of 239 cases. *Epilepsia* 1970;**11**:187–97.
4 Goulon M, Levy-Alcover MA, Nouailhat F. Etat de mal epileptique de l'adulte. Etude epidemiologique et clinique en reanimation. *Rev EEG Neurophysiol* 1985;**14**:277–85.
5 Pilke A, Partinen M, Kovanen J. Status epilepticus and alcohol abuse: an analysis of 82 status epilepticus admissions. *Acta Neurol Scand* 1984;**70**:443-50.
6 Aicardi J, Chevrie JJ. Consequences of status epilepticus in infants and children. In: Delgado-Escueta AV, Wasterlain CG, Treiman DM, Porter RJ, eds. *Status epilepticus: mechanisms of brain damage and treatment. Advances in neurology,* vol 34. New York: Raven Press, 1983:115–25.
7 Bourneville DM. Recherches cliniques et therapeutiques sur l'epilepsie et l'hysterie. Progres Medical. Paris: Delahaye, 1876.
8 Roger J, Lob H, Tassinari C. Status epilepticus. In: Vinken PJ, Bruyn GW, eds. *Handbook of clinical neurology,* Vol 15. New York: Elsevier, 1974:145–88.
9 Treiman DM, Walton NY, Kendrick C. A progressive sequence of electroencephalographic changes during generalised convulsive status epilepticus. *Epilepsy Res* 1990;**5**:49–60.
10 Lothman E. The biochemical basis and pathophysiology of status epilepticus. *Neurology* 1990;**40**(suppl 2):13–22.
11 Simon RP. Physiological consequences of status epilepticus. *Epilepsia* 1985;**26**(Suppl l):S58–66.
12 Brown JK, Hussain IHMI. Status epilepticus. 1: Pathogenesis. *Develop Med Child Neurol* 1991;**33**:3–17.
13 Aminoff MJ, Simon RP. Status epilepticus: causes, clinical features and consequences in 98 patients. *Am J Med* 1980;**69**:657-66.
14 Meldrum BS. Metabolic factors during prolonged seizures and their relation to cell death. In: Delgado Escueta AV, Wasterlain CG, Treiman DM, Porter RJ, eds. *Status epilepticus: mechanisms of brain damage and treatment. Advances in neurology,* vol 34. New York: Raven Press, 1983:261–75.
15 Delgado-Escueta AV, Ward AA, Woodbury DM, Porter RJ, eds. *Basic mechanisms of the epilepsies: molecular and cellular approaches. Advances in neurology,* vol 44. New York: Raven Press, 1986.
16 Delgado-Escueta AV, Wasterlain CG, Treiman DM, Porter RJ, eds. *Status epilepticus: mechanisms of brain damage and treatment. Advances in neurology,* vol 34. New York: Raven Press, 1983.
17 Benowitz NL, Simon RP, Copeland JR. Status epilepticus: divergence of sympathetic activity and cardiovascular response. *Ann Neurol* 1986;**19**:197–9.
18 Young RSK, Fripp RR, Yagel SK, Werner JC, McGrath G, Schuler HG. Cardiac dysfunction during status epilepticus in the neonatal pig. *Ann Neurol* 1985;**18**:291–7.
19 Schmidt D. Diazepam. In: Levy R, Dreifuss FE, Mattson R, Meldrum B, Penry JK, eds. *Antiepileptic drugs,* 3rd ed. New York: Raven Press, 1989:735–64.
20 Schmidt D. Benzodiazepines—an update. In: Pedley TA and Meldrum BS, eds. *Recent advances in epilepsy,* vol 2. Edinburgh: Churchill Livingstone, 1985:125–35.

148

21 Delgado-Escueta AV, Enrile-Bacsal F. Combination therapy for status epilepticus: intravenous diazepam and phenytoin. In: Delgado-Escueta AV, Wasterlain CG, Treiman DM, Porter RJ, eds. *Status epilepticus: mechanisms of brain damage and treatment. Advances in neurology*, vol 34. New York, Raven Press 1983:477–85.

22 Remy C, Jourdil N, Villemain D, Favel P, Genton P. Intrarectal diazepam in epileptic adults. *Epilepsia* 1992;**33**:353–8.

23 Leppik IE, Derivan AT, Homan RW, Walker J, Ramsay RE, Patrick B. Double-blind study of lorazepam and diazepam in status epilepticus. *JAMA* 1983;**249**:1452–4.

24 Dundee JW, Halliday NJ, Harper KW, Brogden RN. Midazolam: a review of its pharmacological properties and therapeutic uses. *Drugs* 1984;**28**:519–43.

25 Galvin GM, Jelinek GA. Midazolam: an effective intravenous agent for seizure control. *Arch Emerg Med* 1987;**4**:169–72.

26 Ghilain S, Van Rijckevorsel-Harmant K, de Barsy TH. Midazolam in the treatment of epileptic seizures. *J Neurol Neurosurg Psychiatry* 1988;**51**:732.

27 Jawad S, Oxley J, Wilson J, Richens A. A pharmacodynamic evaluation of midazolam as an antiepileptic compound. *J Neurol Neurosurg Psychiatry* 1986;**49**:1050–4.

28 Koren G, Butt W, Rajchgot P, Mayer J, Whyte H, Pape K, MacLeod SM. Intravenous paraldehyde for seizure control in newborn infants. *Neurology* 1986;**36**:108–11.

29 Browne TR. Paraldehyde, chlormethiazole, and lidocaine for treatment of status epilepticus. In: Delgado-Escueta AV, Wasterlain CG, Treiman DM, Porter RJ, eds. *Status epilepticus: mechanisms of brain damage and treatment. Advances in neurology*, vol 34. New York: Raven Press, 1983:509–17.

30 Lockman LA. Paraldehyde. In: Levy RH, Dreifuss FE, Mattson RH, Meldrum BS, Penry JK, eds. *Antiepileptic drugs*, 3rd ed. New York: Raven Press, 1989:881–6.

31 Harvey PKP, Higenbottam TW, Loh L. Chlormethiazole in treatment of status epilepticus. *BMJ* 1975;**2**:603–5.

32 Miller P, Kovar I. Chlormethiazole in the treatment of neonatal status epilepticus. *Postgrad Med J* 1983;**59**:801–2.

33 Lingam S, Bertwistle H, Elliston H, Wilson J. Problems with intravenous chlormethiazole (Heminevrin) in status epilepticus. *BMJ* 1980;**i**:155–6.

34 Laxenaire M, Tridon P, Poire P. Effect of chlormethiazole in treatment of delirium tremens and status epilepticus. *Acta Psychiatrica Scand* 1966;**42**(Suppl 192):87–102.

35 Crawford TO, Mitchell WG, Snodgrass SR. Lorazepam in childhood status epilepticus and serial seizures: effectiveness and tachyphylaxis. *Neurology* 1987;**37**:190–5.

36 Sorel L, Mechler L, Harmant J. Comparative trial of intravenous lorazepam and clonazepam in status epilepticus. *Clin Ther* 1981;**4**:326–36.

37 Homan RW, Unwin DH. Benzodiazepines: lorazepam. In: Levy R, Dreifuss FE, Mattson R, Meldrum B, Penry JK, eds. *Antiepileptic drugs*, 3rd ed. New York: Raven Press, 1989:841–54.

38 Mitchell WG, Crawford TO. Lorazepam is the treatment of choice for status epilepticus. *J Epilepsy* 1990;**3**:7–10.

39 Maytal J, Novak GP, King KC. Lorazepam in the treatment of refractory neonatal seizures. *J Child Neurol* 1991;**6**:319–23.

40 Wallis W, Kutt H, McDowell F. IV diphenylhydantoin in treatment of acute repetitive seizures. *Neurology* 1968;**18**:513–25.

41 Leppik IE, Patrick BK, Cranford RE. Treatment of Acute Seizures and Status Epilepticus with Intravenous Phenytoin. In: Delgado-Escueta AV, Wasterlain CG, Treiman DM, Porter RJ, eds. *Status epilepticus: mechanisms of brain damage and treatment. Advances in neurology*, vol 34. New York: Raven Press, 1983:447–52.

42 Cranford RE, Leppik IE, Patrick B, Anderson CB, Kostick B. Intravenous phenytoin: clinical and pharmacokinetic aspects. *Neurology* 1978;**28**:874–80.

43 Shaner DM, McCurdy SA, Herring MO, Gabor AJ. Treatment of status epilepticus: a prospective comparison of diazepam and phenytoin versus phenobarbital and optional phenytoin. *Neurology* 1988;**38**:202–7.

44 Crawford TO, Mitchell WG, Fishman LS, Snodgrass R. Very-high-dose phenobarbital for refractory status epilepticus in children. *Neurology* 1988;**38**:1035–40.

45 Gal P, Toback J, Boer HR, Erkan NV, Wells TJ. Efficacy of phenobarbital monotherapy in treatment of neonatal seizures—relationship to blood levels. *Neurology* 1982;**32**:1401–4.

46 Lockman LA, Kriel R, Zaske D, Thompson T, Virnig N. Phenobarbital dosage for control of neonatal seizures. *Neurology* 1979;**29**:1445–9.

47 Partinen M, Kovanen J, Nilsson E. Status epilepticus treated with barbiturate anaesthesia with continuous monitoring of cerebral function. *BMJ* 1981;**282**:520–1.
48 Young EB, Blume WT, Bolton CF, Warren KG. Anesthetic barbiturates in refractory status epilepticus. *J Can Sci Neurol* 1980;7:291–2.
49 Orlowski JP, Erenberg G, Lueders H, Cruse RP. Hypothermia and barbiturate coma for refractory status epilepticus. *Crit Care Med* 1984;**12**:367–72.
50 Lowenstein DH, Aminoff MJ, Simon RJ. Barbiturate anesthesia in the treatment of status epilepticus: clinical experience of 14 patients. *Neurology* 1988;**38**:395–400.
51 MacKenzie SJ, Kapadia F, Grant IS. Propofol infusion for control of status epilepticus. *Anaesthesia* 1990;**45**:1043–5.
52 De Maria G, Guarneri D, Pasolini MP, Antonini L. Stato di male versivo trattato con Propofol. *Boll Lega Ital Epil* 1991;**74**:191–2.
53 Alia G, Natale E, Mattaliano A, Daniele O. On two cases of status epilepticus treated with propofol. *Epilepsia* 1991;**32**(suppl 1):77 .
54 Wood PR, Browne GPR, Pugh S. Propofol infusion for the treatment of status epilepticus. *Lancet* 1988;**1**:480–1.
55 Levy R, Dreifuss FE, Mattson R, Meldrum B, Penry JK, eds. *Antiepileptic drugs*, 3rd ed. New York: Raven Press, 1989.

7 Raised intracranial pressure

J D PICKARD, M CZOSNYKA

Epidemiology

Raised intracranial pressure is the final common pathway for many intracranial problems (box 1) and has a profound influence on outcome. For example, of the 300 000–500 000 patients with head injury seen in accident and emergency departments in the United Kingdom per annum, 20% are admitted, of whom 10% are in coma (2% of all attenders). Over 50% of these have an intracranial pressure greater than 20 mm Hg.[1 2] A total of 80% of patients with fatal head injuries (4% of all patients with head injuries admitted) show evidence of a significant increase in intracranial pressure at necropsy. Some 35% of those with severe head injuries die and 18% are left severely disabled at enormous financial and emotional cost to the family and community. Similarly, 20 per 100 000 per year are admitted with intracerebral haematoma and 10–12 per 100 000 per annum with subarachnoid haemorrhage. The average regional neurosurgical unit serving a population of two million will manage 200 patients per annum with brain tumours, some 15 patients with chronic subdural haematoma, a similar number of patients with a cerebral abscess, and 50 patients with hydrocephalus.[3] In comatose children the incidence of raised intracranial pressure was 53% of those with head injuries, 23% with anoxic-ischaemia damage, 66% with meningitis, 57% with encephalitis, 100% with mass lesions, and 80% with hydrocephalus.[4] There is a considerable

Box 1—Some common causes of raised intracranial pressure

Head injury
Intracranial haematoma (extradural, subdural, and intracerebral)
Diffuse brain swelling
Contusion

Cerebrovascular
Subarachnoid haemorrhage
Intracerebral haematoma
Hydrocephalus
Cerebral venous thrombosis
Major cerebral infarct
Hypertensive encephalopathy (malignant hypertension, eclampsia)

Hydrocephalus
Congenital or acquired
Obstructive or communicating

Craniocerebral disproportion
Brain "tumour" (cysts; benign or malignant tumours)
Secondary hydrocephalus
Mass effect
Oedema

"Benign" intracranial hypertension
  CNS infection
  Meningitis
  Encephalitis
  Abscess
    Cerebral malaria
    Secondary hydrocephalus

  Metabolic encephalopathy
  Hypoxic–ischaemic
  Reye's syndrome etc.
  Lead encephalopathy
  Hepatic coma
  Renal failure
  Diabetic ketoacidosis
    Burns
    Near drowning
  Hyponatraemia

Status epilepticus

(Adapted from references 4, 5, 6, 7)

risk in all such patients of secondary brain damage with long term severe disability if raised intracranial pressure is not recognised and managed appropriately.

Pathophysiology

Resting intracranial pressure represents that equilibrium pressure at which CSF production and absorption are in balance, and is associated with an equivalent equilibrium volume of CSF. CSF is actively secreted by the choroid plexus at about 0·35 ml/minute and production remains constant provided cerebral perfusion pressure is adequate. CSF absorption is a passive process through the arachnoid granulations and increases with rising CSF pressure:[22]

$$\text{CSF drainage} = \frac{\text{CSF pressure} - \text{Sagittal sinus pressure}}{\text{Outflow resistance}}$$

The "four-lump" concept describes most simply the causes of raised intracranial pressure: the mass, CSF accumulation, vascular congestion, and cerebral oedema (box 2).[5-7] The description of a patient with raised intracranial pressure as having cerebral congestion, vasogenic oedema, etc can only be a working approximation, albeit useful, until our rather crude methods of assessment are refined. In adults, the normal intracranial pressure under resting conditions is between 0 and 10 mm Hg with 15 mm Hg being the upper limit of normal. Active treatment is normally instituted if intracranial pressure exceeds 25 mm Hg for more than five minutes, although a treatment threshold of 15–20 mm Hg has been suggested to improve outcome.[8] In the very young, the upper limit of normal intracranial pressure is up to 5 mm Hg.[49] Small increases in mass may be compensated for by reduction in CSF volume and cerebral blood volume but, once such mechanisms are exhausted, intracranial pressure rises with increasing pulse pressure and the appearance of spontaneous waves (plateau and B waves).[10] There is an exponential relationship between increase in volume of an intracranial mass and the increase in intracranial pressure at least within the clinically significant range.

cerebral blood flow. One interesting phenomenon revealed by transcranial Doppler (which reflects flow in large vessels) and laser Doppler (which reflects tissue perfusion) sonography, is the change in flow and perfusion during the cardiac cycle: diastolic perfusion pressure may be below the normal limit of autoregulation whereas systolic is above (see below).

Total cerebral blood flow may be increased or decreased in areas with absent reactivity. Hyperaemia is non-nutritional "luxury perfusion" where cerebral blood flow is in excess of the brain's metabolic requirements[13] and accompanied by early filling veins on angiography and "red veins" at operation. Cerebral vasodilators such as carbon dioxide will dilate "normal" arterioles, increase intracranial pressure, and may run the risk of reducing flow to damaged areas of brain (intracerebral "steal'). Inverse "steal" is one reason for the treatment of raised intracranial pressure by hyperventilation: an acute reduction of $PaCO_2$ vasoconstricts normal cerebral arterioles, thereby directing blood to focally abnormal areas.

Normally, cerebral blood flow is coupled to cerebral oxidative metabolism via multiple mechanisms involving local concentrations of hydrogen ions, potassium, and adenosine, for example. Status epilepticus leads to gross cerebral vasodilatation and intracranial hypertension as a result of greatly increased cerebral metabolism and local release of endogenous vasodilator agents. Depression of cerebral energy metabolism by anaesthesia and hypothermia may reduce cerebral blood flow and intracranial pressure where there is a large area of the brain with reasonable electrical activity[14] and where normal flow–metabolism coupling mechanisms are intact as indicated by a reasonable cerebral blood flow carbon dioxide reactivity.[15]

Spontaneous waves of intracranial pressure are associated with cerebrovascular dilatation. Cerebral blood volume increases during plateau waves (intracranial pressure >50 mm Hg for more than five minutes) and may be the result in some cases of inappropriate autoregulatory vasodilatation in response to a critical fall in cerebral perfusion pressure, although certainly not in all cases (fig 2).[16] Transcranial Doppler examination has revealed that middle cerebral artery flow velocity increases at the same rate as B waves (0·5–2/minute) of intracranial pressure (fig 3).[17]

Finally, gradients of intracranial pressure may develop when herniation occurs—transtentorial, subfalcine, and foramen

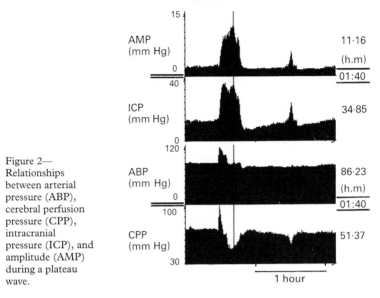

Figure 2—
Relationships
between arterial
pressure (ABP),
cerebral perfusion
pressure (CPP),
intracranial
pressure (ICP), and
amplitude (AMP)
during a plateau
wave.

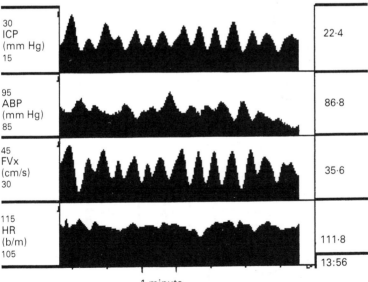

Figure 3—B waves of intracranial pressure in a head injured patient and their
relationship to similar variations in middle cerebral artery flow velocity compared
with fluctuations in arterial blood pressure (ABP) and heart rate (HR).

157

magnum. Blockage to the free flow of CSF between intracranial compartments leads to a much greater and more rapid rise in intracranial pressure in the compartment harbouring the primary pathology and hence to the final common sequence of transtentorial and foramen magnum coning. When intracranial pressure equals arterial blood pressure, angiographic pseudo-occlusion occurs, and reverberation, systolic spikes, or no flow may be seen on transcranial Doppler sonography (fig 4). Patients will often satisfy the formal clinical criteria for brainstem death, for which transcranial Doppler examination is not a substitute.[18][19]

There is a complex interaction between the properties of the CSF and the cerebral circulations that may be modelled (fig 5).[20][21] The relative contributions of abnormalities of CSF absorption and cerebral blood volume may be approximated by calculating the proportion of CSF pressure attributable to CSF outflow resistance and venous pressure from Davson's equation: (intracranial pressure = CSF formation rate × outflow resistance + sagittal sinus pressure.[22] Phenomena such as the interaction of autoregulation to changing cerebral perfusion pressure with $PaCO_2$ may be quantified.[23]

Monitoring techniques

Clinical features

In the non-trauma patient, there may or may not be a clear history of novel headache, vomiting, and visual disturbance suggestive of papilloedema or a sixth cranial nerve palsy. The absence of

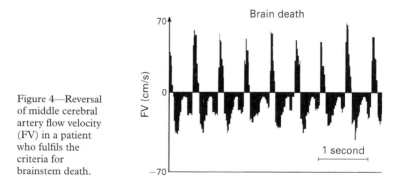

Figure 4—Reversal of middle cerebral artery flow velocity (FV) in a patient who fulfils the criteria for brainstem death.

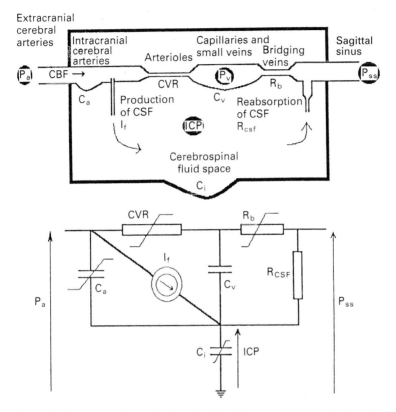

Figure 5—Hydrodynamic model of cerebral blood flow and CSF circulation with the electrically equivalent circuit (for details, see Czosnyka *et al*[21]). P_a = internal carotid artery blood pressure; P_v = cerebral venous pressure; P_{ss} = sagittal sinus blood pressure; ICP = intracranial pressure; I_f = CSF formation rate; CVR = resistance of cerebral arterial bed; R_b = resistance of bridging veins; R_{CSF} = resistance to CSF reabsorption; C_a = compliance of cerebral arterial bed; C_v = compliance of cerebral venous bed; C_i = compliance of lumbar CSF compartment.

papilloedema does not exclude raised intracranial pressure in patients with acute or chronic problems: disc swelling was found in only 4% of head injured patients, 50% of whom had raised intracranial pressure on monitoring.[6] Even in the 1990s, it is regrettable that a clear history of raised intracranial pressure may be misinterpreted until the final denouement of disturbance of consciousness and pupillary abnormality or apnoea presents. Only slowly has the danger of lumbar puncture in the differential diagnosis of neurological patients been appreciated by the non-expert. Many of the later signs of raised intracranial pressure are the result of herniation: monitoring should detect raised intracranial pressure at an earlier stage and hence should be treated before irreversible damage occurs.

CT scanning

CT scanning may reveal not only a mass, hydrocephalus, or cerebral oedema but also evidence of diffuse brain swelling such as absent perimesencephalic cisterns, compressed third ventricle, and midline shift.

Invasive methods of intracranial pressure monitoring including CSF infusion tests

The gold standard of intracranial pressure monitoring, which was first introduced before 1951,[10][24] still remains the measurement of intraventricular fluid pressure either directly or via a CSF reservoir, with the opportunity to exclude zero drift. Subdural fluid-filled catheters are reasonably accurate below 30 mm Hg. A total of 25 mm Hg for more than five minutes is the usual threshold level at which treatment should be instigated. Risk of infection, epilepsy, and haemorrhage is less with subdural than with intraventricular catheters but even the latter should be less than 5% overall. Catheter tip transducers are very useful particularly for waveform analysis, whether placed intraventricularly, subdurally, or intracerebrally. Ventricular catheters permit the therapeutic drainage of CSF in cases of ventricular dilatation. In more chronic conditions of ventricular dilatation, where intracranial pressure is not greatly raised, obstruction to CSF absorption may be confirmed by CSF infusion tests (ventricular or lumbar) taking care to adapt the technique to the site of any obstruction.[25-27] Twenty four hour intracranial pressure monitoring in patients with so-called normal pressure hydrocephalus may reveal a high incidence of B waves during sleep which is a very helpful prognostic sign for the outcome following shunting.[28][29] Benign intracranial hypertension seldom requires more than CSF pressure monitoring through a lumbar catheter or needle for an hour.

Considerable effort continues into the close analysis of the intracranial pressure trace to determine whether it is possible to reveal the mechanism of raised intracranial pressure and whether autoregulatory reserve remains intact.[30] It has been proposed[7] that congestion or vascular brain swelling may be present when the ratio of the amplitudes of the pulse and respiratory components of the intracranial pressure trace exceeds two, when there is an increase in the high-frequency centroid or when there is a high-amplitude transfer function for the fundamental harmonic from arterial pressure to intracranial pressure. Such a transfer function is calculated from the first Fourier transform of the digitised signal. Continuous multimodality monitoring is required to draw any safe conclusions, however, and should include some measure of cerebral blood flow (for example, transcranial Doppler sonography) and cerebral metabolism (for example, EEG, jugular venous oxygen). Indices of imminent decompensation would be very helpful but volume–pressure responses,[31] pressure–volume indices, or definition of the contribution of CSF outflow resistance to intracranial pressure[22] are not suitable for routine clinical use.

Non-invasive intracranial pressure monitoring

It would be very helpful to monitor intracranial pressure or cerebral perfusion pressure without invasive catheters. Transcranial Doppler examination, tympanic membrane displacement and even skull compliance studies have been advocated. It would be very helpful to have answers to the following questions: What is the cerebral perfusion pressure at any given time? What is the relative contribution of each possible mechanism to raised intracranial pressure? What features may predict decompensation? Is it possible to have an online assessment of cerebrovascular reactivity either to changes in cerebral perfusion pressure (autoregulation) or to carbon dioxide? Which therapy or cocktail is best suited to the sum of that individual's "split-brain" problems?

A non-invasive method which monitored continuously both cerebral perfusion pressure and cerebral blood flow autoregulatory reserve would be very helpful in refining management of the swollen brain.

Transcranial Doppler—Aaslid's description of transcranial Doppler sonography in 1982 permitted bedside monitoring of one index of cerebral blood flow, non-invasively, repeatedly, and even continuously.[32 33] The problem has been that it is a big tube technique which measures flow velocity in branches of the circle of Willis, most commonly the middle cerebral artery. Changes in velocity may reflect either changes in blood flow or in diameter of the insonated artery. Unfortunately, diameter and flow may not change in complementary directions and great care must be taken with the interpretation.[34] Low velocity may indicate low flow or arterial dilatation at constant flow. High velocity may indicate high flow or arterial constriction/vasospasm at constant flow. Considerable ingenuity has been expended in analysis of a transcranial Doppler waveform (fig 6). The amplitude of the flow velocity pulse wave (FV_a) reflects pulsatile changes in regional cerebral blood flow and is dependent on the amplitude of the arterial pressure wave, regional cerebrovascular resistance, the elastance of the capillary bed, and the basal cerebral arteries. Aaslid suggested that an index of cerebral perfusion pressure

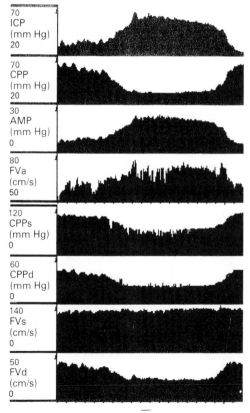

Figure 6—Relationship among intracranial pressure, cerebral perfusion pressure, intracranial pressure amplitude (AMP), and flow velocity (systolic FV_s, diastolic FV_d, and amplitude FV_a) during a plateau wave. AMP increases with increases in intracranial pressure and decreases in cerebral perfusion pressure: flow velocity amplitude increases as a result of the fall in diastolic flow velocity.

1 minute

could be derived from the ratio of the amplitudes of the first harmonics of the arterial blood pressure and the middle cerebral artery velocity (detected by transcranial Doppler sonography) multiplied by mean flow velocity. There is a reasonable correlation between the pulsatility index (peak systolic − end diastolic FVs/time averaged FV_m) of middle cerebral artery velocity and cerebral perfusion pressure after head injury but absolute measurements of cerebral perfusion pressure cannot be extrapolated.[35] Nelson et al [36] have provided both experimental and theoretical modelling evidence for three haemodynamic phases as cerebral perfusion pressure falls. Above the lower limit of autoregulation, falls in cerebral perfusion pressure are masked by arteriolar dilatation, a fall in cerebrovascular resistance and gradual increase in FV_a so that cerebral blood flow and FV_m remain stable. During the transitional phase, cerebral blood flow and FV_m start to fall gradually: cerebral perfusion pressure in diastole is close to or below the critical closing pressure of the capillaries so that the fall in FV in diastole is greater and FV_a increases further. Finally autoregulation becomes exhausted with a rapid fall in cerebral blood flow and FV_m, a sharp decrease in FV_a, and an increase in cerebrovascular resistance. Where autoregulation is impaired throughout, cerebral blood flow and FV_m fall pressure-passively as cerebral perfusion pressure is reduced, and there is no increase in FV_a. The correlation coefficient between FV_a and arterial pressure may provide a continuous online index of autoregulatory reserve: as autoregulation becomes exhausted, correlation rapidly moves from negative to positive. The response of the cerebral circulation to stress, such as a period of hypotension, hypercapnia, or transient carotid compression may also be assessed.[21 33] Hence, autoregulation and cerebrovascular reactivity may be assessed within the vascular territory supplied by the insonated artery. Comparison of the changes in blood flow velocity in a number of branches of the circle of Willis with that in the cervical internal carotid artery and with cerebral arteriovenous oxygen difference may help to distinguish vasospasm from hyperaemia at least on a global basis. Vasospasm defined by transcranial Doppler examination has been associated with delayed cerebral ischaemia after trauma.[37-39] Such techniques cannot yet define the proportional contributions of both vasospasm and hyperaemia in the same or different parts of the brain in patients who may have both. Depressed cerebral blood flow carbon dioxide reactivity was found in one study to correlate with very severe brain injury or with extensive focal lesions in middle cerebral artery distribution. Knowledge of the integrity of the cerebral blood flow carbon dioxide response was helpful in determining the potential effectiveness of hyperventilation or barbiturates for intracranial pressure control.[40]

Tympanic membrane displacement—Intracranial pressure is transmitted via the cochlear aqueduct to the perilymph of the cochlea providing that the aqueduct is patent. Perilymphatic pressure may be assessed indirectly by recording displacement of the tympanic membrane during stapedial reflex contractions elicited by a loud sound.[41] High perilymphatic pressure displaces the resting position of the stapes footplate laterally, thereby allowing a higher degree of motion in a medial direction, and results in a more inward going tympanic membrane displacement on stapedial contraction. Low perilymphatic pressure will have an opposite effect. A transducer probe attached to a head set is placed in the patient's external auditory meatus and computer based instrumentation allows small movements of the tympanic membrane to be measured when 1000 Hz of increasing sound pressure level induces stapedial contraction. This very ingenious technique is useful in younger patients with hydrocephalus or benign intracranial hypertension on a sequential basis, provided that a skilled audiologist is available. It does not provide an absolute measure of intracranial pressure. It is of no value in patients on ventilators receiving muscle relaxants. The patency of the cochlear aqueduct decreases with age and should be checked with a postural test.

Cerebral venous oxygen[42 43]

Cerebral arteriovenous oxygen content difference should normally be 5–7 ml/dl. Values below 4 ml/dl indicate cerebral hyperaemia whereas values above 9 ml/dl indicate global cerebral ischaemia. Jugular bulb oxygen saturation may be monitored, preferably continuously, with an indwelling catheter. Single measurements of jugular venous oxygen are of little value given the many fluctuations during the day. Overenthusiastic treatment, which on occasion may induce cerebral ischaemia, may be monitored with this technique. Hyperventilation and barbiturate-induced falls in cerebral perfusion pressure have been shown in individual patients to be counterproductive. An index of regional oxygen metabolism is required. Transcutaneous, transcranial,

164

near infrared spectroscopy is completely non-invasive.[44] Unfortunately, it is well proven only in neonates and younger children and not yet in older age groups.

Cerebral electrical activity

The compressed EEG (cerebral function monitoring) is helpful in deciding whether cerebral metabolic depressants may be indicated in the treatment of intracranial hypertension.[14] Such drugs will obviously not be helpful if the EEG is flat or greatly reduced in amplitude.

Management strategies

Emergency resuscitation and diagnosis

Patients who are rapidly deteriorating or already in coma require immediate resuscitation if necessary with intubation and ventilation followed by a diagnostic CT scan. An intravenous bolus of mannitol (0·5 g/kg over 15 minutes) may be required if there is evidence of coning such as pupillary dilatation. Acute ventricular dilatation demands immediate ventricular drainage—bilateral if the lesion is midline. Hyperacute ventricular dilatation following subarachnoid haemorrhage or in association with a third ventricular lesion need not be gross to cause death. Surgical clots require removal and abscesses require tapping.

Postacute management

Many neurosurgical units worldwide still manage patients without the help or hindrance of intracranial pressure monitoring. The nihilistic argument is that such monitoring has not been clearly shown to improve outcome and sequential CT provides sufficient information. Treatment for raised intracranial pressure has not greatly advanced over the past two decades and can be applied pragmatically. The alternative school of thought argues that monitoring should be selective (box 3) based in part on the initial CT scan. In addition, however, such monitoring is very educational and greatly assists general nursing and medical care; transport of a patient between intensive care and CT too often involves well documented risks of hypoxia and hypotension; intracranial pressure therapy should not be used as a blunderbuss but needs to be selectively targeted if it is not to be counterproductive; and new treatments are emerging very rapidly. Clinical trials based on

Box 3—Indications for intracranial pressure monitoring

Head injury
(a) being artificially ventilated:
—coma with compression of third ventricle and/or reduction in perimesencephalic cisterns on CT
—coma following removal of intracranial haematoma
—coma with abnormal motor response as the best reaction
—coma with midline shift/unilateral ventricular dilatation
—multiple injury including severe chest wall injuries
—early seizures not easily controlled
—refractory hyperpyrexia

(b) uncertainty over surgery for small haematoma/multiple lesions

Intracerebral and subarachnoid haemorrhage
—coma
—postoperatively following intraoperative complications
—hydrocephalus

Coma with brain swelling
—metabolic
—hypoxia/ischaemia
—infective (see box 1)

Hydrocephalus and benign intracranial hypertension
(Adapted from references 4, 7, 42)

outcome studies at six months in such heterogeneous groups of patients may easily miss useful benefits.[45] To treat raised intracranial pressure, it must first be identified, avoidable factors prevented or treated, and finally active treatment instigated, it is to be hoped, based on our understanding of the individual mechanism involved. Intracranial pressure should be treated before herniation occurs—clinical signs particularly in patients on a ventilator are just too crude. Knowledge of intracranial pressure may help with prognosis and counselling of relatives: in one series of diffuse head injuries, where intracranial pressure persistently exceeded 20 mm Hg, almost all the patients died compared with a mortality rate of 20% in those in whom intracranial pressure could be kept below 20 mm Hg with treatment.[46]

Box 4—Potential problems exacerbating raised intracranial pressure

1 Calibration of intracranial pressure and arterial blood pressure transducers and monitors particularly to check the zero reference point

2 Neck vein obstruction —inappropriate position of head and neck—avoid constricting tape around neck

3 Airway obstruction —inappropriate positive end expiratory pressure
—secretions, bronchospasm, etc

4 Inadequate muscle relaxation —breathing against ventilation
—muscle spasms

5 Hypoxia/hypercapnia

6 Further mass lesion—rescan

7 Incomplete analgesia, incomplete sedation, and anaesthesia

8 Seizures

9 Pyrexia

10 Cerebral vasodilating drugs

11 Hypovolaemia

12 Hyponatraemia (often iatrogenic fluid overload)

Prevention of intracranial hypertension: general medical and nursing care—avoidable factors

Simple measures need to be checked (box 4).[7 42] Ideally the position of the patient should minimise any obstruction to cerebral venous drainage by head-up tilt while avoiding any fall in cardiac output or carotid arterial blood pressure. Direct measurement of global cerebral blood flow and cerebral perfusion pressure suggests that head-up tilt of up to 30° is safe but careful scrutiny should be kept of cerebral perfusion pressure in individual patients.[47–50]

Hypovolaemia should be avoided, contrary to some historical teaching. The evidence is most clear cut in patients after subarachnoid haemorrhage: dehydration particularly when coupled with hyponatraemia increases the risk of cerebral infarction.[51] Patients with CT evidence of raised intracranial pressure are already at greater risk of hypovolaemia after subarachnoid haemorrhage.[52] Dehydration increases the risk of hypovolaemia which may be revealed only when the patient is given an anaesthetic

167

agent, for example, for an orthopaedic procedure or as part of a regimen to control raised intracranial pressure. A stable circulation must be maintained,[53] if necessary with colloid and inotropes (dobutamine or dopamine for its renal sparing action). Overenthusiastic hypertensive–hypervolaemic therapy remains very controversial in the context of head injury with its multiple pathology and uncertainty over the integrity of the blood–brain barrier.[54-56] Systemic hypertension should not be treated directly with agents such as sodium nitroprusside. Sodium nitroprusside impairs autoregulation and increases the risk of boundary zone infarction.[57] The cause of hypertension, for example, pain or retention of urine, should be looked for.

Most neurosurgical patients with hyponatraemia do *not* have inappropriate secretion of antidiuretic hormone, and it is unwise to use fluid restriction to treat them even if they do.[51 58] A useful dictum in neurosurgery is that blood volume comes before plasma sodium levels. Moderate hyponatraemia impairs cerebrovascular reactivity experimentally to both hypercapnia and hypotension but does not augment the cerebrovascular effects of experimental subarachnoid haemorrhage.[59] A spectrum of abnormalities gives rise to hyponatraemia following subarachnoid haemorrhage, for example: initial natriuresis leading to volume depletion, antidiuretic hormone secretion stimulated both by stress and volume depletion, antidiuretic hormone-induced water retention, steroid and sympathetic induced effects on the kidney, and possible release of atrial natriuretic factor (both cardiac and cerebral in origin) and digoxin-like substance.

Seizures may be difficult to recognise when the patient is paralysed and ventilated. Episodes of pupillary dilatation with increases in arterial blood pressure and intracranial pressure are suggestive.

Pyrexia not only increases cerebral metabolism and hence cerebral vasodilatation but also cerebral oedema. Severe hypothermia was used historically to treat raised intracranial pressure but it has become clear more recently that mild hypothermia of a few degrees centigrade only will reduce cerebral ischaemia for reasons that are not yet clear.[113] Hyperglycaemia should be avoided. There is considerable evidence that cerebral ischaemia and infarction are made worse by hyperglycaemia, and the use of high glucose solutions is contraindicated unless there is significant evidence of benefit in a particular metabolic encephalopathy.[60 61]

Osmotic diuretics

Intravenous mannitol is invaluable as a first aid measure in a patient with brain herniation as a result of raised intracranial pressure. Its more prolonged use and mechanisms of action remain contentious issues. Osmotherapy began experimentally with hypertonic saline and then urea, entering neurosurgical practice with 30% urea in 1958. A maximum fall in intracranial pressure occurs within 30 minutes of starting urea, and the effect lasts for up to three hours but with the possibility of subsequent rebound.[62] Conceptually, the mechanism was thought to be osmotic extraction of water across the intact blood–brain barrier acting as a semipermeable membrane. Experimentally, urea shrank normal rather than oedematous brain.[63] Entry of urea into the oedematous brain through a "defective" barrier would take water in and thereby account for rebound. Overenthusiastic bolus administration of an osmotic diuretic may cause abrupt systemic hypertension, an increase in cerebral blood volume if autoregulation is defective or its upper limit is exceeded, and promote herniation rather than the reverse.[64]

More recent studies indicate that mannitol, given time, removes water from both normal and oedematous brain, be it ischaemic or interstitial (Marmarou's infusion model).[65-67] The oedematous area around many mass lesions may still have an intact blood–brain barrier at least to the conventional high molecular weight tracers. The time course is slow and does not account for the immediate effect of mannitol on intracranial pressure. In patients with peritumoral oedema, mannitol causes withdrawal of water mainly from brain areas where the barrier is impaired as judged by T1-MRI and in vitro measurements of brain water content.[68] Mannitol, however, may accumulate in oedematous white matter with repeated doses.[69]

The more immediate effects of intravenous mannitol include a fall in whole blood viscosity with reduced red cell rigidity and corpuscular volume, an increase in brain compliance, and possibly cerebral vasoconstriction.[70-72] Experimental perivascular administration of mannitol evokes vasodilatation. The cerebral vasoconstriction with intravascular bolus administration was short-lived—in the cat, both pial arteriolar diameter and intracranial pressure returned to normal within 30 minutes and, thereafter, both increased at the same rate as changes in blood viscosity.[72]

169

Administration over 15 minutes produced no change in pial arteriole or venular diameter in another study.[73] Current studies in patients are using transcranial and laser Doppler sonography to re-examine these conflicting reports. Why should a sudden change in blood viscosity evoke acute transient vasoconstriction? Chronic changes in blood viscosity by plasma exchange, without alterations in haemoglobin or arterial oxygen content, do not change steady-state cerebral blood flow in humans.[74] Patients with high plasma viscosity or with high viscosity due to large numbers of white cells do not have low cerebral blood flow values. In a series of patients with haematological diseases but no evidence of cerebrovascular disease, arterial oxygen content was the major determinant of cerebral blood flow—blood viscosity *per se* had no significant effect on cerebral blood flow.[75] If a single blood vessel is considered, the apparent viscosity of blood diminishes in proportion to its radius as a result of the marginal sheath of low viscosity and axial flow of red cells.[76] The width of this sheath is relatively greatest in small vessels. Furthermore, apparent viscosity increases with falling velocity. Hence with pial arterial dilatation, local blood viscosity will rise both because of the increased proportion of red cells and as a result of the reduction in flow velocity if tissue perfusion flow remains constant. Simplistically, according to Poiseuille, as viscosity is reduced deliberately, so the pressure gradient along the pial arteriole under observation falls. Hence, the distal intravascular pressure increases if the proximal pressure remains constant. The distal end of the arteriole therefore constricts if autoregulatory mechanisms such as the Bayliss effect are intact. "Viscosity" autoregulation should depend on pressure autoregulation unless there is a separate endothelial mechanism that is flow or viscosity sensitive. Alternatively, mannitol may transiently increase cerebral blood flow, increase oxygen delivery and wash out local vasodilators such as adenosine.[72] Vasoconstriction then follows. Extracellular hyperosmolarity is a potent cerebral vasodilator and it is remarkable that the intravenous vasoconstrictor effect of mannitol so completely dominates the acute cerebrovascular effect. If the viscosity mechanism is apposite, it will depend upon the distribution gradient of intravascular pressures along the cerebrovascular tree which may not be easy to predict with different pathologies and cerebral perfusion pressures. Certainly the reported effects of mannitol on cerebral blood flow are not easy to rationalise.[77-80] In patients with severe head injuries, in whom autoregulation was absent, intravenous mannitol caused an increase in cerebral blood flow and no reduction in intracranial pressure.[81] Intracranial pressure was reduced in those patients where autoregulation was intact. In patients with unruptured aneurysms, however, in most of whom autoregulation was presumably intact, mannitol (bolus or infusion) increased cerebral blood flow for many hours.[80] More regional assessments of cerebral blood flow suggest that mannitol may stabilise pH and cerebral blood flow in regions of moderate but not severe ischaemia.[82] Other suggested mechanisms for the effect of mannitol include movement of water from CSF into capillaries and scavenging of free radicals.[83] Plasma hyperosmolality rapidly reverses the interstitial fluid pressure/CSF pressure gradient and there is a rapid volume shift within 30 minutes from CSF into brain tissue.[131]

Many attempts have been made to rationalise how much mannitol may be given and when, for more prolonged effects.[84 85] In practice, mannitol tends to be given as an intermittent bolus whenever the individual patient's intracranial pressure rises significantly above the threshold of 25–30 mm Hg. The effects of mannitol may be potentiated by adding frusemide.[85] It is crucial to avoid dehydration and latent hypotension with careful attention to fluid balance. Colloid with an adequate plasma half life (albumin, hetastarch, for example) should be combined with careful electrolyte replacement. Another dose of mannitol should not be given if osmolarity exceeds 330 mmol/l for fear of tubular damage and renal failure. Repeated doses of mannitol should not be given unless an intracranial pressure monitor is in place. Some authors continue to recommend glycerol for prolonged osmotherapy.[86]

Hyperventilation, the buffer TRIS, and indomethacin

The cerebral vasoconstrictor effect of hypocapnia, induced by hyperventilation, does not persist much beyond a day, probably in part because the bicarbonate buffering mechanisms within the brain and cerebrovascular smooth muscle themselves readjust to return extracellular and intracellular pH nearer to the original values.[87] This phenomenon has now been confirmed in vivo in normal subjects by magnetic resonance spectroscopy. Neurosurgical patients with healthy lungs and systemic circulation often hyperventilate spontaneously down to a $PaCO_2$ of 30 mm Hg.[6 42] More enthusiastic hyperventilation may precipitate cerebral ischaemia with EEG slowing, CSF lactic acidosis, and a cerebral arteriovenous oxygen content difference of more than 9 ml/dl. Arterial blood pressure may be reduced by the combination of dehydration and aggressive hyperventilation. Finally, weaning from the ventilator may be more difficult and prone to "rebound" intracranial hypertension: the brain's buffering mechanisms have to readjust back again. Finally, cerebrovascular reactivity to carbon dioxide may be absent in some patients after head injury, but such reactivity is seldom measured before hyperventilation is started. Transcranial Doppler examination is a simple way of assessing carbon dioxide reactivity. In one study, controlled hyperventilation used prophylactically did not improve outcome but did prolong the recovery phase.[88] Hence there is growing awareness that hyperventilation be used sparingly, for example, to treat persistent intracranial pressure waves.

CSF lactate accumulation and CSF acidosis occur after head injury.[89 90] Both severity of injury and the proportion of patients with a poor outcome are related to high and increasing CSF lactate levels. Cerebral tissue lactic acidosis is related to secondary brain damage following a primary insult such as cerebral ischaemia even if moderate acidosis *per se* has no persisting effect on normal neurons. Akiota *et al*[91] found that the intravenous buffer tris(hydroxymethyl)aminomethane (TRIS) ameliorated both the CSF acidosis and brain swelling following epidural balloon compression of the brain in dogs. In 1970, Gordan and Rossanda[92] suggested that hyperventilation might be beneficial as the result of compensation of CSF acidosis but only at very low $PaCO_2$ (20–25 mm Hg) which is now proposed to produce severe cerebral vasoconstriction and, in some individuals, cerebral ischaemia. TRIS, after intravenous administration, equilibrates with the intracellular and extracellular spaces in the body as well as with CSF. Evidence is accumulating both experimentally and in humans that TRIS is at least as effective as mannitol in reducing experimental oedema in the brain and lowering intracranial pressure after head injury.[93 94] TRIS reduces the demand for mannitol and CSF drainage. In the most recently published randomised prospective clinical trial,[94] a total of 149 patients with severe head injury (Glasgow Coma Scale $\leqslant$ 8) were randomly assigned to either a control or a TRIS group. Both groups of patients matched in terms of clinical parameters including age, sex, number of surgical mass lesions, number in each Glasgow scale stratum, and the first intracranial pressure measurement. All patients were treated by standard management protocols, intubated, mechanically ventilated, and maintained in the Pacarbon dioxide range of 32–35 mm Hg for five days. TRIS was administered as a 0·3 mol/l solution in an initial loading dose (body weight × blood acidity deficit, average 4·27 ml/kg hourly) given over two hours, followed by constant infusion of 1 ml/kg hourly for five days. Outcome was measured at three, six, and 12 months postinjury. Although analysis indicated no significant difference between these two groups at three months, six months, or one year, there was a difference regarding intracranial pressure. The time that intracranial pressure was above 20 mm Hg in the first 48 hours after injury was less in patients treated with TRIS. Also the number of patients requiring barbiturate coma was significantly less in the TRIS group (5·5% versus 18·4%). The authors concluded that TRIS ameliorated the deleterious effects of prolonged hyperventilation, was beneficial in intracranial pressure control, and further study of dose and timing of administration was warranted.

The cerebrovascular response to hypercapnia may be manipulated in other ways. It has been known since 1973 that the cerebrovascular carbon dioxide response is blocked by indomethacin in doses that partly inhibit brain cyclo-oxygenase activity in vivo.[95] Cerebral venous pressure is very significantly reduced suggesting that intracranial pressure is reduced. That observation was not used clinically because of fear that indomethacin was inhibiting production of prostacyclin and that might be counterproductive. Certainly, cerebral oxygen delivery is seriously impaired when indomethacin is given to very young animals or to very early preterm infants undergoing treatment for patent ductus arteriosus.[96] In five patients with injury with cerebral contusion and oedema, in whom it was not possible to control intracranial pressure by hyperventilation and barbiturate sedation, indomethacin (bolus injection of 30 mg followed by 30 mg/hour for seven hours) reduced intracranial pressure below 20 mm Hg for several hours.[97] Cerebral blood flow was reduced at two hours without any changes in cerebral arteriovenous oxygen or lactate differences. Rectal temperature also fell from 38·6 to 37·3°C. Hence a more substantial trial of indomethacin appears warranted, perhaps avoiding young children until further experience is accumulated. Inhibition of nitric oxide synthesis also blocks the cerebrovascular carbon dioxide response but may also increase focal cerebral infarction in the rat middle cerebral artery occlusion model.

Continuous CSF drainage and surgical decompression

External ventricular drainage via a catheter or reservoir is a rapid procedure in an emergency in a patient with hydrocephalus. Biventricular drainage is required for third ventricular lesions which occlude both foramina of Munro. Colloid cysts are best dealt with as the primary procedure unless the patient is in extremis. Patients with communicating hydrocephalus or benign intracranial hypertension may be temporarily controlled by lumbar drainage through an indwelling catheter. It is unkind, unnecessary, and less effective to use repeated lumbar punctures. It is becoming recognised that permanent CSF drainage via lumbar peritoneal shunts may be complicated by secondary descent of the cerebellar tonsils in patients with no previous evidence of a Chiari malformation.[98] In all cases of external drainage, CSF should be drained gradually against a positive pressure of 15–25 cm H_2O to avoid unrestrained drainage. In the case of a posterior fossa tumour, upward coning may be precipitated if the supratentorial ventricles are drained too precipitously. In patients with a hemisphere mass causing midline shift and contralateral hydrocephalus, drainage of that ventricle may make the shift worse. In patients with diffuse brain swelling, the ventricles are small and not always easy to cannulate. Stereotactic techniques are useful but not appropriate in an emergency. Even where intracranial pressure is controlled by drainage against a pressure 15–25 cm H_2O, such a ventricular catheter readily becomes blocked and is seldom a satisfactory technique *per se*. CSF drainage alone is the optimal method of controlling intracranial hypertension in patients with subarachnoid haemorrhage where the cause is often disturbance of the CSF circulation, but there is probably an increased risk of rebleeding. CSF drainage is used as a diagnostic technique to assess patients in the poorer grades of subarachnoid haemorrhage. When they improve early surgery should be considered.

Removal of bone flaps or subtemporal decompressions are

174

performed much less frequently nowadays.[99] Patients with large meningiomas may have a smoother postoperative course if a flap is removed electively at the end of the operation rather than as an emergency a few hours later. Benign intracranial hypertension can be treated by a combination of optic nerve sheath fenestration and lumbar peritoneal or cisternoperitoneal shunting: subtemporal decompressions are rarely indicated. Babies with complex forms of craniosynostosis may require craniofacial surgery to expand the volume of the skull. Slit ventricle syndrome for shunt-induced CSF overdrainage may be managed by use of siphon control devices or programmable valves—subtemporal decompression is seldom required. This procedure was sometimes followed by temporal lobe epilepsy.

There is a very restricted place for decompressive craniotomy following head injury and there is the potential to do considerable harm.[99 100] With a very tight brain, opening the dura induces herniation through the defect. Cerebral venous drainage from the herniated brain obstructs and further brain swelling ensues with infarction. Experimentally, craniectomy facilitates formation of hydrostatic brain oedema as might be expected from consideration of Starling's equation.[101] Craniectomy may be considered in young patients without evidence of diffuse axonal injury (high Glasgow Coma Scale score on admission) and evidence of diffuse swelling.[102] For paediatric encephalopathies, Kirkham makes a case for performing decompression earlier rather than later, and certainly before the EEG disappears.[103]

Steroids, free radical scavengers, and the lazaroids

The mechanism of the remarkable effect of glucocorticoids such as dexamethasone on focal, relatively chronic, cerebral lesions remains incompletely understood. Patients deteriorating with a cerebral tumour or an abscess rapidly improve within 24 hours. It is not yet proven whether steroids help traumatic cerebral contusions. Intracranial pressure waves and compliance improve together although mean intracranial pressure and water content take days longer to subside. Brain biopsy for tumour is much safer after at least three days of dexamethasone (10–20 mg loading dose; 4 mg four times a day thereafter) particularly when combined with stereotactic biopsy techniques. Care should be taken to counsel patients about the side effects of steroids even with short courses.

Much controversy has surrounded the use of very high dose steroids in head injury but careful controlled trials have shown no benefit and in one study the outcome of the treatment group was worse.[104-108] Even higher doses started within a few hours of injury are currently under scrutiny. This rationale is based on trials in spinal cord injury of methylprednisolone (30 mg/kg daily) which showed a modest benefit in the group where it was started within eight hours of injury.

One purported mechanism of action for steroids involves lipid peroxidation and free radicals.[109 110] Oxygen is needed for aerobic life but it has toxic properties. All organisms are subject to oxidative stress as up to 2% of oxygen consumed by the brain, for example, is used to form semi-reduced oxygen intermediates: superoxide, hydrogen peroxide, and hydroxyl free radicals. These may be used as part of normal biochemistry or if the safety mechanisms fail—superoxide dismutase, catalase, glutathione peroxidase, glutathione, vitamin E, and ascorbate—then such reactive oxygen species may attack nucleic acids, proteins, carbohydrates, and particularly lipids in the brain. Ferrous iron from blood clots is also active along with such reactive oxygen species. Cerebrovascular effects of acute hypertension and subarachnoid haemorrhage may involve free radical mechanisms damaging the endothelium. Non-glucocorticoid steroid analogues of methylprednisolone as well as methylprednisolone itself weakly inhibit lipid peroxidation. The 21-amino-steroids (the antioxidant family known as the lazaroids) are potent inhibitors of lipid peroxidation and have a vitamin E sparing effect.[111] Various experimental models of head and spinal injury and focal or global ischaemia have shown a variable degree of protection after treatment with the lazaroid U-74006F, so that it is now undergoing large scale clinical trials in head injury and subarachnoid haemorrhage. Recently, the steroid component of the lazaroid molecule has been replaced by the antioxidant ring structure of vitamin E. U-78517F has greater in vitro lipid antioxidant properties than U-74006F. It is interesting that the iron chelator desferrioxamine may be helpful in treating the coma of cerebral malaria and experimental vasogenic oedema. Early results in severe head injuries with the oxygen radical scavenger—polyethylene glycol conjugated superoxide dismutase—have recently been reported but a much larger trial is required to establish efficacy.[112]

Cerebral metabolic depressants: excitotoxic amino acid antagonists

The cerebral metabolic depressant effect of deep hypothermia is now seldom used except during cardiopulmonary bypass and total circulatory arrest. Such a technique may be used for complex basilar aneurysms where interventional radiological techniques are inappropriate. Brain energy metabolism is depressed more conveniently by hypnotic agents including barbiturates, etomidate, propofol, althesin, and γ-hydroxybutyrate. Unfortunately all such agents have side effects, the most relevant of which is systemic hypotension, often compounded by dehydration or hypovolaemia. It is essential to maintain a normal arterial blood pressure and not allow cerebral perfusion pressure to fall. Central venous pressure monitoring is required. One factor maintaining cerebral perfusion pressure in patients with raised intracranial pressure may be the Cushing mechanism—lower the intracranial pressure and cerebral perfusion pressure falls.

Hypnotic agents depress cerebral oxidative metabolism and hence lower cerebral blood flow and volume, and intracranial pressure. Cerebral electrical activity and normal coupling mechanisms between metabolism and flow must be present if barbiturates are to lower intracranial pressure.[14 15 42] Normal flow metabolism coupling mechanisms may be assessed by the cerebrovascular response to carbon dioxide. Short term protection during aneurysmal surgery with barbiturate or propofol is widely used. Synergy with even moderate hypothermia may be helpful provided mean arterial pressure is maintained.[42] After initial reports of the effectiveness of short acting barbiturates in lowering intracranial pressure after head injury, three controlled trials have failed to show any overall significant improvement of outcome or reduction in number of patients dying with intracranial hypertension.[114-116] Such trials involved heterogeneous groups of patients, however, and a treatment benefit in a subgroup may have been missed.

In the United Kingdom, althesin has been withdrawn even though its idiosyncratic allergic problems would not have been a contraindication in the intensive care environment. Etomidate blocks steroidogenesis but it is apparently still used in the United States as an intraoperative protection agent by combining it with dexamethasone postoperatively for a few days.[117] γ-Hydroxybutyrate lowers blood pressure and its administration involves a considerable sodium load.[118] Propofol (di-isopropylphenol) is widely used but care has to be taken to avoid hypotension. Propofol also has free radical scavenging effects.[119] The ideal hypnotic agent awaits development. In the patient with cardiovascular instability, intravenous lignocaine (1·5 mg/kg) may have a place in lowering intracranial pressure.[120] This dose is as effective as intravenous thiopentone (3 mg/kg).

Epilepsy has long been known to increase intracranial pressure and increase the risk of cerebral ischaemia as a result of a massive increase in cerebral electrical activity and oxidative metabolism: both metabolic demand and cerebral perfusion pressure are embarrassed. Seizures must be treated aggressively. Over the last decade, however, a more focal phenomenon has been revealed: inappropriate hypermetabolism in small areas of the brain in association with local release or failed reuptake of excitotoxic amino acids such as glutamate.[121 122] For example, subdural haemorrhage in the rat is accompanied by increased glutamate concentrations in the hippocampus with increased local cerebral glucose utilisation and late ischaemic brain damage. N-methyl-D-aspartate antagonists will protect against such damage[123] just as they reduce delayed neuronal loss and the volume of cerebral infarction after middle cerebral artery occlusion, provided such agents are given prophylactically or in some cases within an hour of occlusion.[124 125] The therapeutic window of opportunity is very short unless it is surmised that glutamate release occurs at various times after a head injury, not just at the moment of impact. Such impressive experimental data has led to phase I and II trials of glutamate receptor antagonists in patients after severe head injury. The results are awaited with keen interest. Ironically, that old fashioned treatment for severe head injuries—rectal magnesium chloride—is now known to be a non-competitive N-methyl-D-aspartate receptor antagonist and reduces the infarct volume after middle cerebral occlusion in the rat.[126]

Targeted therapy

It is clear that there are many causes of raised intracranial pressure. The Edinburgh school has attempted[7] to define which therapy should be selected for each cause of intracranial hypertension.

They suggest that hypnotic agents may be most logically targeted at younger patients with diffuse congestive brain swelling with preserved cerebral electrical activity, jugular venous oxygen saturation over 75%, a pulse–respiratory ratio in the intracranial pressure trace of over 2, preserved cerebral blood flow carbon dioxide reactivity, and absence of a diastolic notch on transcranial Doppler recordings of middle cerebral artery velocity. Mannitol may be best used in patients of any age with focal lesions, a low cerebral perfusion pressure, and reasonably preserved autoregulation. If arterial blood pressure is low despite colloid then inotropic agents such as dobutamine or dopamine should be used. Subarachnoid haemorrhage with raised intracranial pressure is best managed by CSF drainage accepting that there is probably an increased risk of rebleeding.

Children

The management of raised intracranial pressure in childhood must take account of a number of factors.[4 127] The critical values for intracranial pressure, arterial pressure, and cerebral perfusion pressure are lower, the younger the child. The normal intracranial pressure in the newborn is probably of the order of 2–4 mm Hg. Arterial pressure at birth is about 40 mm Hg, 80/55 by one year and 90/60 during the early school years. Cerebral perfusion pressure rises from 28 mm Hg at 28–32 weeks of gestational age to 37·5 mm Hg at normal full term. In the neonate, much lower cerebral blood flow values may be tolerated for longer. Many of the pathologies differ from the adult including birth asphyxia, posthaemorrhagic ventricular dilatation, craniocerebral disproportion, and the many metabolic and infective encephalopathies. Hyperaemia plays a greater role as a cause of raised intracranial pressure in children after head injury than in adults.[128 129] The NIH Traumatic Data Bank of severe head injuries revealed that diffuse brain swelling occurs twice as often in children (aged 16 years or younger) as in adults. A total of 53% of children with diffuse swelling died compared with a mortality rate of 16% in those without. The skull may expand in children where fusion of the sutures has not occurred. Controlled trials of therapy in the various conditions are made difficult by the very small numbers of patients seen in each centre. As with adults, there is a wide diversity of opinion on the use of barbiturate coma, steroids and mannitol. Even fluid restriction still has its advocates in the neonates, and for inappropriate secretion of antidiuretic hormone. The dangers of fluid restriction, based on assuming that the syndrome of inappropriate secretion of antidiuretic hormone is the common cause of hyponatraemia after intracranial insults, have been documented very clearly in studies of adults after subarachnoid haemorrhage.

Conclusions

This review has been written at an unfortunate time. Novel questions are being asked of the old therapies and there is an abundance of new strategies both to lower intracranial pressure and to protect the brain against cerebral ischaemia. In the United Kingdom, the problem is to ensure that appropriate patients continue to be referred to centres where clinical trials of high quality can be undertaken. One of the success stories of the past decade has been the decline in the number of road accidents as a result of seat belt legislation, improvements in car design, and the drink/driving laws. Hence, fortunately there are fewer patients with head injuries to treat and it is even more important that patients are appropriately referred if studies to assess efficacy of the new strategies are not to be thwarted. The nihilistic concept that intensive investigation with intracranial pressure monitoring for patients with diffuse head injury or brain swelling following evacuation of a haematoma or a contusion has no proven beneficial effect on outcome, requires revision. A cocktail of treatment may be required that can be created only when patients are monitored in sufficient detail to reveal the mechanisms underlying their individual intracranial pressure problem.

Ethical problems may arise over how aggressively therapy for intracranial hypertension should be pursued and for how long. There has always been the concern that cranial decompression or prolonged barbiturate coma may preserve patients but with unacceptably severe disability. Some patients may be salvaged from herniating with massive cerebral infarction with the use of osmotherapy, but is the outcome acceptable?[130 131] Similar considerations apply to some children with metabolic encephalopathies. Where such considerations have been scrutinised in patients with severe head injury, the whole spectrum of outcomes appears to be

Management of raised intracranial pressure

Conscious patient
● Diagnosis based on suspicious history (novel headaches, nausea, vomiting, visual blurring/obscurations, diplopia) with or without papilloedema on examination
Any patient with drowsiness or fluctuation in conscious level or visual obscurations merits emergency referral to neurosurgery

● Definitive investigation by CT scan combined with general medical assessment including chest radiograph
Never perform a lumbar puncture in a patient with suspected raised intracranial pressure, even if papilloedema is absent, until a CT scan has shown no evidence of either a mass lesion or diffuse brain swelling

● Management depends on the presumptive diagnosis after CT and proceeds in consultation with neurosurgery—for example, space-occupying lesion
　—tumours: dexamethasone, tissue diagnosis and excision, radiotherapy, chemotherapy as appropriate
　—abscess: aspiration/excision

● Hydrocephalus: CSF shunt with or without prior intracranial pressure monitoring/CSF infusion studies

● Benign intracranial hypertension: referral to combined neurosurgery/neuro-ophthalmology service for CSF monitoring, diuretics/steroids/diet for mild cases. CSF shunt/optic nerve sheath fenestration for severe/refractory cases

Unconscious patient where intracranial catastrophe suspected (for causes see box 1)

Emergency resuscitation for patients no longer obeying commands
● Intubation and ventilation

● Intravenous mannitol (0·5 g/kg) where patient deteriorating

● Definitive investigation
　—CT scan in combination with general medical assessment and consideration of any available history
　—intracranial pressure monitoring

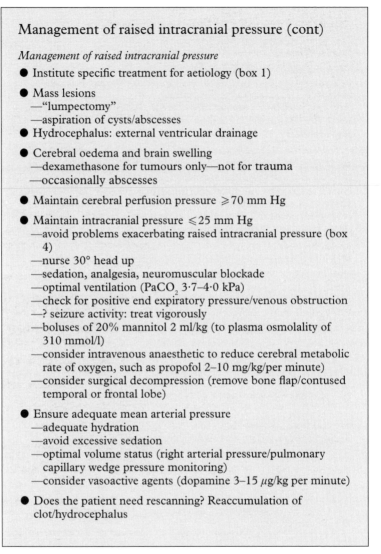

Management of raised intracranial pressure (cont)

Management of raised intracranial pressure

● Institute specific treatment for aetiology (box 1)

● Mass lesions
  —"lumpectomy"
  —aspiration of cysts/abscesses
● Hydrocephalus: external ventricular drainage

● Cerebral oedema and brain swelling
  —dexamethasone for tumours only—not for trauma
  —occasionally abscesses

● Maintain cerebral perfusion pressure ⩾70 mm Hg

● Maintain intracranial pressure ⩽25 mm Hg
  —avoid problems exacerbating raised intracranial pressure (box 4)
  —nurse 30° head up
  —sedation, analgesia, neuromuscular blockade
  —optimal ventilation ($PaCO_2$ 3·7–4·0 kPa)
  —check for positive end expiratory pressure/venous obstruction
  —? seizure activity: treat vigorously
  —boluses of 20% mannitol 2 ml/kg (to plasma osmolality of 310 mmol/l)
  —consider intravenous anaesthetic to reduce cerebral metabolic rate of oxygen, such as propofol 2–10 mg/kg/per minute)
  —consider surgical decompression (remove bone flap/contused temporal or frontal lobe)

● Ensure adequate mean arterial pressure
  —adequate hydration
  —avoid excessive sedation
  —optimal volume status (right arterial pressure/pulmonary capillary wedge pressure monitoring)
  —consider vasoactive agents (dopamine 3–15 μg/kg per minute)

● Does the patient need rescanning? Reaccumulation of clot/hydrocephalus

shifted so that the number of severe disabilities and persistent vegetative states are not increased. It is important to be sensitive to such issues, however, based on experience of the particular cause of raised intracranial pressure in a given age group.

We are indebted to Dr J M Turner, Mr E Guazzo and Mr P Kirkpatrick for their comments on the manuscript.

1 Jennett B, Teasdale G. *Management of head injuries.* Philadelphia: F A Davies, 1981.
2 Miller JD, Jones PA, Dearden NM, Tocher JL. Progress in the management of head injury. *Br J Surg* 1992;**79**:60–4.
3 Pickard JD, Bailey S, Sanderson H, Rees M, Garfield JS. Steps towards cost-benefit analysis of regional neurosurgical care. *BMJ* 1990;**301**:629–35.
4 Minns RA. Problems of intracranial pressure in childhood. *Clinics in developmental medicine* **113/114**. London: Mac Keith Press, 1991:1–458.
5 Langfitt TW. Increased intracranial pressure. *Clin Neurosurg* 1969;**16**:436–71.
6 Miller JD. Normal and increased intracranial pressure. In: Miller JD, ed. *Northfield's surgery of the central nervous system* 2nd ed, London: Blackwell, 1987:7–57.
7 Miller JD, Dearden NM. Measurement, analysis and the management of raised intracranial pressure. In: Teasdale GM, Miller JD, eds. *Current neurosurgery.* Edinburgh: Churchill Livingstone, 1992:119–56.
8 Saul TG, Ducker TB. Effect of intracranial pressure monitoring and aggressive treatment on mortality in severe head injury. *J Neurosurg* 1982;**56**:498–503.
9 Welch K. The intracranial pressure in infants. *J Neurosurg* 1980;**52**:693–9.
10 Lundberg N. Continuous recording and control of ventricular fluid pressure in neurosurgical practice. *Acta Psych Neurol Scand* 1960;**36**(Suppl 149):1–193.
11 Avezaat CJJ, von Eijndhoven JHM, Wyper DJ. Cerebrospinal fluid pulse pressure and intracranial volume-pressure relationships. *J Neurol Neurosurg Psychiatry* 1979;**42**:687–700.
12 Czosnyka M, Laniewski P, Batorski L, *et al.* Remarks on amplitude-pressure characteristic phenomenon. In: Hoff JT, Betz AL, eds. *Intracranial pressure VII.* Berlin: Springer Verlag 1989:255–9.
13 Obrist WD, Langfitt TW, Jaggi JL, *et al.* Cerebral blood flow and metabolism in comatose patients with acute head injury. Relationship to intracranial hypertension. *J Neurosurg* 1984;**61**:241–55.
14 Bingham RM, Procaccio F, Prior PF, Hinds CJ. Cerebral electrical activity influences the effects of etomidate on cerebral perfusion pressure in traumatic coma. *Br J Anaesth* 1985;**57**:843–8.
15 Nordstrom CH, Messeter K, Sundbarg G, *et al.* Cerebral blood flow, vasoreactivity and oxygen consumption during barbiturate therapy in severe traumatic brain lesions. *J Neurosurg* 1988;**68**:424–31.
16 Rosner MJ, Becker DP. Origins and evolution of plateau waves. Experimental observations and theoretical model. *J Neurosurg* 1984;**60**:312–24.
17 Newell DW, Aaslid R, Stooss R, Reulen HJ. The relationship of blood flow velocity fluctuations to intracranial pressure B waves. *J Neurosurg* 1992;**76**:415–21.
18 Kirkham FJ, Levin SD, *et al.* Transcranial pulsed Doppler ultrasound findings in brainstem death. *J Neurol Neurosurg Psychiatry* 1987;**50**:1504–13.
19 Hassler W, Steinmetz H, Pirschel J. Transcranial Doppler study of intracranial circulatory arrest. *J Neurosurg* 1989;**71**:195–201.
20 Marmarou A, Shulman K, Larmorgese J. Compartmental analysis of compliance and outflow resistance of the cerebrospinal fluid outflow system. *J Neurosurg* 1975;**43**:523–34.
21 Czosnyka M, Pickard JD, Whitehouse H, Piechnik S. The hyperaemic response to a transient reduction in cerebral perfusion pressure—a modelling study. *Acta Neurochir (Wien)* 1992;**115**:90–7.
22 Marmarou A, Maset AL, Ward JD, *et al.* Contribution of CSF and vascular factors to elevation of intracranial pressure in severely head-injured patients. *J Neurosurg* 1987;**66**:883–90.
23 Czosnyka M, Harris NG, Pickard JD. carbon dioxide cerebrovascular reactivity as a function of perfusion pressure—a modelling study. *Acta Neurochir (Wien)* 1993;**121**:159–65.
24 Guillaume J, Janny P. Manometrie intracranienne continué interet de la methode et premiers resultats. *Revue Neurologique* 1951;**84**:131–42.
25 Katzman R, Hussey F. A simple constant-infusion manometric test for measurement of CSF absorption. I Rationale and method. *Neurology* 1970;**20**:534–44.
26 Borgesen SE, Gjerris F. The predictive value of conductance to outflow of CSF in normal pressure hydrocephalus. *Brain* 1982;**105**:65–86.
27 Czosnyka M, Batorski L, Laniewski P, Maksymowicz W, Koszewski W, Zaworski W. A computer system for the identification of the cerebrospinal compensatory model. *Acta Neurochir (Wien)* 1990;**105**:112–16.
28 Symon L, Dorsch NWC, Stephens RJ. Pressure waves in so-called low-pressure hydro-

cephalus. *Lancet* 1972;**2**:1291–2.

29 Pickard JD. Teasdale GM, Matheson M, Wyper DJ, *et al.* Intraventricular pressure waves—the best predictive test for shunting in normal pressure hydrocephalus. In: Shulman K, *et al*, eds. *Intracranial pressure IV.* Berlin: Springer-Verlag 1980:498–500.

30 Laniewski P, Czosnyka M, Maksymowicz W. Continuous analysis of the intracranial pressure waveform as a method of autoregulatory reserve assessment. *Intracranial pressure VIII.* Berlin: Springer Verlag 1993:376–81.

31 Miller JD, Garibi J, Pickard JD. Induced changes in cerebrospinal fluid volume. Effects during continuous monitoring of ventricular fluid pressure. *Arch Neurol* 1973;**28**:265–9.

32 Aaslid R, Markwalder T-M, Nornes H. Non-invasive transcranial Doppler ultrasound recording of flow velocity in basal cerebral arteries. *J Neurosurg* 1982;**57**:769–74.

33 Newell DW, Aaslid R. *Transcranial Doppler.* New York: Raven Press, 1992.

34 Martin JL, Perry S, Pickard JD. Cerebral blood flow and Doppler flow velocity: different responses to three vasodilators. *J Cereb Blood Flow Metab* 1991;**11**(suppl 2):S455.

35 Chan KH, Miller JD, Dearden NM, Andrews PJD, Midgley S. The effect of cerebral perfusion pressure upon changes in middle cerebral artery flow velocity and jugular venous bulb oxygen saturation after severe head injury. *J Neurosurg* 1992;**77**:55–61.

36 Nelson RJ, Czosnyka M, Pickard JD, Maksymowicz W, Perry S, Martin JL, Lovick AHJ. Experimental aspects of cerebrospinal hemodynamics: the relationship between blood flow velocity waveform and cerebral autoregulation. *Neurosurgery* 1992;**31**:705–10.

37 Chan KH, Dearden NM, Miller JD. The significance of posttraumatic increase in cerebral blood flow velocity: a transcranial Doppler ultrasound study. *Neurosurgery* 1992; **30**:697–700.

38 Chan KH, Dearden NM, Miller JD, Midgley S, Piper IR. Transcranial Doppler waveform differences in hyperemic and nonhyperemic patients after severe head injury. *Surg Neurol* 1992;**38**:433–6.

39 Chan KH, Miller JD, Dearden NM. Intracranial blood flow velocity after head injury: relationship to severity of injury, time, neurological status and outcome. *J Neurol Neurosurg Psychiatry* 1992;**55**:787–91.

40 Schalen W, Messeter R, Nordstrom CH. Cerebral vasoreactivity and the prediction of outcome in severe traumatic brain lesions. *Acta Anaesthesiol Scand* 1991;**35**:113–22.

41 Reid A, Marchbanks RJ, Martin R, Pickard JD, Bateman N, Brightwell R. Mean intracranial pressure monitoring by an audiological technique—a pilot study. *J Neurol Neurosurg Psychiatry* 1989;**52**:610–12.

42 Campkin TV, Turner JM. *Neurosurgical anaesthesia and intensive care,* 2nd ed. London: Butterworth, 1986.

43 Robertson CS, Narayan RH, Gokaslan ZL, *et al.* Cerebral arteriovenous oxygen difference as an estimate of cerebral blood flow in comatose patients. *J Neurosurg* 1989;**70**: 222–30.

44 Wyatt JS, Cope M, Delpy DT, Wray S, Reynolds EOR. Quantification of cerebral oxygenation and haemodynamics in sick newborn infants by near infrared spectroscopy. *Lancet* 1986;**2**:1063–6.

45 Jennett B, Teasdale G, Galbraith S, *et al.* Severe head injuries in three countries. *J Neurol Neurosurg Psychiatry* 1977;**40**:291–8.

46 Miller JD, Butterworth JF, Gudeman SK, *et al.* Further experience in the management of severe head injury. *J Neurosurg* 1981;**54**:289–99.

47 Ropper AH, O'Rourke D, Kennedy SK. Head position, intracranial pressure and compliance. *Neurology* 1982;**32**:1288–91.

48 Rosner MJ, Coley IB. Cerebral perfusion pressure, intracranial pressure and head elevation. *J Neurosurg* 1986;**65**:636–41.

49 Feldman Z, Kanter MJ, Robertson CS, *et al.* Effect of head elevation on intracranial pressure, cerebral perfusion pressure and cerebral blood flow in head injured patients. *J Neurosurg* 1992;**76**:207–11.

50 Kanter MJ, Robertson CS, Sheinberg MA, *et al.* Changes in cerebral hemodynamics with head elevated vs head flat. In: Avezaat C, ed. *Intracranial pressure VIII.* Berlin: Springer-Verlag, 1993:429–32.

51 Hasan D, Vermeulen M, Wijdicks EFM, *et al.* Effect of fluid intake and hypertensive treatment on cerebral ischaemia after subarachnoid haemorrhage. *Stroke* 1989;**20**: 1511–15.

52 Nelson RJ, Roberts J, Rubin C, Walker V, Ackery DM, Pickard JD. Association of hypovolaemia after subarachnoid haemorrhage with computer tomographic scan evidence of raised intracranial pressure. *Neurosurgery* 1991;**29**:178–82.

53 Marmarou A, Anderson RL, Ward JD, et al. Impact of intracranial pressure instability and hypotension on outcome in patients with severe head trauma. *J Neurosurg* 1991; 75:S59–66.

54 Muizelaar JP. Induced arterial hypertension in the treatment of high intracranial pressure. In: Hoff JT, Betz AL, ed. *Intracranial pressure VII*. Springer-Verlag, 1989:508–10.

55 Rosner MJ, Rosner SD. Cerebral perfusion pressure management of head injury. In: Avezaat C, ed. *Intracranial pressure VIII*. Berlin: Springer-Verlag, 1993:540–3.

56 Shimoda M, Oda S, Tsugane R, Sato O. Intracranial complications of hypervolemic therapy in patients with delayed ischemic deficit attributed to vasospasm. *J Neurosurg* 1993;78:423–9.

57 Fitch W, Pickard JD, Tamura A, Graham DI. Effects of hypotension induced with sodium nitroprusside on the cerebral circulation before, and one week after, the subarachnoid injection of blood. *J Neurol Neurosurg Psychiatry* 1988;51:88–93.

58 Nelson PB, Seif SM, Maroon JC, Robinson AG. Hyponatraemia in intracranial disease: perhaps not the syndrome of inappropriate secretion of antidiuretic hormone (SIADH). *J Neurosurg* 1981;55:938–41.

59 Nelson RJ, Perry S, Burns ACR, Roberts J, Pickard JD. The effects of hyponatraemia and subarachnoid haemorrhage on the cerebral vasomotor responses of the rabbit. *J Cereb Blood Flow Metab* 1991;11:661–6.

60 Myers RE. Anoxic brain pathology and blood glucose. *Neurology* 1976;34:345.

61 Marie C, Bralet J. Blood glucose level and morphological brain damage following cerebral ischaemia. *Cerebrovasc Brain Metab Rev* 1991;3:29–38.

62 Reed DJ, Woodbury DM. Effect of hypertonic urea on cerebrospinal fluid pressure and brain volume. *J Physiol (Lond)* 1963;164:252–64.

63 Pappius HM, Dayes LA. Hypertonic urea—its effect on the distribution of water and electrolytes in normal and edematous brain tissue. *Arch Neurol* 1965;13:395–402.

64 Ravassin P, Abou-Madi M, Archer D, Chiolero R, Freeman J, Trop D, de Tribolet N. Changes in CSF pressure after mannitol in patients with and without elevated CSF pressure. *J Neurosurg* 1988;69:869–76.

65 James HE, Harbaugh RD, Marshall LF, Shapiro HM. The response to multiple therapeutics in experimental vasogenic edema. In: Shulman K, Marmarou A, Miller JD, et al, eds. *Intracranial pressure IV*. Berlin, Springer-Verlag. 1980:272–6.

66 Rosenberg GA. *Brain fluids and metabolism*. Oxford: Oxford University Press, 1990.

67 Inao S, Kuchiwaki H, Wachi A, et al. Effect of mannitol on intracranial pressure—volume status and cerebral haemodynamics in brain oedema. *Acta Neurochir (Wien)* 1990;Suppl 51:401–3.

68 Bell BA, Smith MA, Kean DM, et al. Brain water measured by magnetic resonance imaging: correlation with direct estimation and change following mannitol and dexamethasone. *Lancet* 1987;1:66–9.

69 Kaufmann AM, Cardoso ER. Delayed cerebral accumulation of mannitol in vasogenic edema. In: Avezaat C, ed. *Intracranial pressure VIII*. Berlin: Springer-Verlag, 1993:592–5.

70 Burke AM, Quest DO, Chien S, et al. The effects of mannitol on blood viscosity. *J Neurosurg* 1981;55:550–3.

71 Miller JD, Leech P. Effects of mannitol and steroid therapy in intracranial volume pressure relationships. *J Neurosurg* 1975;42:274–81.

72 Muizelaar JP, Wei EP, Kontos HA, Becker DP. Mannitol causes compensatory cerebral vasoconstriction and vasodilatation in response to blood viscosity changes. *J Neurosurg* 1983;59:822–8.

73 Auer LM, Haselsberger K. Effect of intravenous mannitol on cat pial arteries and veins during normal and elevated intracranial pressure. *Neurosurgery* 1987;21:142–6.

74 Harrison MJG. Influence of haemocrit in the cerebral circulation. *Cerebrovasc Brain Metab Rev* 1989;1:55–67.

75 Brown MM, Wade JPH, Marshall J. Fundamental importance of arterial oxygen content in the regulation of cerebral blood flow in man. *Brain* 1985;108:81–93.

76 Purves MJ. *The Physiology of the cerebral circulation*. Cambridge: Cambridge University Press, 1972.

77 Bruce DA, Langfitt TW, Miller JD, et al. Regional cerebral blood flow, intracranial pressure, and brain metabolism in comatose patients. *J Neurosurg* 1973;38:131–44.

78 Johnston IH, Harper AM. The effect of mannitol on cerebral blood flow. An experimental study. *J Neurosurg* 1973;38:461–71.

79 Mendelow AD, Teasdale GM, Russell T, et al. Effect of mannitol on cerebral blood flow and cerebral perfusion pressure in human head injury. *J Neurosurg* 1985;63:43–8.

80 Jafar JJ, Johns LM, Mullan SF. The effect of mannitol on cerebral blood flow. *J Neurosurg* 1986;**64**:754–9.

81 Muizelaar JP, Lutz HA, Becker DP. Effect of mannitol on intracranial pressure and cerebral blood flow and correlation with pressure autoregulation in severely head-injured patients. *J Neurosurg* 1984;**61**:700–6.

82 Meyer FB, Anderson RE, Sundt TM, Yaksh TL. Treatment of experimental focal cerebral ischaemia with mannitol. Assessment by intracellular pH, cortical blood flow and EEG. *J Neurosurg* 1987;**66**:109–15.

83 Takagi H, Saito T, Kitahara T, Morii SM, Ohwada J, Yada K. The mechanism of the intracranial pressure reducing effect of mannitol. In: Ishii S, Nagai H, Brock M, eds. *Intracranial pressure V*. Berlin: Springer-Verlag, 1983:729–33.

84 Smith HP, Kelly DL, McWhorter JM, *et al*. Comparison of mannitol regimes in patients with severe head injury undergoing intracranial pressure monitoring. *J Neurosurg* 1986; **65**:820–4.

85 Roberts PA, Pollay M, Engles C, Pendleton B, Reynolds E, Stevens FA. Effect on intracranial pressure of furosemide combined with varying doses and administration rates of mannitol. *J Neurosurg* 1987;**66**:440–6.

86 Smedema RJ, Gaab MR, Heissler HE. A comparison study between mannitol and glycerol therapy in reducing intracranial pressure. In: Avezaat, ed. *Intracranial pressure VIII*. Berlin: Springer-Verlag, 1993:605–8.

87 Muizelaar JP, van der Poel HG, Li Z, Kontos HA, Levasseur JE. Pial arteriolar vessel diameter and CO_2 reactivity during prolonged hyperventilation in the rabbit. *J Neurosurg* 1988;**69**:923–7.

88 Ward JD, Choi S, Marmarou A, *et al*. Effect of prophylactic hyperventilation on outcome in patients with severe head injury. In: Hoff IT, Betz AL, eds. *Intracranial pressure VII*. Berlin: Springer-Verlag, 1989:630-4.

89 Enevoldsen EM, Cold G, Jensen FT, *et al*. Dynamic changes in regional cerebral blood flow, intraventricular pressure, CSF pH and lactate levels during the acute phase of head injury. *J Neurosurg* 1976;**44**:191–214.

90 De Salles AAF, Kontos HA, Becker DP, *et al*. Prognostic significance of ventricular CSF lactic acidosis in severe head injury. *J Neurosurg* 1986;**65**:615–24.

91 Akiota T, Ota K, Matsumato A, *et al*. The effect of THAM on acute intracranial hypertension. An experimental and clinical study. In: Beks JWF, Bosch DA, Brock M, eds. *Intracranial pressure III*. Berlin: Springer-Verlag, 1976:219–33.

92 Gordan E, Rossanda M. Further studies in cerebrospinal fluid acid-base status in patients with brain lesions. *Acta Anaesth Scand* 1970;**14**:97–109.

93 Gaab MR, Seegers K, Goetz C. THAM (tromethamine, "tris-buffer"): effective therapy of traumatic brain swelling. In: Hoff JT, Betz AL, eds. *Intracranial pressure VII*. Berlin: Springer-Verlag, 1989:616-19.

94 Wolf AL, Levi L, Marmarou A, *et al*. Effect of THAM upon outcome in severe head injury: a randomized prospective clinical trial. *J Neurosurg* 1993;**78**:54–9.

95 Pickard JD, Mackenzie ET. Inhibition of prostaglandin synthesis and the response of baboon circulation to carbon dioxide. *Nature New Biol* 1973;**245**:187–8.

96 Edwards AD, Wyatt JS, Richardson C, *et al*. Effects of indomethacin on cerebral haemodynamics in very preterm infants. *Lancet* 1990;**335**:1491–5.

97 Jensen K, Öhrstrom J, Cold GE, Astrup J. The effects of indomethacin on intracranial pressure, cerebral blood flow and cerebral metabolism in patients with severe head injury and intracranial hypertension. *Acta Neurochir (Wien)* 1991;**108**:116–21.

98 Sullivan LP, Stears JC, Ringer SP. Resolution of syringomyelia and chiari malformation by ventriculo-atrial shunting in a patient with pseudotumour cerebri and a lumbo-peritoneal shunt. *Neurosurgery* 1988;**22**:744-7.

99 Editorial. Cranial decompression. *Lancet* 1988;**1**:1204.

100 Gower DJ, Lee KS, McWhorter JM. Role of subtemporal decompression in severe closed head injury. *Neurosurgery* 1988;**23**:417–22.

101 Umezewa H, Shima K, Chigasaki H, Ishii S. Effects of the pressure gradient on hydrostatic brain edema. In: Hoff JT, Betz AL, eds. *Intracranial pressure VII*. Berlin: Springer-Verlag, 1989:953-6.

102 Rittierodt M, Gaab MR. Traumatic brain swelling and operative decompression: a prospective investigation. In: Avezaat C, *et al*, ed. *Intracranial pressure VIII*. Berlin: Springer-Verlag,1993.

103 Kirkham FJ, Neville BGR. Successful management of severe intracranial hypertension by surgical decompression. *Dev Med Child Neurol* 1986;**28**:506–9.

186

104 Cooper PR, Moody S, Clark WK, et al. Dexamethasone and severe head injury: a prospective double blind trial. *J Neurosurg* 1979;**51**:307–16.

105 Saul TF, Ducker TB, Salomon M, et al. Steroids in severe head injury. A prospective randomized clinical trial. *J Neurosurg* 1981;**54**:596–600.

106 Braakman R, Schouten HJD, Dishoeck BMV, Minderhoud JM. Megadose steroids in severe head injury: results of a prospective double blind clinical trial. *J Neurosurg* 1983;**58**:326–30.

107 Giannotta SL, Weiss MH, Apuzzo MLJ, Martin E. High dose glucocorticoids in the management of severe head injury. *Neurosurgery* 1984;**15**:497–501.

108 Dearden NM, Gibson JB, McDowall DG, et al. Effect of high dose dexamethasone on outcome from severe head injury. *J Neurosurg* 1986;**64**:81–8.

109 Floyd RA, Carney JM. Protection against oxidative damage to CNS by α-phenyl-tert-butyl nitrone and other spin-trapping agents: a novel series of nonlipid free radical scavengers. In: Marangos PJ, Lal H, eds. *Emerging strategies in neuroprotection*, Boston: Birkäuser, 1992:252–72.

110 Halliwell B, Gutteridge JMC. *Free radicals in biology and medicine*. Oxford: Clarendon Press, 1985.

111 Hall ED. Lazaroids: novel cerebroprotective antioxidants. In: Marangos PJ, Lal H. *Emerging strategies in neuroprotection*. Boston: Birkäuser, 1992:224–37.

112 Muizelaar JP, Marmarmou A, Young HA, et al. Improving the outcome of severe head injury with the oxygen radical scavenger polyethylene glycol-conjugated superoxide dismutase: a Phase II trial. *J Neurosurg* 1993;**78**:375–82.

113 Welsh FA, Sims RE, Harris VA. Mild hypothermia prevents ischemic injury in gerbil hippocampus. *J Cereb Blood Flow Metab* 1990;**10**:557–63.

114 Schwartz M, Tator CH, Rowed DW, et al. The University of Toronto Head Injury Treatment Study: a prospective randomized comparison of pentobarbital and mannitol. *Can J Neurol Sci* 1984;**11**:434–40.

115 Ward JD, Becker DP, Miller JD, et al. Failure of prophylactic barbiturate coma in the treatment of severe head injury. *J Neurosurg* 1985;**62**:383–8.

116 Eisenberg HM, Frankowski RF, Condant CG, et al. High dose barbiturate control of elevated intracranial pressure in patients with severe head injury. *J Neurosurg*1988;**69**:15–23.

117 Batjer HH. Cerebral protective effects of Etomidate: experimental and clinical aspects. *Cerebrovasc Brain Metab Rev* 1993;**5**:17–32.

118 Leggate JRS, Dearden NM, Miller JD. The effects of gammahydroxybutyrate and thiopentone on intracranial pressure in severe head injury. In: Miller JD, Teasdale GM, et al eds. *Intracranial pressure VI*. Berlin: Springer-Verlag, 1986:754-9.

119 Murphy PG, Myers DS, Davies MJ, et al. The antioxidant potential of propofol (2,6-diisopropylphenol). *Br J Anaesth* 1992;**68**:613–18.

120 Bedford RF, Persing JA, Pobereskin L, Butler A. Lidocaine or thiopental for rapid control of intracranial hypertension? *Anaesth Analg* 1980;**59**:435-7.

121 Meldrum B. Protection against ischaemic neuronal damage by drugs acting on excitatory neurotransmission. *Cerebrovasc Brain Metab Rev* 1990;**2**:27–57.

122 Choi DW. Methods of antagonizing glutamate neurotoxicity. *Cerebrovasc Brain Metab Rev* 1990;**2**:105–47.

123 Inglis FM, Kuroda Y, Bullock R. Glucose hypermetabolism after acute subdural haematoma is ameliorated by a competitive NMDA antagonist. *J Neurotrauma* 1992;**9**:75–84.

124 Gill R, Foster AC, Woodruff GN. MK801 is neuroprotective in gerbils when administered during the post-ischaemic period. *Neuroscience* 1988;**25**:847–56.

125 Park CK, Nehls DG, Graham DI, Teasdale GM, McCulloch J. The glutamate antagonist MK801 reduces focal ischaemic brain damage in the rat. *Ann Neurol* 1988;**24**:543–55.

126 Izumi Y, Roussel S, Pinard E, Seylaz J. Reduction of infarct volume by magnesium after middle cerebral artery occlusion in rats. *J Cereb Blood Flow Metab* 1991;**11**:1025–30.

127 Levene M. *Neonatal neurology*. Edinburgh: Churchill Livingstone, 1987.

128 Bruce DA, Alavi A, Bilaniuk, et al. Diffuse cerebral swelling following head injuries in children: the syndrome of "malignant brain edema". *J Neurosurg* 1981;**54**:170–8.

129 Aldrich EF, Eisenberg HM, Saydjari C, et al. Diffuse brain swelling in severely head-injured children. *J Neurosurg* 1992;**76**:450–4.

130 Harrison MJG. Is shrinking the brain a good thing after cerebral infarction? In: Warlow C, Garfield J, eds. *Dilemmas in the management of the neurological patient*. Edinburgh: Churchill Livingstone, 1984:62–73.

131 Pullen RGL, De Pasquale M, Cserr HF. Bulk flow of cerebrospinal fluid into brain in response to acute hyperosmolality. *Am J Physiol* 1987;**253**:538–45.

8 Management of subarachnoid haemorrhage

THOMAS A KOPITNIK, MICHAEL HOROWITZ, DUKE S SAMSON

Overview

The brain is unique in its structure and development. Unlike other organs, as the cerebral blood vessels penetrate the cranial cavity, the vessels form a collateral network along the base of the brain with only the smaller vessels penetrating the brain substance. The larger vessels are contained within the subarachnoid space, a well formed compartment which contains circulating CSF.[1-3] Sheets of arachnoid partition the subarachnoid space into distinct chambers called cisterns which provide a fragile barrier to migration of CSF, infection, and blood. It is within this fragile network of arachnoidal reflections that a subarachnoid haemorrhage may occur.

Subarachnoid haemorrhage is a condition, not a disease, which can be produced by a multitude of aetiologies. The phase I report of the 1966 Cooperative Study recorded 6368 patients experiencing spontaneous subarachnoid haemorrhage over an eight year period, of whom 51% had cerebral aneurysms.[4] Stehbens reviewed 11 series from 1950 to 1969 and found aneurysmal subarachnoid haemorrhage in 18–76% of the cases.[5] Other causes included trauma, cerebral and spinal vascular malformations, intrinsic and extrinsic cranial and spinal neoplasms, pathological and iatrogenic coagulopathy, vasculitis, collagen vascular disease, sickle cell anaemia, cerebral infarction, and drug misuse. The true incidence of subarachnoid haemorrhage varies considerably on a geographical basis. In the United States it is the cause of death in 16 per 100 000,[6] whereas Japan reports rates of 25 deaths per 100 000 people.[7] Rhodesia reports only 3·5 deaths from subarachnoid haemorrhage per 100 000 people per year.[8]

In the 1966 Cooperative Study of intracranial aneurysms and subarachnoid haemorrhage, Locksley found that 50% of 2627 patients with aneurysmal subarachnoid haemorrhage were female. Under the age of 40 the condition occurs more commonly in men but over the age of 50 it is more common in women.[9] Regardless of the aetiology, subarachnoid haemorrhage most often occurs between the ages of 40 and 60, with the peak frequency between 55 and 60 years of age. The peak incidence attributed to aneurysms occurred at slightly older ages than subarachnoid haemorrhage from arteriovenous malformation with 63% of first haemorrhagic episodes from arteriovenous malformation occurring between the ages of 30 and 40.[10] Whereas subarachnoid haemorrhage does not seem to have a consistent seasonal prevalence,[11] some authors have reported an increased incidence in spring and autumn.[12] [13] Ohno and Chyahe et al reported a peak seasonal incidence in Japan in the winter months.[14–17]

A third of the patients who develop subarachnoid haemorrhage do so while they are asleep, a third during routine daily activities, and a third during strenuous activity. Bending and lifting activities have the highest association with subarachnoid haemorrhage among those activities considered strenuous.[10]

Death rates from the initial haemorrhage range from 40–60%.[18] Freytag reported 250 consecutive deaths from subarachnoid haemorrhage and found that 60% were immediate whereas 20% were within 24 hours of the ictus; only 11% of the patients lived beyond 24 hours.[19] Ruptured cerebral aneurysm is the most common cause of non-traumatic subarachnoid haemorrhage, although hypertensive subarachnoid haemorrhage was the most common cause of early death in the Cooperative Study. Hypertensive subarachnoid haemorrhage accounted for 52% of the deaths, whereas aneurysmal subarachnoid haemorrhage accounted for 36%. Ninety per cent of all patients dying within 72 hours had an intracranial haematoma.[20]

For the purposes of discussion we will divide subarachnoid haemorrhage into distinct categories of aneurysmal and non-aneurysmal. Although some overlap exists in the medical management of subarachnoid haemorrhage in both categories, aneurysmal subarachnoid haemorrhage presents unique surgical management circumstances that will be discussed separately.

Diagnosis

Signs and symptoms

Headaches occur in 85–95% of patients with subarachnoid haemorrhage.[21-23] At least a third of patients will have a minor leak, referred to as a sentinel haemorrhage. This may occur hours or days before a major aneurysmal haemorrhage.[24] Many authors have emphasised that a sudden minor, but unusual, headache may herald a haemorrhage in the near future.[21-27] In 2621 cases reviewed by the 1966 Cooperative Study for premonitory symptoms, the following were present immediately before a major subarachnoid haemorrhage: headache (48%), orbital pain (7%), diplopia (4%), ptosis (3%), visual loss (4%), seizures (4%), motor or sensory deficit (6%), dysphasia (2%), bruit (3%), dizziness (10%), and other (13%).[10 20]

A significant subarachnoid haemorrhage usually presents with the sudden onset of intense headache followed by pain radiating into the occipital or cervical region. As blood flows into the spinal canal, cervical pain or nuchal rigidity develops. The duration and intensity of the nuchal rigidity usually depend on the magnitude of the subarachnoid haemorrhage but may vary between patients. Signs and symptoms similar to infectious meningitis are typically seen, due to an inflammatory reaction of the leptomeninges to extravasated blood. Kernig's or Laségue's sign may be present if substantial meningeal irritation exists. Other symptoms include photophobia, nausea, vomiting, lethargy, and alteration in mental status. If we include patients that die, brief or permanent loss of consciousness occurs in most patients with subarachnoid haemorrhage. After the haemorrhage the patient may regain normal mentation or may remain lethargic, confused, or obtunded. Altered level of consciousness is related to haematoma formation, hydrocephalus, increased intracranial pressure, vasospasm, or reduced cerebral blood flow.[28] Other signs of neurological involvement may include motor or sensory deficits, upper motor neuron reflex

190

changes, visual field deficits, abnormal brain stem reflexes, and abnormal motor posturing. Unlikely causes of motor deficits include emboli from the aneurysm sac, brain compression by a large or giant aneurysm, or seizures. Seizures occur at the time of subarachnoid haemorrhage in about 10% of patients.[29-32] Other clinical signs that often accompany the presenting symptoms include mild hyperpyrexia, hypertension, and ophthalmological findings. Intraocular haemorrhages may occur in the vitreous fluid or retina, but subhyaloid or preretinal haemorrhages are more indicative of subarachnoid haemorrhage.[33-34] Subhyaloid haemorrhages appear as bright red, sharply demarcated regions adjacent to the optic disc. Cranial nerve palsies can be seen, especially in cases of posterior communicating and superior cerebellar artery aneurysms; less often with aneurysms of the carotid and basilar bifurcation and the posterior cerebral and anterior choroidal arteries. Third cranial nerve palsy associated with aneurysmal subarachnoid haemorrhage or aneurysm induced compression typically results in a dilated pupil, ptosis, or deficits in ocular motility. Compression of the third nerve within the cavernous sinus may present with a midpoint pupil secondary to compression of sympathetic fibres en route to the iris. Pain in the trigeminal distribution can result from subarachnoid haemorrhage or aneurysmal nerve compression, but is rare and more commonly seen in association with cavernous carotid aneurysms. Abducens nerve palsy is often seen after subarachnoid haemorrhage and is thought to be related to increased intracranial pressure and subsequent nerve traction from downward brainstem herniation during the haemorrhage.

It is important to be very aware of the possibility of subarachnoid haemorrhage. Shields noted that minor bleeds were often misdiagnosed as influenza, migraine, sinusitis, headache, stiff neck, and malingering.[35] Nearly a half of all patients with subarachnoid haemorrhage enrolled in a recent international cooperative study had delays in excess of three days from onset to transfer to a neurosurgical centre.[36] Kassell *et al* studied 150 consecutive patients with known ruptured aneurysms and found that only 38% were referred to neurosurgeons within 48 hours of the first symptoms. The most common cause for delay was misdiagnosis by physicians (37%), followed by administrative delays in referral (23%).[37] Because delayed referral to a neurosurgical centre seriously affects patient outcome, education of primary care physicians towards rapid diagnosis and prompt referral seems warranted.

Diagnostic tests

Brain CT is the procedure of choice for the diagnosis of subarachnoid haemorrhage. This can demonstrate the magnitude and location of the haemorrhage, give clues to probable location of an aneurysm, and assess ventricular size. The success in detecting subarachnoid haemorrhage by CT is dependent on the length of time between the haemorrhage and the scan. If the scan is obtained within five days of the haemorrhage, the probability is high that it can confirm the diagnosis. Eighty five per cent of patients scanned within 48 hours of subarachnoid haemorrhage and 75% of patients scanned within five days will have detectable subarachnoid blood on CT.[38-41] The distribution of blood on the scan may suggest the probable location of the aneurysm. Acute blood within the interhemispheric and supratentorial ventricular system is often the consequence of a ruptured aneurysm of the anterior communicating artery. Focal blood within the fourth ventricle suggests an aneurysm of the vertebral or posterior inferior cerebellar artery. Intracerebral haematomas are most often seen with ruptured aneurysms of the middle cerebral artery, internal carotid bifurcation, or distal anterior cerebral artery. Inferior frontal lobe and interhemispheric flame shaped haematomas commonly occur with ruptured anterior communicating artery aneurysms and are a highly accurate CT finding for localising the source of the subarachnoid haemorrhage.[42-43]

Fisher *et al* developed a grading scale for the CT appearance of subarachnoid haemorrhage dependent on the severity and location of subarachnoid blood (box 1).[44] The Fisher grading system is used to relate the amount of subarachnoid blood on a scan to

---

Box 1—CT grading of subarachnoid haemorrhage

Grade	CT criteria
I	No blood detected
II	Diffuse deposition or thin layer with all vertical layers of blood less than 1 mm thick
III	Localised clots with or without vertical layers of blood 1 mm or greater in thickness
IV	Diffuse or no subarachnoid blood with intracerebral or intraventricular clots

---

the probability of developing delayed ischaemia secondary to vasospasm. Patients in Grades I, II, and IV had no or minimal incidence of clinically significant vasospasm whereas patients in grade III had a 95·8% incidence. These findings implicate the breakdown products of subarachnoid clot in the genesis of cerebral vasospasm. The greater the magnitude of subarachnoid clot, the higher the likelihood that delayed cerebral ischaemia from vasospasm will occur.

Visual examination of CSF obtained by lumbar puncture can confirm the diagnosis of subarachnoid haemorrhage when CT is negative. In 1901, Sicard found that yellow discolouration of CSF after centrifugation was a reliable diagnostic sign of previous subarachnoid haemorrhage.[45] The term xanthochromia (*xanthochromie*) was first used in 1902 to describe the yellow colour of CSF in a case of pneumococcal meningitis, and was later used in the 1920s to refer to the colour of CSF several hours after subarachnoid haemorrhage.[46-50] The CSF supernatant does not demonstrate discolouration immediately after subarachnoid haemorrhage, but only after red blood cells haemolyse and release oxyhaemoglobin. Xanthochromia can usually be detected four hours after subarachnoid haemorrhage; it becomes maximum one week later, and is usually undetected at three weeks.[51] If xanthochromia is present in the CSF, subarachnoid haemorrhage has probably occurred. If a traumatic lumbar puncture is suspected, partial or total clearing of the CSF may occur during collection. If bloody CSF is allowed to stand undisturbed in a test tube a clot will not usually form if the blood is from a subarachnoid haemorrhage. Repeat lumbar puncture hours after a traumatic tap will be of little diagnostic value, as blood contaminating the CSF will also show xanthochromia. Lumbar puncture after subarachnoid haemorrhage is not without risk. Duffy reviewed 54 patients undergoing lumbar puncture after spontaneous haemorrhage. Thirteen per cent had significant neurological deterioration afterwards. Six of the seven patients who deteriorated had evidence of brain shifts on follow up CT.[52] Whether or not these changes were directly related to the lumbar puncture is unknown. However, because lumbar puncture carries the risk of brain herniation or aneurysm rebleeding, the procedure should only be performed if the diagnosis remains in question after CT, or when CT is unavailable. Lumbar puncture is also useful in ruling out infectious meningitis, which may mimic symptoms of subarachnoid haemorrhage.

193

After making a diagnosis of subarachnoid haemorrhage, four vessel cerebral angiography should be performed as soon as possible. The angiographic investigation should visualise the full course of all intracranial vessels, including the posterior inferior cerebellar arteries, in at least two planes. The angiographer's goal is to demonstrate the cause of the subarachnoid haemorrhage, define the aneurysm's neck and projection, delineate the vessels arising adjacent to the aneurysm, determine if multiple aneurysms are present (20% incidence), and assess the degree of any concomitant vasospasm. In 1977, Nibbelink *et al* reported a significant complication rate for cerebral angiography in acute subarachnoid haemorrhage.[53] Complications and their frequencies were: transient hemiparesis, 2%; permanent neurological deficits, 2·5%; death, 2·6%; worsening of ischaemic deficit, 3%; and aneurysmal rebleeding, 1·5%. The present day complication rate for cerebral angiography should be less than 1% if carried out by an experienced neuroradiologist.[54] Aneurysm rupture during angiography has been reported, but is fortunately an infrequent occurrence.[55-59]

Brain MRI is not useful in the acute diagnosis of subarachnoid haemorrhage because blood is difficult to visualise on early scans. It has, however, proved valuable in the localisation of subarachnoid clot beyond the time the blood is detectable with CT.[60] We have found MRI invaluable in the evaluation of giant intracranial aneurysms. Because giant aneurysms are often partially thrombosed, they incompletely opacify during angiography and MRI can demonstrate the magnitude and location of these lesions. We have used magnetic resonance angiography, and occasionally CT angiography, to follow the size of such untreated giant aneurysms.[61-65]

Serial CT is performed periodically for several days after subarachnoid haemorrhage to detect hydrocephalus or rebleeding. Hydrocephalus may symptomatically present with headache, drowsiness, confusion, or agitation. The incidence of acute hydrocephalus after subarachnoid haemorrhage varies extensively among reported series. Bohn and Hugosson found that 1% of their patients operated on for ruptured cerebral aneurysms ultimately required shunting for hydrocephalus.[66] Modesti and Binet found a 63% incidence of abnormal ventricular enlargement on CT within 24 hours of haemorrhage.[67] Van Gijn *et al* reported a series of 174 patients with subarachnoid haemorrhage. Thirty four (20%) developed acute hydrocephalus within 72 hours of the haemorrhage. Although intraventricular blood was closely associated with development of hydrocephalus, the extent of cisternal haemorrhage was not. The mortality among those patients with acute hydrocephalus was significantly higher than for those without this complication.[68] If hydrocephalus develops after subarachnoid haemorrhage, clinical judgment should be used to assess its severity and the need for diversion of CSF. We have found that some patients will exhibit transient, asymptomatic ventricular enlargement after subarachnoid haemorrhage, which usually resolves spontaneously. If hydrocephalus causes clinical manifestations, continuous external ventricular drainage is instituted until the ventricular size and intracranial pressure normalise CSF. One exception to this strategy is the existence of an unsecured aneurysm. In such an instance CSF drainage, if required, should be carefully controlled so as not to reduce ventricular size or intracranial pressure to a point that the tamponade effect on the aneurysm is lost and rerupture is promoted.[69] Continuous external ventricular drainage can usually be performed with little additional morbidity or mortality.[70] If the external ventriculostomy cannot be weaned without the recurrence of hydrocephalus, an internal ventriculoperitoneal shunt is placed.

Clinical classification

After the diagnosis of subarachnoid haemorrhage has been established, patients are assigned a clinical grade based on one of the accepted grading systems. Grading systems for subarachnoid haemorrhage have been reported since the 1930s, when Bramwell graded patients as either apoplectic or paralytic.[71] Botterell *et al* introduced a useful grading scale in 1956 which has undergone several modifications, including one in 1973 by Lougheed and Marshall.[72 73] One of the more universally accepted grading scales for patients with subarachnoid haemorrhage is that of Hunt and Hess (1968),[74] which was later modified by Hunt and Kosnik in 1974[75] (box 2). Both Botterell and Hunt grading scales put the patient into the next worse grade if serious systemic disease or vasospasm is present. Attention to the name and date of the classification system used is important to ensure comparability of various patients or patient series reported.[76]

Box 2—Clinical grading of subarachnoid haemorrhage

Adapted from Hunt and Hess[74] and Hunt and Kosnik[75].

Grade

0	Unruptured aneurysm without symptoms
I	Asymptomatic or minimal headache and slight nuchal rigidity
Ia	No acute meningeal or brain reaction, but with fixed neurological deficit
II	Moderate to severe headache, nuchal rigidity, no neurological deficit other than cranial nerve palsy
III	Drowsy, confused, or mild focal deficit
IV	Stupor, moderate to severe hemiparesis, possible early decerebrate rigidity, and vegetative disturbances
V	Deep coma, decerebrate rigidity, moribund appearance

Non-aneurysmal subarachnoid haemorrhage

About 75% of patients who have a non-traumatic, spontaneous subarachnoid haemorrhage will have a cerebral aneurysm.[77] Arteriovenous malformation will be discovered in 5%, and 20% of patients will have various other causes to which the haemorrhage is attributed, or no cause found. When the initial angiogram does not demonstrate the cause of the haemorrhage, further investigation with repeat angiography is controversial. Earlier studies found that a significant number of patients had an aneurysm demonstrated on a second angiogram or at necropsy that was not evident on the initial study.[78-80] As angiographic techniques have improved, the yield of repeat angiography has decreased. Forster *et al* reported only one patient in whom a second angiogram diagnosed a previously occult cerebral aneurysm out of 56 patients with initially negative studies.[81] Others have reported higher diagnostic yields of 3–22%.[82-85] It has been our policy to tailor each diagnostic evaluation to the patient's specific findings. If the initial angiogram fails to demonstrate a cause of the haemorrhage, but shows focal vasospasm, the angiogram is also repeated in five to seven days. We also advocate repeat angiography if a portion of the cerebral vasculature is not adequately visualised on the initial study or in patients who have a large amount of subarachnoid blood visualised on CT.

The differential diagnoses that must be considered in non-aneurysmal subarachnoid haemorrhage are extensive. Trauma is the most frequent cause and at times, it can be difficult to determine if the haemorrhage was the result or the cause of the patient's injuries. Other causes include angiographically demonstrable and angiographically occult vascular malformations, coagulopathic conditions, granulomatous angiitis, venous thrombosis, small arterial and venous tears, CNS infection, intra-axial and extra-axial tumours, hypertension, drug misuse, and various aetiologies within the spinal canal.[86-88] Subarachnoid haemorrhage of spinal origin occurs most commonly from spinal arteriovenous malformations, but may also be related to spinal neoplasms or use of systemic anticoagulants.

Subarachnoid haemorrhage is a condition not amenable to immediate intervention to lessen the severity of the initial haemorrhage. The management goals in spontaneous subarachnoid haemorrhage are similar to those in patients with head trauma—namely, to diagnose the condition and minimise the potential for further injury. The treatment of subarachnoid haemorrhage of unknown aetiology is aimed at preventing secondary injury and providing relief of symptoms. Patients are initially placed at bed rest under close observation. Blood pressure is controlled with antihypertensive drugs and the patients are well hydrated. Headache and cervical pain are treated with analgesics as needed and prophylactic anticonvulsants are given. Corticosteroids in the form of dexamethasone (4 mg every six hours) are used to alleviate symptoms and signs of blood induced meningitis. We also administer an oral calcium channel blocking agent nimodipine (60 mg every four hours) to reduce the effects of cerebral vasospasm, should it occur. Symptomatic vasospasm occurs in a small percentage of patients who present with subarachnoid haemorrhage of undetermined aetiology. The incidence is less than in those patients found to have aneurysmal subarachnoid haemorrhage, and is related to the magnitude of the haemorrhage seen on the presenting CT.[83] We have noted angiographic vasospasm in non-aneurysmal subarachnoid haemorrhage, although clinically symptomatic vasospasm in this specific group of patients is rare in our experience. The treatment of symptomatic vasospasm will be further discussed in the section to follow on aneurysmal subarachnoid haemorrhage.

Patients who present with non-aneurysmal subarachnoid haemorrhage are typically in better neurological condition than those patients with subarachnoid haemorrhage from ruptured aneurysms.[89-92] Although the source of subarachnoid haemorrhage remains undiscovered in 20% of patients, the mortality for this group of patients is less than 3%. The incidence of rebleeding is 4% in the first six months and ranges from 0·2–0·86% per year after six months.[93] Reported series concerning subarachnoid haemorrhage with negative angiography indicate that 80% of patients with subarachnoid haemorrhage of undetermined aetiology have a good outcome and return to gainful employment, as opposed to less than 50% of patients with aneurysmal subarachnoid haemorrhage.[77 92] The patient's clinical status usually corresponds to the amount of subarachnoid blood present on CT.[84] The magnitude of the haemorrhage seen on CT relates to the development of complications secondary to the haemorrhage. These include cerebral vasospasm, hydrocephalus, seizures, memory disturbances, headache, and psychological disturbances. Stober *et al* have reviewed the blood distribution on CT after both aneurysmal and non-aneurysmal subarachnoid haemorrhage and determined that subarachnoid haemorrhage of unknown aetiology is unlikely to result in blood in the sylvian or interhemispheric fissures.[94] The interpeduncular or perimesencephalic cisterns often demonstrate focal blood collection when subarachnoid haemorrhage of unknown aetiology occurs.[43]

Aneurysmal subarachnoid haemorrhage

General considerations

Ruptured cerebral aneurysms constitute 77% of the cases of subarachnoid haemorrhage.[95] Chason and Hindman found 137 cerebral aneurysms, a 5% incidence, in a necropsy study of 2786 patients who died of causes unrelated to the haemorrhage. They also showed that 42% of these aneurysms had ruptured previously.[96] This is consistent with other reports, which have shown a history of previous haemorrhage in 60% of aneurysms discovered in people under 60 years of age.[97] Necropsy studies will demonstrate a higher incidence of ruptured aneurysms than clinical or radiological studies because aneurysm rupture is a frequent cause of sudden death. Although many series reflect widely variable epidemiological statistics, an approximate occurrence rate for aneurysm rupture is 10 per 100 000 population per year. There is an average prevalence rate of unruptured aneurysms of 5% in the adult population.

There are three basic theories for the pathogenesis of cerebral aneurysms. One theory proposes that a congenital weakness in the muscular layer of cerebral arteries allows the intimal layer to herniate and eventually distend and destroy the elastic membrane, leading to outpouching of an aneurysmal sac. Other theories have attributed aneurysm formation to postnatal degeneration within the vessel wall, which leads to deterioration of the internal elastic lamina and resultant aneurysm formation. Others have postulated that it is a combination of congenital and degenerative effects that lead to aneurysm formation.[98] The law of LaPlace relates wall stress to radius and transmural pressure and can be used to show that as the radius of the aneurysm enlarges, significantly less force is required to cause further enlargement or rupture of the sac.[99]

Aneurysms tend to occur at vascular bifurcations although they sometimes occur unassociated with vessel branches.[100] Forbus used a rigid glass model to demonstrate that the point of greatest stress on the artery wall occurs at the apex of a vascular bifurcation in line with the direction of flow.[101]

The average size of ruptured aneurysms is 7·5 mm. Two per cent of aneurysms under 5 mm rupture, in contrast with 40% of those between 6 mm and 10 mm in external diameter.[102] Unruptured but symptomatic giant aneurysms (>2·5 cm) carry a grave prognosis related to both mass effect and future rupture. The commonly held perception that giant aneurysms do not bleed and can be managed conservatively is dangerously misleading. Between 30% and 70% of giant aneurysms that become symptomatic are associated with subarachnoid haemorrhage.[103 104]

About 20% of patients will have multiple aneurysms.[6] This makes it imperative to visualise all cerebral vessels on diagnostic angiography when subarachnoid haemorrhage is investigated. The presence of multiple aneurysms will significantly affect surgical planning. When multiple aneurysms are present, the most proximal, the most irregularly shaped, and the largest will be the most likely sources of haemorrhage.[105] Aneurysms with small secondary outpouchings are thought to be particularly prone to rupture, and these outpouchings may actually be false sacs from previous haemorrhages.[106] DuBoulay has hypothesised that secondary aneurysm loculations are regions where the aneurysm wall is most unstable. Asymptomatic aneurysms rarely had secondary loculations. He also found the mortality of such aneurysms to be twice that of smooth walled lesions.[107]

Examinations that are helpful in determining which of the multiple aneurysms is the most likely source of subarachnoid haemorrhage include the history of the ictal event, clinical examination, CT, angiogram, and MRI study. The patient may be able to lateralise the initial headache when bilateral aneurysms are present, and the clinical examination may demonstrate unilateral weakness or cranial nerve palsy. When multiple aneurysms are diagnosed, CT localisation of subarachnoid blood, ventricular shift, and the site of an intraparenchymal haematoma are helpful findings. Local vasospasm may be present near the ruptured lesion on angiography. The aneurysm most likely to have bled will often be the largest, have the most irregular contour, or have a nipple-like secondary loculation. Nehls *et al* found statistical evidence that aneurysms associated with the anterior communicating complex, the basilar apex, and the posterior inferior cerebellar artery-vertebral junction were the most likely aneurysms to bleed when multiple aneurysms were diagnosed.[108] MRI can be valuable in detecting subarachnoid clot beyond the time clot is visible on CT and in localising the causative source of haemorrhage in cases with multiple aneurysms. Focal increased signal intensity is often found around a ruptured aneurysm.[60]

After the diagnosis of ruptured cerebral aneurysm has been confirmed as the cause of subarachnoid haemorrhage, treatment plans need to be considered. The treatment for subarachnoid haemorrhage secondary to a ruptured aneurysm is primarily surgical although the development of Guglielmi detachable coils (Target Therapeutics, Fremont, CA, USA) has made interventional neuroradiological management a viable option in selected cases.[109-116] The primary surgical approach is aimed at repairing the ruptured lesion and treating any asymptomatic aneurysms that are accessible through the surgical exposure. There seems to be a poorly understood phenomenon of enlargement and rupture of previously asymptomatic aneurysms in patients who undergo surgery to clip the ruptured lesion. Others have noted an increased frequency of asymptomatic aneurysm rupture after treatment of the symptomatic aneurysm.[117 118] A possible explanation may relate to increased haemodynamic stress in the perioperative period producing an increase in the transmural pressure gradient within asymptomatic aneurysms. Despite these statements, haemorrhage from a previously asymptomatic aneurysm after surgery to treat the ruptured aneurysm is an extremely rare occurrence in our experience. Others have reported that postoperative volume expansion and induced hypertension after surgery for a ruptured aneurysm are both safe and efficacious, and do not seem to promote rupture of asymptomatic lesions.[119 120]

Non-operative or non-interventional treatment is reserved for those patients in the poorest grades who are not expected to survive. Nevertheless, some authors have reported good results in moribund patients.[121] Yasargil retrospectively compared surgical and non-surgical management in patients with ruptured aneurysms in a specific region of Switzerland. Of 624 proved ruptured aneurysms, 349 (55·9%) underwent operation, with five (1·4%) deaths. A total of 275 (44·1%) patients did not undergo surgery and only four (0·6%) patients survived, resulting in a mortality rate of 98·5% in the non-operated patients.[122] Therefore, subarachnoid haemorrhage from a ruptured cerebral aneurysm has a high mortality and non-operative management is rarely indicated. In our opinion, expectant management should be confined to poor grade patients who are not expected to survive.

Patient selection and timing of treatment are important factors determining outcome. The dilemma of which patient should undergo surgery and when surgery should be performed in relation to the onset of subarachnoid haemorrhage or vasospasm remains an unresolved issue. Current trends in neurosurgery and our own results support early intervention in patients with good clinical grades. Early surgery is performed to secure the ruptured aneurysm, to prevent rebleeding, and to remove as much subarachnoid clot as possible to reduce the risk of vasospasm. We generally offer surgery to those patients in Hunt-Hess grades I-III[76] as soon as they are fully radiologically evaluated and medically prepared. Poor grade patients, grades IV and V,[76] are treated non-surgically until their clinical condition improves. Patients with Hunt and Hess grades 0–III are selected for coiling on a case by case basis depending on their medical history and aneurysm geometry and location. Diagnosis and treatment of acute posthaemorrhagic hydrocephalus by external ventricular drainage will often result in patients improving by one grade. In a similar fashion, patients who are in a poor grade, but harbour a significant intraparenchymal haematoma, may show significant improvement with surgery to obliterate the aneurysm and reduce mass effect from the haematoma.

The rationale for conservative management of poor grade patients stems from previous studies evaluating surgical results related to the patient's preoperative status. Hunt and Hess categorised patients into grades to investigate prognosis of the preoperative neurological status, and found that operative mortality approached 75% in poor grade (grades IV and V) patients.[74] The explanation for dismal surgical results in poor grade patients is probably multifactorial. A combination of raised intracranial pressure, reduced cerebral blood flow, poor tissue tolerance to manipulation, and poor tolerance to temporary occlusion, all contribute to poor surgical results. Some have seen encouraging results with aggressive surgical treatment of poor grade patients,[121] although our experience and that of others[102] has reaffirmed that in general, these patients have poor surgical outcomes.

Once a patient with aneurysmal subarachnoid haemorrhage is deemed a candidate for surgery, timing of surgery becomes an important issue. The overall management morbidity and mortality must be a consideration in the surgical planning. The major factors that must be considered are: (a) rate of aneurysm rebleeding, (b) delayed ischaemia deficit due to vasospasm, and (c) technical considerations of the operative procedure. The predominant historical opinion has been that if surgery was intentionally delayed for 1–2 weeks after subarachnoid haemorrhage, the surgical outcomes were much more favourable compared with those of early surgery. Norlen and Olivecrona published the results of 100 consecutive aneurysms of the anterior communicating artery managed in this fashion and reported a remarkable 3% mortality.[123] It was presumed that technical difficulties associated with early surgery would negate any potential benefit of early surgery in preventing rebleeding and facilitating the management of vasospasm. There was also concern that early surgery could worsen the effects of vasospasm in the face of disturbed autoregulation.[124 125] Because of improvements in neuroanaesthesia, neurosurgical instrumentation, and the advent of the operative microscope, investigators have reconsidered the optimal timing of aneurysm surgery.

Recent studies investigating the timing of surgery for ruptured intracranial aneurysms have shown that early surgery was not significantly more difficult than delayed surgery from a technical standpoint, as perceived by the operating surgeons. Although the results of surgery delayed until after postbleed day 10 were superior to results of early surgery, the morbidity and mortality of rebleeding, and other complications associated with delayed surgery, negated any benefit of delaying the procedure. Early surgery did result in a decreased incidence of aneurysm rebleeding, but did not significantly affect the incidence of subsequent vasospasm.[36 126] The overall results of these contemporary cooperative studies show that overall management morbidity and mortality of early versus delayed surgical therapy are not significantly different. However, such studies included patients treated before the advent of triple-H therapy (haemodilution, hypervolaemia, hypertension), calcium channel blockers, and non-steroidal medications, all of which may improve the patient's outcome. The possible exception may be the patients who are alert and in excellent grade on admission; this group has had the most favourable results with early surgery. The surgeon must weigh all factors, including his or her technical capabilities, the risk of rebleeding, and potential management difficulties, including vasospasm, when deciding on the best time to perform the surgical procedure. Timing may be less of an issue for aneurysm coiling as this procedure may be performed at little increased risk during the diagnostic arteriogram, thus theoretically securing the aneurysm immediately on presentation.

Subarachnoid haemorrhage from aneurysms is further complicated by a concurrent pregnancy. Because surgical management reduces both maternal and fetal death, it is generally recommended. In cases of unruptured aneurysms, caesarian section has not been shown to reduce the risk of subarachnoid haemorrhage.[127]

Preoperative management of aneurysmal subarachnoid haemorrhage

Evaluation

We recommend early surgical repair of ruptured aneurysms followed by aggressive medical therapy, if necessary, for vasospasm. It is preferable that patients be transferred to a neurosurgical centre as soon as possible after their haemorrhage. The idea that patients need to be observed for a period before transfer to a neurosurgical centre is an erroneous concept and only serves to delay transfer unnecessarily and to place patients at risk for rebleeding. We have found that immediate transfer once the diagnosis is suspected provides the best chance for optimal patient outcome. It is imperative that pertinent radiographic studies, including arteriograms, be sent to the neurosurgeon along with the patient. Sending poor quality copies of radiographs or not sending the complete angiogram because of hospital administrative policy results in needless and dangerous repetition of vital diagnostic examinations.

We admit patients directly to the surgical intensive care unit, where further assessment is performed. Patients are graded according to the Hunt-Hess grading scale, and accompanying radiographic studies are evaluated.[74 75] If not previously obtained, angiography is performed as soon as possible after admission, individualised for each patient. Early angiography is beneficial for early diagnosis, even if patients are not offered immediate surgery. An angiogram obtained early after haemorrhage will confirm the diagnosis, and preoperative planning or immediate surgery or coil embolisation can be undertaken. Preoperative preparation usually includes routine blood tests, type and crossmatch of packed red blood cells, placement of central venous access and radial arterial monitoring catheters, and premedication.

Medical management

Preoperative medication and fluid management are important aspects of care of patients with subarachnoid haemorrhage. We initially attempt to normalise the patient's intravascular volume status and do not prophylactically induce hypervolaemia. Prophylactic hypervolaemia has been shown to be hazardous and offers no clear benefit.[128] Medications include anticonvulsants, corticosteroids, calcium channel blockers, antihypertensive drugs, and analgesics. Strict attention to control of blood pressure before aneurysm surgery has been shown to reduce the rate of aneurysm rebleeding.[129] The effect of calcium channel blockers on outcome is less clear. Reports show that prophylactic use of these agents does not prevent angiographic vasospasm, but may decrease the overall management morbidity after subarachnoid haemorrhage.[130-134] In the light of the reports on calcium channel blocking agents, we give all patients one of these drugs immediately on admission to the hospital. Further studies need to be performed on this important issue.

The administration of antifibrinolytic drugs designed to minimise clot lysis is controversial.[135 138] ε-Aminocaproic acid (Amicar) is one of the more widely used antifibrolytic drugs, which primarily act to inhibit the conversion of plasminogen into plasmin, the main function of which is to digest fibrin and aid in clot lysis. Intravenous injection of ε-aminocaproic acid provides a peak plasma concentration 20 minutes after injection, and 75% will be excreted unchanged in the urine within 12 hours. The drug crosses the blood-brain barrier and achieves maximal antifibrinolytic activity within the CSF 48 hours after therapy is initiated.[139] Patients are given 2 g/hour intravenously for 48 hours, then 1·5 g/hour for the duration of therapy or until surgery is performed. Review of the 1966 cooperative study found a decreased incidence of aneurysm rebleeding and death at 14 days from 21% to 10% with the use of antifibrinolytics.[140] Although antifibrinolytic therapy lessens the incidence of rebleeding by 50% during the first two weeks after haemorrhage, there is an increase in associated medical complications. The most frequent of these is diarrhoea, occurring in 24% of patients. Communicating hydrocephalus is 25% more frequent with antifibrinolytic therapy according to the report of Park.[140a] The greatest concern over use of antifibrinolytic agents is the associated increase in ischaemic neurological deficits that has negated its benefits in some studies.[135] Our view is that antifibrinolytics have little part to play in acute aneurysmal subarachnoid haemorrhage if surgery is anticipated within two days of admission. These agents may be of value if an operative procedure is delayed longer than 48 hours. Their efficacy when used in conjunction with calcium channel blockers has yet to be studied.

Surgical planning

Aneurysm rebleeding is a catastrophic event that may occur relatively soon after the initial bleed.[119] The frequency of aneurysm rebleeding is 4% within the first 48 hours after the initial haemorrhage and 1·5% each day for the next 12 days. The mortality from aneurysm rebleeding is at least 70%. Surgical or interventional treatments offer the best protection against this highly lethal complication.

Some neurosurgeons are concerned that surgery soon after acute subarachnoid haemorrhage is technically difficult due to brain swelling and obscuration of vital structures by acute blood within the subarachnoid space. Despite this most of our grade I–III patients undergo surgery early to minimise the incidence of rebleeding. Although this surgery can be technically more demanding, we have not found patient morbidity and mortality to be adversely affected. We have found intraoperative ventricular puncture and aggressive gravity drainage of CSF to be an extremely useful adjunct in overcoming an initially swollen brain soon after subarachnoid haemorrhage.[141] The results of the most recent cooperative study confirm that although most surgeons report that the brain is significantly more swollen during early surgery, most thought that surgery is not significantly more difficult.[126] In this cooperative study, early surgery reduced the incidence of rebleeding, but had no effect in decreasing the incidence of vasospasm, which theoretically might have been expected by early subarachnoid clot removal.[142-145] However, most patients were treated before the widespread use of triple-H therapy and calcium channel blockers.

Surgical considerations and complications

The goals of aneurysm surgery after subarachnoid haemorrhage are: (*a*) aneurysm obliteration with preservation of normal vasculature, (*b*) minimisation of brain tissue disruption, and (*c*) removal of as much subarachnoid and intraparenchymal clot as is safely feasible. Our patients undergoing uncomplicated aneurysm repair after subarachnoid haemorrhage had morbidity and mortality of about 10%. When intraoperative rupture occurred, the morbidity and mortality increased to about 20%. Factors such as the phase of the dissection, the use of blunt versus sharp dissection techniques, and complete aneurysm neck dissection play key roles in minimising intraoperative aneurysm rupture. Adequate depth of anaesthesia, strict blood pressure control, ventricular drainage at the time of surgery, aggressive sphenoid wing removal, and appropriately situated craniotomies which permit minimal brain retraction, will aid in reducing the incidence of aneurysm rupture before arachnoid dissection.

The most frequent time for intraoperative aneurysm rupture is during arachnoid dissection before clip application.[146-148] In our experience, ill-advised blunt dissection techniques are the most frequent cause of intraoperative rupture. Aneurysm rupture produced by blunt dissection typically produces a large tear at the aneurysm sac-neck junction, and the amount of bleeding is usually torrential. Bleeding from sharp dissection is usually from punctate holes and, therefore, more controllable. To reduce the risk of rupture, dense clot surrounding the vessels and the aneurysm should be sharply divided with microscissors or microarachnoid knives. Dissection should also follow the normal vasculature when working in the vicinity of the aneurysm. Early proximal and distal vascular control before aneurysm dissection is mandatory in all cases. Definitive neck dissection before clip application will also reduce the likelihood of clip-induced rupture of the aneurysm, which is similar to aneurysm rupture from blunt dissection.

Intraoperative aneurysm rupture is an inevitable complication of intracranial aneurysm surgery. Close blood pressure control, basal craniotomy flaps, minimal brain retraction, strict use of sharp dissection techniques, dissection along normal vascular anatomy, temporary occlusion of parent vessels, and appropriate use of available clips, can potentially minimise the incidence of intraoperative rupture and provide the optimal chance for a good surgical outcome.

In the event of intraoperative aneurysm rupture, we have found several techniques useful. Temporary occlusion of afferent and efferent vessels involved in the aneurysm is one of the most useful measures. We use etomidate or pentothal induced electroencephalographic burst suppression during temporary occlusion to theoretically optimise cerebral protection.[149] We do not use induced hypotension to control intraoperative aneurysm rupture because of the theoretically deleterious effects of hypotension on patients specifically susceptible to either acute or delayed ischaemia. Giannotta et al found that induced hypotension negatively influenced outcomes when used to control intraoperative aneurysm rupture.[148]

We attempt to remove as much subarachnoid clot as is deemed safe. The variable consistency of acute and subacute subarachnoid blood at various stages of fibrinolysis renders the success of clot removal unpredictable. Previous reports have found some potential benefit in preventing vasospasm or lessening its severity by aggressive subarachnoid clot removal.[143 144] Recent reports have focused on the use of topical thrombolytic agents such as tissue-type plasminogen activator (tPA) instilled into the subarachnoid space during surgery. Use of tPA has been reported to show some

207

effect on chemical thrombolysis of subarachnoid clot in the post-operative period.[137 140 150-153] In our limited experience, tPA does seem to aid in the clearance of subarachnoid blood seen on CT. Whether this chemically induced thrombolysis will be beneficial in decreasing the morbidity and mortality of vasospasm remains to be demonstrated. The addition of tPA at surgery carries some risk of increased bleeding in the operative site postoperatively.

Management of aneurysms using Guglielmi detachable coils

Background

The Guglielmi detachable coil system was developed by the Italian neurosurgeon Guglielmi and Target Therapeutics, Fremont, California. The device provides the interventionalist with the ability to insert a coil into an aneurysm or blood vessel, assess its position, and withdraw it if the result is not satisfactory.[109-116] Other coil systems are not detachable but rather are pushed or injected into position. Once these coils leave the catheter they are difficult, if not impossible, to retrieve.

To treat an aneurysm with Guglielmi detachable coils, the interventionalist must first place a microcatheter into the aneurysm fundus. Once properly positioned a coil is inserted through the catheter and into the aneurysm. If the operator does not approve of the configuration he or she can remove it and reposition it or choose another size coil. The system consists of a soft platinum coil soldered to a stainless steel delivery wire. When the coil is properly positioned within the fundus a 1 mA current is applied to the delivery wire. The current dissolves the stainless steel delivery wire proximal to the platinum coil by electrolysis. At the same time, the positively charged platinum theoretically attracts the negatively charged blood elements such as white and red blood cells, platelets, and fibrinogen thus inducing an intra-aneurysmal thrombosis. Once electrolysis occurs the delivery wire can be removed leaving the coil in place. Another coil can now be introduced into the fundus. The process is continued until the aneurysm is densely packed with platinum and no longer opacifies during diagnostic contrast injections.

The mechanism by which Guglielmi detachable coils occlude aneurysms is still debated. We have made observations at surgery on recently coiled aneurysms that lead us to question the theory that the positive charge within the aneurysm during electrolysis produces significant thrombus formation. Coils likely provide immediate protection against rebleeding by reducing blood flow within the aneurysm sac, buffering arterial pulsations within the fundus, and sealing the weak portion of the wall or hole. Eventually organised thrombus forms within the aneurysm and the aneurysm is excluded from the parent vessel by the formation of endothelial connective tissue that covers the ostium of the neck. This has been demonstrated by Mawad *et al*[112] in experimental dog models and in our own human necropsy studies.

Indications for the use of Guglielmi coils is increasing as interventionalists become more skilled in their placement. They tend to be most successful in aneurysms with small necks or necks that are smaller in diameter than the maximal aneurysm diameter and aneurysms without appreciable intrafundal thrombus. Decisions concerning their applications are made on a case by case basis and few dogmatic rules exist.

Outcomes

In 1995 Vinuela reviewed the USA Multicenter GDC Study Group's results with 753 aneurysms treated in 715 patients. Complete occlusion of small aneurysms with small necks occurred in 62% of cases and complete occlusion in small aneurysms with wide necks was 33%. Large aneurysms with small necks and giant aneurysms with thrombus each had a 37% occlusion rate and giant aneurysms alone had 35% occlusion rates. Technical complications occurred in 11% of cases and included aneurysm perforation (1·5%), parent artery narrowing (0·5%), parent artery occlusion (3·8%), embolisation (3·7%), and coil migration (1·1%). Complications that had permanent clinical implications, however, occurred in only 4·4% of cases. The mortality related to procedure was 1·12% and the overall mortality for the entire study population was 5·2%. Aneurysm haemorrhage rate after embolisation was 1·26%. Aneurysm recanalisation occurred in 7·7% of small aneurysms, 15% of large aneurysms, 29% of giant aneurysms, and 31% of giant and partially thrombosed lesions. Since 1994, results have improved as different sized and less traumatic coils have become available. These advances allow for denser fundus packing and improved obliteration rates with reduction in delayed recanalisation.

Aneurysm embolisation using the Guglielmi detachable coil system offers an alternative to traditional surgical clipping in certain patients. The results of such treatment, as shown in Vinuela's review are not yet as effective as those of open surgery. Nevertheless, in certain instances coiling is a viable option. Decisions must be made on a case by case basis. At our institution considerations include patient age, medical condition, aneurysm geometry, and location. The individual surgeon's and interventionalist's relative skills are not particularly relevant at institutions where both disciplines are practised at the highest level, but they should be considered in the choice of treatment when discrepancies exist.

Postoperative management

Patient care after surgery to obliterate a ruptured cerebral aneurysm is complex and must be based on many considerations. Major problems in the immediate postoperative period include brain swelling, bleeding into the operative site, fluid and electrolyte disturbances, hydrocephalus, and the onset of cerebral vasospasm. Also, many postoperative complications present with similar symptoms but require entirely different treatments. Along with the neurological examination, frequent CT, evaluation of vital signs, blood electrolyte determination, transcranial Doppler evaluations, and cerebral blood flow determinations are particularly helpful in differentiating between these various complications.

Patients who have had surgery to repair a ruptured aneurysm are predisposed to develop brain swelling and oedema. Irritation of the brain surface and vessels by subarachnoid clot, disturbance of cerebral vascular autoregulation, raised intracranial pressure, and infarction related to iatrogenic vessel occlusion or vasospasm all contribute to postoperative brain swelling. Patients are typically maintained on dexamethasone (16 mg/day) during the first operative week. Although no studies have proved that patients with subarachnoid haemorrhage derive any benefit from corticosteroid therapy, we think that the inhibitory effects of corticosteroids on phospholiphase A2, complement activation, leucocyte migration, and lymphocyte function may be beneficial in the prevention of vasospasm.[154] Intravascular volume status is closely assessed with either venous access monitors or pulmonary artery catheters, depending on the patient's condition. Judicious fluid management can minimise cerebral swelling by avoiding systemic overload. At the time of surgery the degree of brain swelling and the necessity of frontal or temporal lobectomy are assessed. In a similar fashion, lobectomy is considered postoperatively if clinical deterioration occurs concomitant with CT evidence of brain swelling.

Fluid and electrolyte disturbances are relatively common after subarachnoid haemorrhage and surgery to repair a ruptured aneurysm. Takaku *et al* found an 8·8% incidence of electrolyte disturbances after aneurysm surgery.[155] Hyponatraemia is the most common abnormality, occurring in 53%, whereas hypernatraemia had the highest mortality (42%). Hyponatraemia can be due to either inappropriate secretion of antidiuretic hormone or true natriuresis due to cerebral salt wasting.[156 157] Both syndromes are characterised by a decrease in plasma sodium concentrations and osmolality, associated with increased urinary concentration greater than 25 mmol/l. Clinical differentiation of these syndromes is important because patients with primary salt wasting syndrome are hypovolaemic and require sodium and fluid replacement. Conversely, true inappropriate antidiuretic hormone secretion is treated with fluid restriction.

As previously discussed, communicating hydrocephalus both before and after surgery can be seen in patients with subarachnoid haemorrhage. There have been some reports that early operation and subarachnoid clot removal may decrease the incidence of postoperative hydrocephalus.[158] Others have proposed that preoperative antifibrinolytic drugs contribute to the development of hydrocephalus.[159] Regardless of the cause, hydrocephalus should be ruled out in any patient with a decline in mental status before or after aneurysm surgery.

Delayed ischaemic deficit secondary to cerebral vasospasm is the greatest cause of morbidity in patients surviving the initial haemorrhage. Angiographic vasospasm occurs in 70% of patients with subarachnoid haemorrhage, with 20–30% of patients having clinically significant narrowing. Cerebral vasospasm has a peak incidence around the sixth to eighth day after subarachnoid haemorrhage, although it can occur at any time up to about 14 days afterwards; beyond this it is extremely rare.[160 161] When vasospasm develops, it may last for several days to several weeks.[160 162] The most reliable predictor of those patients predisposed to develop vasospasm is the amount and distribution of subarachnoid blood seen on CT. Thick layers of blood in the basal cisterns carry a higher risk of vasospasm than diffuse or focal loculations. Lobar haematomas and interhemispheric blood are associated with a low risk of vasospasm. Subarachnoid blood in the sylvian fissure seems to carry a risk of intermediate vasospasm.[163 164] Clinical vasospasm develops gradually over hours or days, and is typically associated with gradual, progressive decline in neurological status. Headache, fever, and leukocytosis are often present and may herald the onset of vasospasm before neurological deterioration. Permanent neurological deficit or death occurs in about 12% of patients who develop severe clinical vasospasm.[160 165]

At present, the mainstay of treatment for clinically significant cerebral vasospasm is the induction of hypervolaemia and systemic hypertension, often referred to as hyperdynamic therapy. The neurological deficits seen with vasospasm are the result of arterial narrowing and increased cerebrovascular resistance. Because autoregulation is usually impaired after subarachnoid haemorrhage, manoeuvres that increase cerebral perfusion pressure can increase cerebral blood flow in the ischaemic regions.[166 167] Patients undergoing induced hypertension and intravascular volume expansion are best treated in an intensive care unit with arterial and central venous pressure monitoring. An indwelling arterial catheter is used to assess blood pressure and a Swan-Ganz catheter is used to monitor pulmonary capillary wedge pressure. Transcutaneous pulse oximeters are used to monitor oxygen saturation. Desaturations may indicate early pulmonary decompensation from hypervolaemic therapy. Fluid balance is assessed hourly.

The initial therapy for symptomatic vasospasm consists of volume expansion with plasma protein fractionate to create a positive fluid balance of 1–2 litres. The pulmonary artery wedge pressure is usually maintained between 14 and 18 mm Hg, and the central venous pressure is kept at about 10 mm Hg. If clinical improvement is not seen soon after volume expansion, arterial blood pressure is raised with dopamine, dobutamine, or levophed and typically maintained with systolic pressures between 180 and 220 mm Hg. Kassell et al have reported 58 patients treated for cerebral vasospasm with volume expansion and induced arterial hypertension, with reversal of neurological symptoms in 75%. They found neurological improvements to be permanent in 74% and temporary in 7%.[119] As intravascular volume is expanded, patients may undergo a secondary diuresis which can make artificially increasing the pulmonary capillary wedge pressure difficult. Use of low dose vasopressin can help minimise the diuresis and maintain an increased intravascular fluid volume. Hypervolaemic and hypertensive therapy is continued until the neurological symptoms resolve or complications from therapy require re-evaluation of the risk/benefit ratio of continuing this type of treatment. Complications include pulmonary oedema, congestive heart failure, brain oedema, hypertensive cerebral haemorrhage, systemic complications of prolonged vasopressor use, and myocardial infarction. Relative contraindications to hyperdynamic therapy include cerebral oedema, cerebral infarction, myocardial dysfunction, pulmonary oedema, adult respiratory distress syndrome, and increased intracranial pressure.[168]

When hyperdynamic therapy has proved unsuccessful or is contraindicated, we have found other manoeuvres helpful. Selective intra-arterial infusion of papaverine hydrochloride (300 mg in 100 ml normal saline over one hour) into the symptomatic vascular territory may reverse angiographic vasospasm in some patients. The results of this therapy can be clinically dramatic, but in a similar fashion may be extremely fleeting or unsuccessful. Further investigation needs to be performed to clarify the role of intra-arterial infusions of vasolidators for treatment of cerebral vasospasm.[169 170]

Another potentially useful adjunct in the treatment of posthaemorrhagic cerebral vasospasm is transluminal balloon angioplasty of the large intracranial vessels (internal carotid artery, M1 segment of the middle cerebral artery, vertebral and basilar arteries). Some investigators have reported encouraging results with the use of this technique.[171-173] We have witnessed considerable improvement in cerebral circulation after transluminal angioplasty but have also seen fatal complications due to vessel dissection or rupture. Linskey *et al* reported a fatal subarachnoid haemorrhage that was produced by a rupture of a residual aneurysm neck by the angioplasty catheter.[174] The use of such adjunctive treatment modalities should be undertaken with caution until the safety and efficacy of these procedures is better established.

New pharmaceutical products may improve the outcome of patients with subarachnoid haemorrhage. Calcium channel blockers have been discussed earlier (nimodipine, 60 mg orally every four hours for 10–21 days). Their efficacy in reducing the detrimental effects of vasospasm have been shown in controlled studies,[130-134] although the true mechanism of action remains elusive. A second drug currently under intense investigation is the free radical scavenger 21-aminosteroid U74006F (Tirilizad, Upjohn Co, Kalamazoo, MI, USA). Four controlled studies have shown a reduction in morbidity after subarachnoid haemorrhage in men given this medication.[175-178] Additional studies are needed to prove efficacy in men and women.

Management after hospital discharge

Patients who have survived subarachnoid haemorrhage and are ultimately discharged from the hospital require close follow up to detect and treat latent complications. Communicating hydrocephalus—manifested by increasing headache, lethargy, confusion, or regression of a previously improving neurological status—may develop after discharge. Fluid and electrolyte disturbances may not become evident until after discharge, and may only be suspected with a patient history of abnormal fluid intake coupled with changes in mental status. Seizures after subarachnoid haemorrhage occur in 10–30% of patients, with the highest incidence associated with middle cerebral artery aneurysms. Most occur within 18 months of the haemorrhage and 83% of patients have fewer than three events. The most important risk factors determining the development of a seizure disorder are poor neurological grade and focal neurological deficits. There is no evidence that seizures during the initial haemorrhage are likely to persist or recur. Hart *et al* was unable to demonstrate benefit of prophylactic anticonvulsant therapy after acute subarachnoid haemorrhage.[31] Because our belief is that postoperative seizures are socioeconomically stigmatising, patients in our practice with subarachnoid haemorrhage are usually placed on prophylactic anticonvulsants when they present to the hospital, and are postoperatively maintained on medications for three to six months.

Important considerations in survivors of subarachnoid haemorrhage are the disease's neuropsychiatric sequelae.[179 180] Even patients with good Glasgow outcome scores will have deficits 12 months after the haemorrhage. Short term memory is reduced in 53% and long term memory is reduced in 21%. Visuospatial construction and memory, mental flexibility, and psychomotor speed remain abnormal in 28–62%. Ten per cent have dysphasic language performance and up to 50% remain unemployed.

Because latent complications may develop, our protocol is to follow patients on a monthly basis after discharge with CT and laboratory testing as necessary. Patients are weaned from anticonvulsant drugs three to six months postoperatively and are followed up with clinic visits until they are neurologically stable for one year.

Management of subarachnoid haemorrhage

Subarachnoid haemorrhage is a complex medical event that affects a significant number of people each year. The causes can be multifactorial, but most commonly relate to bleeding from a cerebral aneurysm. The optimal management of this life threatening condition relies on a systematic and organised approach leading to the correct diagnosis and the timely referral to a neurosurgeon capable of treating this condition. The following is a brief summary of the steps that should be initiated when subarachnoid haemorrhage is suspected.

● The clinician should have a high index of suspicion that a sudden, severe, unexplained headache in any patient could represent an acute subarachnoid haemorrhage.

● Brain CT should be done immediately after the diagnosis is suspected.

● If the CT is positive, lumbar puncture is unnecessary and dangerous due to the risks of aneurysm rebleeding or transtentorial brain herniation. If the CT is negative, lumbar puncture may be helpful if the history of the ictal headache is not typical of subarachnoid haemorrhage, insidious in onset, or of migrainous character. If the patient relates a history typical of subarachnoid haemorrhage, a cerebral anteriogram should be performed despite negative CT. Up to 15% of scans obtained within 48 hours of subarachnoid haemorrhage will be negative.

● Once the diagnosis is confirmed by CT, a neurosurgeon who can ultimately treat the patient should be immediately contacted. It is often best to allow the surgeon who will be caring for the patient to arrange for the diagnostic arteriogram to be performed at the institution where the patient will undergo surgery to repair the aneurysm. Arteriography performed by institutions rarely treating subarachnoid haemorrhage may be technically inadequate and require repetition on transfer to the neurosurgeon. Digital arteriography and magnetic resonance angiography does not as yet have the resolution necessary to adequately evaluate acute subarachnoid haemorrhage.

• After the diagnosis of ruptured cerebral aneurysm is confirmed, immediate transfer to a neurosurgical centre for treatment is of paramount importance. Delays in transfer may prove fatal because of the potential for aneurysm rebleeding before operative intervention.

• Blood pressure must be closely monitored and controlled after subarachnoid haemorrhage. Hypertension will increase the chance of catastrophic rebleeding. Blood pressure control should be initiated immediately on diagnosis.

• Preoperative medications include prophylactic anticonvulsants, calcium channel blockers, corticosteroids, and antihypertensive drugs as needed. We do not initiate antifibrinolytic therapy unless surgery is not considered within 48 hours of the initial bleed. Medications that can be initiated before transfer to a neurosurgeon include dexamethasone (4 mg intravenously, six hourly), nimodipine (60 mg, four hourly by mouth), and phenytoin (10 mg/kg intravenous load, then 100 mg by mouth eight hourly). A frequent source of diagnostic difficulty for the neurosurgeon lies in the use of excessive amounts of narcotic analgesics before transfer to the neurosurgical service. Although pain control facilitates blood pressure control, the ability to accurately grade the patient's level of consciousness has significant impact on the timing of surgery. Clinical grading obscured by large doses of narcotic analgesics makes surgical planning more difficult.

• Send all radiographs, MRI, and laboratory work with the patient to avoid needless repetition.

• We perform surgery or endovascular coiling to obliterate the ruptured aneurysm as soon as possible after the onset of subarachnoid haemorrhage. Patients with poor grades, IV and V, are treated non-surgically or neurointerventionally until their clinical condition improves.

• Postoperative care is directed towards supportive care and complication recognition and treatment. Frequent postoperative complications include brain oedema, bleeding into the operative site, fluid and electrolyte disturbances, hydrocephalus, and cerebral vasospasm.

• Cerebral vasospasm may occur at any time, with a peak incidence around the sixth to eighth day after subarachnoid haemorrhage, and should be suspected for any unexplained decline in neurological status.

• Brain CT is useful to detect haematomas, acute hydrocephalus, or the development of subclinical ischaemic infarcts.

• Current treatments for cerebral vasospasm include induced hypervolaemia and systemic hypertension, transluminal angioplasty, intra-arterial vasodilator infusion, and investigational systemic medications such as tirilizad mesylate.

Despite therapeutic and surgical advances over the past two decades, a percentage of patients with subarachnoid haemorrhage will ultimately die or be neurologically injured, as long as subarachnoid haemorrhage remains a condition that is not widely preventable. Physicians who diagnose and manage patients with acute subarachnoid haemorrhage would be well advised to remain up to date on the ever changing developments in the management of this ubiquitous and catastrophic condition that may strike healthy and unsuspecting people at any time.

1 Clemente CD. *Anatomy, a regional atlas of the human body*, 3rd ed. Baltimore; Urban and Schwarzenberg, 1987:572–3.

2 Liliequist B. The subarachnoid cisterns. An anatomic and roentgenologic study. *Acta Radiol (Stockholm)* 1959;suppl:185.

3 Haines DE, Harkey HL, Al-Mefty O. The "subdural" space: a new look at an outdated concept. *Neurosurg* 1993;**32**:111–20.

4 Sahs AL. Randomized treatment study. Introduction. In: Sahs AL, Nibbelink DW, Turner JC, eds. *Aneurysmal subarachnoid hemorrhage. Report of the Cooperative Study*. Baltimore: Urban and Schwarzenberg, 1981:19–20.

5 Stehbens WE. Subarachnoid hemorrhage. *Pathology of the cerebral blood vessels*. St Louis: CV Mosby, 1972:252–83.

6 Sahs A, Perret GE, Locksley HB, Nishioka H. *Intracranial aneurysms and subarachnoid hemorrhage*. Philadelphia: J B Lippincott, 1969.

7 Shokichi U, Masumichi I, Munesuke S, Masayoshi S. Subarachnoid hemorrhage as a cause of death in Japan. *Z Rechtsmed* 1973;**72**:151–60.

8 Levy LE, Rachman L, Castle WM. Spontaneous primary subarachnoid hemorrhage in Rhodesian Africans. *Afr J Med Sci* 1973;**4**:77–86.

9 Locksley HB. Report on the cooperative study of intracranial aneurysms and subarachnoid hemorrhage, Sect 5, P1. Natural history of subarachnoid hemorrhage, intracranial aneurysms, and arteriovenous malformations. *J Neurosurg* 1966;**25**:219–39.

10 Locksley HB. Natural history of subarachnoid hemorrhage, intracranial aneurysms and arteriovenous malformations. Pt 1. In: Sahs AL, Perret GE, Locksley HB, Nishioka H, eds. *Intracranial aneurysms and subarachnoid hemorrhage. A cooperative study*. Philadelphia: Lippincott, 1969:37–57.

11 Talbot S. Epidemiological features of subarachnoid and cerebral haemorrhages. *Postgrad Med J* 1973;**49**:300–4.

12 Crompton MR. The coroner's cerebral aneurysm: a changing animal. *J Forensic Sci Soc* 1975;**15**:57–65.

13 Murphy JP. Subarachnoid hemorrhage; intracranial aneurysm. *Cerebrovascular disease*. Chicago: Year Book, 1954:199–241.

14 Ohno Y. Biometeorologic studies on cerebrovascular diseases. I. Effects of meteorologic factors on the death from cerebrovascular accident. *Jpn Circ J* 1969;**33**:1285–98.

15 Ohno Y. Biometeorologic studies on cerebrovascular diseases. II. Seasonal observation on effects of meteorologic factors on the death from cerebrovascular accident. *Jpn Circ J* 1969;**33**:1299–308.

16 Ohno Y. Biometeorologic studies on cerebrovascular diseases. III. Effects by the combination of meteorologic changes on the death from cerebrovascular accident. *Jpn Circ J* 1969;**33**:1309–14.

17 Chyahe D, Chen T, Bronstein K, Brass LM. Seasonal fluctuation in the incidence of intracranial aneurysm rupture and its relationship to changing climate conditions. *J Neurosurg* 1994;**81**:525–30.

18 Pakarinen S. Incidence, aetiology, and prognosis of primary subarachnoid hemorrhage. *Acta Neurol Scand* 1967;**29**(suppl):1–128.

19 Freytag E. Fatal rupture of intracranial aneurysms. Survey of 250 medicolegal cases. *Arch Pathol* 1966;**81**:418–24.

20 Locksley HB. Natural history of subarachnoid hemorrhage, intracranial aneurysms and arteriovenous malformations. Part II. In: Sahs AL, Perret GE, Locksley HB, Nishioka H, eds. *Intracranial aneurysms and subarachnoid hemorrhage. A cooperative study.* Philadelphia: Lippincott, 1969:58–108.

21 Adams HP, Jergenson DD, Sahs AL. Pitfalls in the recognition of subarachnoid hemorrhage. *JAMA* 1980;**244**:794–6.

22 Leblanc R. The minor leak preceding subarachnoid hemorrhage. *J Neurosurg* 1987;**66**:35–9.

23 Leblanc R, Winfield JA. The warning leak in subarachnoid hemorrhage and the importance of its early diagnosis. *Can Med Assoc J* 1984;**131**:1235–6.

24 Calvert JM. Premonitory symptoms and signs of subarachnoid hemorrhage. *Med J Aust* 1966;**53**:651–7.

25 Richardson JC, Hyland HH. Intracranial aneurysm. A clinical and pathological study of subarachnoid and intracerebral hemorrhage caused by berry aneurysms. *Medicine* 1984;**20**:1–83.

26 Berman AJ. The problem of the intracranial aneurysm. *Angiology* 1958;**9**:136–53.

27 Gillingham FJ. The management of ruptured intracranial aneurysm. *Ann Roy Coll Surg* 1958;**23**:89–117.

28 Ito Z, Matsuoka S, Moriyama T, *et al.* Factors related to level of consciousness in the acute stage of ruptured intracranial aneurysms. *Brain Nerve (Tokyo)* 1975;**27**:895–901.

29 Austin DC. A review of intracranial aneurysms. *Henry Ford Hosp Med Bull* 1964;**12**:251–71.

30 Fisher CM. Clinical syndromes in cerebral thrombosis, hypertensive hemorrhage, and ruptured saccular aneurysm. *Clin Neurosurg* 1975;**22**:117–47.

31 Hart RG, Byer JA, Slaughter JR, *et al.* Occurrence and implications of seizures in subarachnoid hemorrhage due to ruptured intracranial aneurysms. *Neurosurgery* 1981;**8**:417–21.

32 Sarner M, Rose FC. Clinical presentation of ruptured intracranial aneurysm. *J Neurol Neurosurg Psychiatry* 1967;**30**:67–70.

33 Tsementzis SA, Williams A. Ophthalmological signs and prognosis in patients with a subarachnoid hemorrhage. *Neurochirurgia* 1984;**27**:133–5.

34 Garfunkle AM, Danys IR, Nicolle DH, Colohan ART, Brem S. Terson's syndrome: a reversible cause of blindness following subarachnoid hemorrhage. *J Neurosurg* 1992;**76**:766–71.

35 Shields CB. Current trends in management of cerebral aneurysms. *J Kentucky Med Assoc* 1977;**75**:529–35.

36 Kassell NF, Torner JC, Haley C, *et al.* The international cooperative study on the timing of aneurysm surgery. Part 1: Overall management results. *J Neurosurg* 1990;**73**:18–36.

37 Kassell NF, Kongable GL, Torner JC, Adams HP, Mazuz H. Delay in referral of patients with ruptured aneurysms to neurosurgical attention. *Stroke* 1985;**16**:587–90.

38 Kendall BE, Lee BC, Claveria E. Computerized tomography and angiography in subarachnoid hemorrhage. *Br J Radiol* 1976;**49**:4873–501.

39 Liliequist B, Lindquist M, Valdimarsson E. Computed tomography and subarachnoid hemorrhage. *Neuroradiology* 1977;**14**:21–6.

40 Modesti LM, Binet EF. Value of computed tomography in the diagnosis and management of subarachnoid hemorrhage. *Neurosurgery* 1978;**3**:151–6.

41 Scotti G, Ethler R, Melancon D, *et al.* Computed tomography in the evaluation of intracranial aneurysms and subarachnoid hemorrhage. *Radiology* 1977;123:85–90.

42 Weir B, Miller J, Russell D. Intracranial aneurysms: a clinical, angiographic, and computerized tomographic study. *Can J Neurol Sci* 1977;4:99–105.

43 Jafar JJ, Weiner HL. Surgery for angiographically occult cerebral aneurysms. *J Neurosurg* 1993;79:674–9.

44 Fisher CM, Kistler JP, Davis JM. Relation of cerebral vasospasm to subarachnoid hemorrhage visualized by computerized tomographic scanning. *Neurosurgery* 1980;6:1–9.

45 Sicard J-A. Chromodiagnostid cu liquide cephalorachidien dans les hemorragies du nevraxe. Valeur de la teinte jaunatre. *CR Soc Biol* 1901;53:1050-3.

46 Milian G. Chiray, Méiningite à pneumocoques. Zanthochromie du liquide cephal-rachidien. *Bull Soc Anat Paris* 1902;4:550-2.

47 Froin G. *Les Hemorragies Sous-Arachnoidiennes et le Mecanisme de l'Hematolyse en general* Paris: Steinheil, 1904.

48 Collier J, Adie WJ. Cerebral vascular lesions. In: Price FW, ed. *A textbook of the practice of medicine.* London: Henry Frowde and Hodder and Stoughton, 1922:1348–65.

49 Symondo CP. Spontaneous subarachnoid hemorrhage. *Q J Med* 1924–25;18:93–122.

50 Greenfield JG, Carmichael EA. *The cerebrospinal fluid in clinical diagnosis* London: Macmillan, 1925:50-2.

51 Barrows LJ, Hunter FT, Banker BQ. The nature and clinical significance of pigments in the cerebrospinal fluid. *Brain* 1955;78:59–80.

52 Duffy GP. Lumbar puncture in spontaneous subarachnoid hemorrhage. *BMJ* 1982;285:1163–4.

53 Nibbelink DW, Torner J, Henderson WG. Intracranial aneurysms and subarachnoid hemorrhage. *Stroke* 1977;8:202–18.

54 Hesselink JR. Investigation of intracranial aneurysm. In: Fox JL, ed. *Intracranial aneurysms, vol. 1.* New York: Springer-Verlag, 1983:497–548.

55 Teal JS, Wade PJ, Bergeron RT, *et al.* Ventricular opacification during carotid angiography secondary to rupture of intracranial aneurysm. *Radiology* 1973;106:581–3.

56 Vines FS, Davis DO. Rupture of intracranial aneurysm at angiography. *Radiology* 1971;99:353–4.

57 Goldstein SL. Ventricular opacification secondary to rupture of intracranial aneurysm during angiography. *J Neurosurg* 1967;27:265–7.

58 Komiyama M. Aneurysmal rupture during angiography. *Neurosurgery* 1993;33:798–803.

59 Saitoh H, Hayakawa K, Nishimura K, Okuno Y, Teraura T, Yumitori K, Ohumura A. Rerupture of cerebral aneurysms during angiography. *AJNR Am J Neuroradiol* 1995;16:539–42.

60 Hackney DB, Lesnick JE, Zimmerman RA, Grossman RI, Goldberg HI, Bilaniuk LT. MR identification of bleeding site in subarachnoid hemorrhage with multiple intracranial aneurysms. *J Comput Assist Tomogr* 1986;10:878–80.

61 Hope JKA, Wilson JL, Thomson FJ. Three dimensional CT angiography in the detection and characterization of intracranial berry aneurysms. *AJNR Am J Neuroradiol* 1996;17:439–45.

62 Ogawa T, Okudera T, Nogushi K, Sasaki M, Inugama A, Uemura K, Yashui N. Cerebral aneurysms: evaluation with three dimensional CT angiography. *AJNR Am J Neuroradiol* 1996;17:447–54.

63 Hsiang JNK, Liang EY, Lam JMK, Zhu XL, Poon WS. The role of computed tomographic angiography in the diagnosis of intracranial aneurysms and emergent aneurysm clipping. *Neurosurgery* 1996;38:481–7.

64 Tampier D, Leblanc R, Oleszek J, Pokrupa R, Melancor D. Three dimensional computed tomographic angiography of cerebral aneurysms. *Neurosurgery* 1995;36:749–55.

65 Huston J, Nichols DA, Leutmer PH, *et al.* Blinded prospective evaluation of sensitivity of MR angiography to known intracranial aneurysms: importance of aneurysm size. *AJNR Am J Neuroradiol* 1994;15:1607–14.

66 Bohn E, Hugosson R. Experiences of surgical treatment of 400 consecutive ruptured cerebral aneurysms. *Acta Neurochir (Wien)* 1978;49:33–43.

67 Modesti LM, Binet EF. Value of computed tomography in the diagnosis and management of subarachnoid hemorrhage. *Neurosurgery* 1978;3:151–6.

68 Van Gijn J, Hijdra A, Wijdicks EF, Vermeulen M, Crevel HV. Acute hydrocephalus after aneurysmal subarachnoid hemorrhage. *J Neurosurg* 1985;63:355–62.

69 Parc L, Delfino R, Leblanc R. The relationship of ventricular drainage to aneurysmal

rebleeding. *J Neurosurg* 1992;**76**:422–7.

70 Bogdahn U, Lau W, Hassel W, Gunreben G, Mertens HG, Brawanski A. Continuous-pressure controlled, external ventricular drainage for treatment of acute hydrocephalus—Evaluation of risk factors. *Neurosurgery* 1992;**31**:898–904.

71 Bramwell E. The etiology of recurrent ocular paralysis (including periodic ocular paralysis and ophthalmoplegic migraine). *Edinburgh Med J* 1933;**40**:209–81.

72 Botterell EH, Lougheed WM, Scott JW, *et al*. Hypothermia, and interruption of carotid, or carotid and vertebral circulation in the surgical management of intracranial aneurysms. *J Neurosurg* 1956;**13**:1–42.

73 Lougheed WM, Marshall BM. Management of aneurysms of the anterior circulation by intracranial procedures. In: Youmans JR, ed. *Neurological surgery, vol. 2*. Philadelphia: WB Saunders, 1973:731–67.

74 Hunt WE, Hess RM. Surgical risk as related to time of intervention, in the repair of intracranial aneurysms. *J Neurosurg* 1968;**28**:14–20.

75 Hunt WE, Kosnik EJ. Timing and perioperative care in intracranial aneurysm surgery. *Clin Neurosurg* 1974;**21**:79–89.

76 Hunt WE. Grading of patients with aneurysms. Letter to the Editor, *J Neurosurg* 1977;**47**:13.

77 Friedman AH. Subarachnoid hemorrhage of unknown etiology. In: Wilkins RH, Rengachary SS, eds. *Neurosurgery update II*, New York: McGraw-Hill, 1991:73–7.

78 Nishioka H, Torner JC, Graf CJ, *et al*. Cooperative study of intracranial aneurysms and subarachnoid hemorrhage: A longterm prognostic study. III. Subarachnoid hemorrhage of undetermined etiology. *Arch Neurol* 1984;**41**:1147–51.

79 Perret G, Nichioka H. Cerebral angiography: diagnostic value and complications of carotid and vertebral angiography. In: Sahs AL, ed. *Intracranial aneurysms and subarachnoid hemorrhage: a cooperative study*. Philadelphia: Lippincott, 1969:109–24.

80 Iwanage H, Wakai S, Ochiai C, Narita J, Inoh S, Nagai M. Ruptured cerebral aneurysms missed by initial angiographic study. *Neurosurgery* 1990;**27**:45–51.

81 Forster DMC, Steiner L, Hakanson S. The value of repeat panangiography in cases of unexplained subarachnoid hemorrhage. *J Neurosurg* 1978;**48**:712–6.

82 Biller J, Toffol GJ, Kassell NF, *et al*. Spontaneous subarachnoid hemorrhage in young adults. *Neurosurgery* 1987;**21**:664–7.

83 Juul R, Fredricksen TA, Ringkjob R. Prognosis in subarachnoid hemorrhage of unknown etiology. *J Neurosurg* 1986;**64**:359–62.

84 Giombini S, Burzzone MG, Pluchino F. Subarachnoid hemorrhage of unexplained cause. *Neurosurgery* 1988;**22**:313–6.

85 Suzuki S, Kayama T, Sakurai Y, *et al*. Subarachnoid hemorrhage of unknown cause. *Neurosurgery* 1987;**21**:310-3.

86 Smith RP, Miller JD. Pathophysiology and clinical evaluation of subarachnoid hemorrhage. In: Youmans JR, ed. *Neurological surgery*. Philadelphia: WB Saunders, 1990:1644–60.

87 Margolis MT, Newton TH. Methamphetamine ("speed") arteritis. *Neuroradiology* 1971;**2**:179–82.

88 Weir B. Medical, neurologic, and ophthalmologic aspects of aneurysms, Pt 2: Neurology of aneurysms and subarachnoid hemorrhage. In: *Aneurysm affecting the nervous system*. Baltimore: Williams and Wilkins, 1987:74–83.

89 Alexander MSM, Dias PS, Uttley D. Spontaneous subarachnoid hemorrhage and negative cerebral panangiography: Review of 140 cases. *J Neurosurg* 1986;**64**:537–42.

90 Andrioli GC, Salar G, Rigobello L, *et al*. Subarachnoid hemorrhage of unknown etiology. *Acta Neurochir (Wien)* 1979;**48**:217–21.

91 Beguelin C, Seiler R. Subarachnoid hemorrhage with normal cerebral panangiography. *Neurosurgery* 1983;**13**:409–11.

92 Brismar J, Sundbarg G. Subarachnoid hemorrhage of unknown origin: prognosis and prognostic factors. *J Neurosurg* 1985;**63**:349–54.

93 Nishioka H, Torner JC, Graf CJ, Kassell NF, Sahs AL, Goettler LC. Cooperative study of intracranial aneurysms and subarachnoid hemorrhage: a long-term prognostic study. II. Ruptured intracranial aneurysms managed conservatively. *Arch Neurol* 1984;**41**:1142–6.

94 Stober T, Emde H, Anstatt T, *et al*. Blood distribution in computer cranial tomograms after subarachnoid hemorrhage with and without an aneurysm on angiography. *Eur Neurol* 1985;**24**:319–23.

95 Pakarinen S. Incidence, aetiology, and prognosis of primary subarachnoid hemorrhage: a study based on 589 cases diagnosed in a defined urban population during a defined period. *Acta Neurol Scand* 1967;**43** (suppl 29):1–128.

96 Chason JL, Hindman WM. Berry aneurysms of the circle of Willis: results of a planned autopsy study. *Neurology* 1958;**8**:41–4.

97 Drake CG. Giant intracranial aneurysms: experience with surgical treatment in 174 patients. *Clin Neurosurg* 1979;**26**:12–95.

98 Sekhar LN, Heros RC. Origin, growth, and rupture of saccular aneurysms: a review. *Neurosurgery* 1981;**8**:248–60.

99 Early CB, Fink LH. Some fundamental applications of the law of LaPlace in neurosurgery. *Surg Neurol* 1976;**6**:185–9.

100 Nakagawa F, Kobayashi S, Takemae T, Sugita K. Aneurysms protruding from the dorsal wall of the internal carotid artery. *J Neurosurg* 1986;**65**:303–8.

101 Forbus WD. On the origin of the miliary aneurysms of the superficial cerebral arteries. *Bull Johns Hopkins Hosp* 1930;**47**:239–84.

102 McCormick WF, Rosenfield DB. Massive brain hemorrhage. A review of 144 cases and an examination of their causes. *Stroke* 1973;**4**:946–54.

103 Sundt TM, Piepgras DG. Surgical approach to giant intracranial aneurysm. Operative experience with 80 cases. *J Neurosurg* 1979;**51**:731–42.

104 Crompton MR. Mechanism of growth and rupture in cerebral berry aneurysms. *BMJ* 1966;**1**:1138–42.

105 Crompton MR. The natural history of cerebral berry aneurysms. *Am Heart J* 1976;**73**:567–9.

106 Stehbens WE. Aneurysms and anatomical variation of cerebral arteries. *Arch Pathol* 1953;**75**:45–64.

107 DuBoulay GH. The significance of loculation of intracranial aneurysms. *Bull Schweiz Akad Med Wiss* 1969;**24**:480–5.

108 Nehls DG, Flom RA, Carter LP, Spetzler RF. Multiple intracranial aneurysms: determining the site of rupture. *J Neurosurg* 1985;**63**:342–8.

109 Mizoi K, Takahashi A, Yoshimoto T, Fujiwara S, Koshu K. Combined endovascular and neurosurgical approach for paraclinoid internal carotid artery aneurysms. *Neurosurgery* 1993;**33**:986–92.

110 Civit T, Anque J, Marchal JC, Bracard S, Picard L, Hepner H. Aneurysm clipping after endovascular treatment with coils: a report of eight patients. *Neurosurgery* 1996;**38**:948–54.

111 Pierot L, Boulin A, Castaings L, Rey A, Moret J. Selective occlusion of basilar artery aneurysms using controlled detachable coils: report of 35 cases. *Neurosurgery* 1996;**28**:948–54.

112 Mawad M, Mawad J, Cartwright J, Eokaslan Z. Long-term histopathologic changes in canine aneurysms embolized with Guglielmi detachable coils. *AJNR Am J Neuroradiol* 1995;**16**:7–13.

113 Graves VB, Strother CM, Duff TA, Perl J. Early treatment of ruptured aneurysms with Guglielmi detachable coils: effect on subsequent bleeding. *Neurosurgery* 1995;**37**:640–8.

114 Guglielmi E. Electrothrombosis of saccular aneurysms via endovascular approach. *J Neurosurg* 1991;**75**:8–14.

115 Guglielmi E. Electrothrombosis of saccular aneurysms via endovascular approach. *J Neurosurg* 1991;**75**:8–14.

116 Guglielmi E, Vinuela F. Endovascular treatment of posterior circulation aneurysms by electrothrombosis using electrically detachable coils. *J Neurosurg* 1992;**77**:514–24.

117 Heiskanen O. The identification of ruptured aneurysm in patients with multiple intracranial aneurysms. *Neurochirurgia (Stuttg)* 1965;**8**:102–7.

118 Pool JL, Potts DG. *Aneurysms and arteriovenous anomalies of the brain. Diagnosis and treatment.* New York: Harper and Row, 1965.

119 Kassell NF, Peerless SJ, Durward QJ, *et al.* Treatment of ischemic deficits from vasospasm with intravascular volume expansion and induced arterial hypertension. *Neurosurgery* 1982;**11**:337–43.

120 Swift DM, Solomon RA. Unruptured aneurysms and postoperative volume expansion. *J Neurosurg* 1992;**77**:908–10.

121 Bailes JE, Speltzer RF, Hadley MN, Baldwin HZ. Management morbidity and mortality of poor-grade aneurysm patients. *J Neurosurg* 1990;**72**:559–66.

122 Yasargil MG. Unoperated cases. In: *Microneurosurgery, vol. 1*. Stuttgart. George Thieme

221

Verlag, 1984:329–30.

123 Norlen G, Olivecrona H. The treatment of aneurysms of the circle of Willis. *J Neurosurg* 1953;**10**:404–15.

124 Weir B, Aronyk K. Management and postoperative mortality related to time of clipping for supratentorial aneurysms. A personal series. *Acta Neurochir (Wien)* 1982;**63**:135–9.

125 Wilkins RH. The role of intracranial arterial spasm in the timing of operations for aneurysm. *Clin Neurosurg* 1977;**24**:185–207.

126 Kassell NF, Torner JC, Jane JA, *et al*. The international cooperative study on the timing of aneurysm surgery. Part 2: surgical results. *J Neurosurg* 1990;**73**:37–47.

127 Dias M, Sekhar LN. Intracranial hemorrhage from aneurysms and arteriovenous malformations during pregnancy and pue-perium. *Neurosurgery* 1990;**72**:855–66.

128 Medlock MD, Dulebohn SC, Elwood PW. Prophylactic hypervolaemia without calcium channel blockers in early aneurysm surgery. *Neurosurgery* 1992;**30**:12–6.

129 Torner JC, Kassell NF, Wallace RB, Adams HP. Preoperative prognostic factors for rebleeding and survival in aneurysm patients receiving antifibrinolytic therapy: Report of the cooperative aneurysm study. *Neurosurgery* 1981;**9**:506–13.

130 Pickard JD, Murray GD, Illingworth R, *et al*. Effect of oral nimodipine on cerebral infarction and outcome after subarachnoid hemorrhage: British Aneurysm Nimopidine Trial. *BMJ* 1989;**298**:636–42.

131 Allen GS, Ahn HS, Preziosi TJ, *et al*. Cerebral arterial spasm: a controlled trial of nimodipine in patients with subarachnoid hemorrhage. *N Engl J Med* 1983;**308**:619–24.

132 Mee E, Dorrance D, Lowe D, *et al*. Controlled study of nimodipine in aneurysm patients treated early after subarachnoid hemorrhage. *Neurosurgery* 1988;**22**:484–91.

133 Pretruk KC, West M, Mohr G, *et al*. Nimodipine treatment in poor grade aneurysm patients. Results of a multicenter double-blind placebo-controlled trial. *J Neurosurg* 1988;**68**:505–17.

134 Barker FG, Ogilvy CS. Efficacy of prophylactic nimodipine for delayed ischemic deficit after subarachnoid hemorrhage: A metaanalysis. *J Neurosurg* 1996;**84**:405–14.

135 Kassell NF, Torner JC, Adams HP. Antifibrinolytic therapy in the acute period following aneurysmal subarachnoid hemorrhage: preliminary observations from the cooperative aneurysm study. *J Neurosurg* 1984;**61**:225–30.

136 Adams HP Jr. Current status of antifibrinolytic therapy of patients with subarachnoid hemorrhage. *Stroke* 1982;**13**:256–9.

137 Mizoi K, Yoshimoto T, Fujiwara S, Sugawara T, Takahashi A, Koshu K. Prevention of vasospasm by clot removal and intrathecal bolus injection of tissue-type plasminogen activator: preliminary report. *Neurosurgery* 1991;**28**:807–13.

138 Findlay JM, Weir BKA, Steinke D, Tanabe T, Gordon P, Grace M. Effect of intrathecal thrombolytic therapy on subarachnoid clot and chronic vasospasm in a primate model of SAH. *J Neurosurg* 1988;**69**:723–35.

139 Burchiel JK, Hoffman JN, Bakay FAR. Quantitative determination of plasma fibrinolytic activity in patients with ruptured intracranial aneurysms who are receiving ε-aminocaproic acid: relationship of possible complications of therapy to the degree of fibrinolytic inhibition. *Neurosurgery* 1984;**14**:57–63.

140 Adams HP, Nibbelink DW, Torner JC, Sahs AL. Antifibrinolytic therapy in patients with aneurysmal subarachnoid hemorrhage. In: Sahs AL, Nibbelink DW, Torner JC. eds. *Aneurysmal subarachnoid hemorrhage. Report of the Cooperative study*. Baltimore: Urban Schwarzenberg, 1981:331–9.

140a Park BE. Spontaneous subarachnoid hemorrhage complicated by communicating hydrocephalus: Epsilon amino caproic acid as a possible predisposing factor. *Surg Neurol* 1979;**11**:73–80.

141 Paine JT, Batjer HH, Samson DS. Intraoperative ventricular puncture—technical note. *Neurosurgery* 1988;**22**:1107–9.

142 Kassell NF, Torner JC. Aneurysmal rebleeding: a preliminary report from the cooperative study. *Neurosurgery* 1983;**13**:479–81.

143 Mizukami M, Kawase T, Usami T, *et al*. Prevention of vasospasm by early operation with removal of subarachnoid blood. *Neurosurgery* 1982;**10**:301–7.

144 Sano K, Saito I. Early operation and washout of blood clots for prevention of cerebral vasospasm. In: Wilkins RH, ed. *Cerebral arterial spasm*. Baltimore: Williams and Wilkins, 1980:510–3.

145 Taneda M. Effect of early operation for ruptured aneurysm on prevention of delayed ischemic symptoms. *J Neurosurg* 1982;**57**:622–8.

146 Batjer HH, Samson D. Intraoperative aneurysmal rupture: incidence, outcome, and suggestions for surgical management. *Neurosurgery* 1986;**18**:701–6.

147 Yasargil MG. *Microsurgery, vol 2*. Stuttgart, George Thieme Verlag, 1984:58–9.

148 Giannotta SL, Oppenheimer JH, Levy ML, Zelman V. Management of intraoperative rupture of aneurysm without hypotension. *Neurosurgery* 1991;**28**:531–6.

149 Batjer HH, Frankfurt AI, Purdy PD, *et al*. Use of etomidate, temporary arterial occlusion, and intraoperative angiography in surgical treatment of large and giant cerebral aneurysms. *J Neurosurg* 1988;**68**:234–40.

150 Seifert V, Eisert WG, Stolke D, Goetz C. Efficacy of single intracisternal bolus injection of recombinant tissue plasminogen activator to prevent delayed cerebral vasospasm after experimental subarachnoid hemorrhage. *Neurosurgery* 1989;**25**:590–8.

151 Findlay JM, Weir RILA, Kassell NF, Disney LB, Grace MGA. Intracisternal recombinant tissue plasminogen activator after aneurysmal subarachnoid hemorrhage. *J Neurosurg* 1991;**75**:181–8.

152 Sasaki T, Ohta T, Kikuchi H, Takakura K, Usui M, Ohnishi H. A phase II clinical trial of recombinant human tissue-type plasminogen activator against vasospasm after aneurysmal hemorrhage. *Neurosurgery* 1994;**35**:597–605.

153 Usui M, Saito N, Hoya K, Todo T. Vasospasm prevention with postoperative intrathecal thrombolytic therapy: a retrospective comparison of urolenase, tissue plasminogen activator, and cisternal drainage alone. *Neurosurgery* 1994;**34**:235–45.

154 Lee SH, Heros RC. Principles of management of subarachnoid hemorrhage: steroids. In: Ratctieson RA, Wirth FP, eds. *Concepts in neurosurgery. Ruptured cerebral aneurysms: perioperative management*. Baltimore: Williams and Wilkins, 1994:77–83.

155 Takaku A, Tanaka S, Mori T, Suzuki J. Postoperative complications in 1,000 cases of intracranial aneurysms. *Surg Neurol* 1979;**12**:137–44.

156 Nelson PB, Sief SM, Maroon JC, Robinson AE. Hyponatremia in intracranial disease: perhaps not the syndrome of inappropriate secretion of antidiuretic hormone (SIADH). *J Neurosurg* 1981;**55**:938–41.

157 Harrigan MR. Cerebral self wasting syndrome: a review. *Neurosurgery* 1996;**38**:152–60.

158 Yamamoto I. Early operation for ruptured intracranial aneurysms: comparative study with computerized tomography. Presented at the *32nd Annual Meeting, Congress of Neurological Surgeons*, Toronto, 1982.

159 Park BE. Spontaneous subarachnoid hemorrhage complicated by communicating hydrocephalus: epsilon amino caproic acid as a possible predisposing factor. *Surg Neurol* 1979;**11**:73–80.

160 Heros R, Zarvas N, Varsos V. Cerebral vasospasm after subarachnoid hemorrhage: an update. *Ann Neurol* 1983;**14**:599–608.

161 Ropper AH, Zervas NT. Outcome 1 year after SAH from cerebral aneurysm. Management, morbidity, mortality, and functional status in 112 consecutive good risk patients. *J Neurosurg* 1984;**60**:909–15.

162 Weir BK. Pathophysiology of vasospasm. *Int Anesthesiol Clin* 1982;**10**:39–43.

163 Pasqualin A, Rosta L, Da Pian R, Cavazzani P, Scienza R. Role of computed tomography in the management of vasospasm after subarachnoid hemorrhage. *Neurosurgery* 1984;**15**:344–53.

164 Kistler JP, Crowell RM, Davis KR, *et al*. The relation of cerebral vasospasm to the extent and location of subarachnoid blood visualized by CT scan. A prospective study. *Neurology* 1983;**33**:424–36.

165 Fisher CM, Roberson GH, Ojemann RG. Cerebral vasospasm with ruptured saccular aneurysm—the clinical manifestations. *Neurosurgery* 1977;**1**:245–8.

166 Symon L. Disordered cerebro-vascular physiology in aneurysmal subarachnoid hemorrhage. *Acta Neurochir (Wien)* 1979;**41**:7–22.

167 Pritz MB, Giannotta SI, Kindt GW, McGillicuddy JE, Prager RL. Treatment of patients with neurological deficits associated with cerebral vasospasm by intravascular volume expansion. *Neurosurgery* 1978;**3**:364–8.

168 Shimoda M, Oda S, Tsugane R, Sato O. Intracranial complications of hypervolemic therapy in patients with a delayed ischemic deficit attributed to vasospasm. *J Neurosurg* 1993;**78**:423–9.

169 Kaku Y, Yonekawa T, Tsukahara T, Kazekawa K. Superselective intra-arterial infusion of papaverine for the treatment of cerebral vasospasm after subarachnoid hemorrhage. *J Neurosurg* 1992;**77**:842–7.

170 Kassell NF, Helm G, Sommons N, Phillips CD, Cail WS. Treatment of cerebral

vasospasm with intra-arterial papaverine. *J Neurosurg* 1992;**77**:848–52.

171 Higashida RT, Halbach W, Cahan LD, *et al*. Transluminal angioplasty for treatment of intracranial arterial vasospasm. *J Neurosurg* 1989;**71**:648–53.

172 Newell DW, Eskridge JM, Maybery MR, *et al*. Angioplasty for the treatment of symptomatic vasospasm following subarachnoid hemorrhage. *J Neurosurg* 1989;**71**:654–60.

173 Zubkov YN, Nikiforov BM, Shustin VA. Balloon catheter technique for dilatation of constricted cerebral arteries after aneurysmal SAH. *Acta Neurochir* 1984;**70**:65–79.

174 Linskey ME, Horton JA, Rao GF, Yonas H. Fatal rupture of the intracranial carotid artery during transluminal angioplasty for vasospasm induced by subarachnoid hemorrhage. *J Neurosurg* 1991;**74**:985–90.

175 Haley EC, Kassell NF, Alves WM, Weir BKA, Hansen CA. Phase II trial of tirilizad in aneurysmal subarachnoid hemorrhage. *J Neurosurg* 1995;**82**:786–90.

176 Matsni T, Asano T. Effects of new 21 amino steroid trilizad mesylate (U74006F) on chronic cerebral vasospasm in a "two hemorrhage" model of beagle dogs. *Neurosurgery* 1994;**34**:1035–9.

177 Smith S, Scherch HM, Hall ED. Protective effects of trilizad mesylate and metabolite U-89678 against blood-brain barner damage after subarachnoid hemorrhage and lipid perxidative neuronal injury. *J Neurosurg* 1996;**84**:229–33.

178 Kassell NF, Haley CE, Hansen C, Alves WM. Randomized, double blind, vehicle controlled trial of tirilyzate mesylate in patients with aneurysmal subarachnoid hemorrhage: a cooperative study in Europe, Australia and New Zealand. *J Neurosurg* 1996;**84**:221–8.

179 Hutter BO, Eislbach JM. Which neuropsychological deficits are hidden behind a good outcome (Glasgow = 1) after aneurysmal subarachnoid hemorrhage? *Neurosurgery* 1993;**33**:999–1006.

180 Ogden JA, Mee EW, Henning M. A prospective study of impairment of cognition and memory and recovery after subarachnoid hemorrhage. *Neurosurgery* 1993;**33**:572–87.

9 Cerebral infection

MILNE ANDERSON

Broadly speaking, infection within the skull can be categorised clinically under three headings: meningitis, encephalitis, and localised space-occupation. These are not mutually exclusive, and commonly, two—or less commonly, all three—clinical syndromes may be found in the same patient. Symptoms and signs that are common to all three are pyrexia, headache, disturbance of conscious level, and focal neurological signs. With meningitis, photophobia, neck stiffness, vomiting, and a variable degree of altered consciousness are found. Encephalitis implies disease of brain parenchyma and, although there are usually signs of meningitis in addition, the findings are of altered mental state earlier in the evolution of the illness, together with more marked deterioration of conscious level, epileptic seizures, and focal neurology. The localised space-occupying syndrome may occur with local suppuration and abscess or granuloma formation, necrotising encephalitis, or with infarction as a result of arteritis or phlebitis. With each syndrome there may or may not be evidence of coexistent systemic or localised infection elsewhere.

Acute meningitis is the most common of the cerebral infection syndromes. Epidemiology, pathogenesis, and evolution are complex, and vary with geography and with age. Presentation occurs within hours, or at most a few days, of the onset of symptoms which, with the signs, are characteristic: headache, fever, photophobia, irritability, neck stiffness, and changed mental state. The causal agent is either a virus or a bacterium. Fungi and parasites cause acute meningitis only in exceptional circumstances. Viral meningitis is a much more benign illness than the bacterial form.

Viral meningitis

The term "acute aseptic meningitis" was coined by Wallgren in 1925[1] to describe acute meningeal irritation, benign and self-limiting, with complete recovery and sterile pleocytic CSF.

It has since become evident that at least 70% of such cases are caused by viruses. CNS viral infections are complications of systemic viral infections, and the virus gains access to the brain by the bloodstream or, less commonly, by travelling up peripheral nerves.[2] Viral meningitis is the result of haematogenous infection and, to enter the CNS, the virus must cross the endothelial cell junctions of the blood–brain barrier, the ability to do this being dependent upon surface adhesion molecules on the cells, surface charges and cellular receptors of the virus, and the property of entering infected cells.[3] Certain viruses preferentially infect the meninges, choroid plexus, and ependyma rather than cerebral parenchyma, causing meningitis; others infect neurons and glia to cause encephalitis. There is, however, considerable overlap, and some viruses may cause meningoencephalitis, incorporating signs of both.

Most cases of viral meningitis occur in children and young adults worldwide. Infections occur throughout the year, with a preponderance in summer and autumn in temperate climates. The annual reported incidence varies from 11 to 27 cases per 100 000,[4][5] and over 7000 cases are reported annually in the United States:[6] the actual number of infections is almost certainly several multiples higher, because of under-reporting. Over half are caused by enteroviruses—coxsackie B or echo, and less commonly by herpes simplex type 1, varicella zoster, mumps, lymphocytic choriomeningitis, and HIV (box 1).

The clinical onset is usually rapid over hours, with pyrexia, malaise, headache, neck stiffness, photophobia, lethargy, myalgia, and irritability. Most cases do not progress further, and the subject can be roused easily and remains coherent. If the conscious level reduces, or focal signs or seizures occur, encephalitis is implied. Resolution begins within a few days and is complete within two weeks in most. A few will have persistent malaise and myalgia for some weeks. The pathogen is seldom identified clinically—parotitis and orchitis may point to mumps, arthralgia and lymphadenopathy to HIV, myalgia and myocarditis to coxsackie virus, and rashes to enteroviruses. The illness is not as severe and prolonged as bacterial meningitis, and the signs are not so marked.

226

Box 1—Viral causes of cerebral infection

Meningitis
Enteroviruses
   Echo
   Polio
   Coxsackie
Herpes simplex 2
Lymphocytic choriomeningitis
Varicella zoster
Mumps
HIV

Encephalitis
Herpes simplex
Varicella zoster
Cytomegalovirus
Epstein–Barr virus
HIV
Mumps
Measles
Rabies
Arboviruses

Differential diagnosis

Conditions from which viral meningitis must be differentiated are the early stages of bacterial meningitis, some cases of subarachnoid haemorrhage and other causes of aseptic meningitis, partially treated bacterial meningitis, meningitis caused by fastidious bacteria, fungi and parasites which do not readily grow in routine culture, parameningeal infection, inflammation or neoplasia, and collagen disease. To confirm the diagnosis, CSF examination is mandatory, but not before dangerously raised intracranial pressure or a space-occupying lesion has been excluded by appropriate imaging. CSF pressure is normal or slightly raised, and the fluid is clear to the naked eye. White cell counts are in the range of up to 500–1000 mm^3, mainly lymphocytes, although, in some, polymorphs may predominate. In such cases it is prudent to re-examine CSF 12–24 hours later to identify a lymphocytosis and exclude a bacterial cause.[7] CSF protein may be slightly raised, glucose is normal or only slightly reduced. Numerous laboratory tests have been applied to CSF with the claim that they differentiate a bacterial from a viral aetiology, but none is sufficiently discriminating to be useful. These include lactate, lysozyme, C-reactive protein, and creatinine kinase estimations. A similar lack of specificity applies to the occasional abnormalities which may be seen in blood counts, blood biochemistry, and the EEG.

In most cases it is not necessary to establish an exact aetiology for treatment purposes, as the disease is benign and self-limiting and, provided other similar treatable diseases have been excluded, symptomatic treatment with analgesics and antiemetics is all that is required. Antibiotics should not be given.

To establish the aetiology, the virus may be isolated from CSF or by serological studies of acute and convalescent serum samples, identification of IgM antibody or viral antigen in CSF. The application of recently developed immunological and DNA probe amplification techniques, including polymerase chain reaction (PCR), to detect viral antigen, is promising.[8] In the UK, their use at present is dictated more by local availability than by clinical need.

Viral encephalitis

Acute viral encephalitis is due to direct invasion of brain parenchyma, and the clinical manifestations are caused by cell dysfunction from this invasion and associated inflammatory change. At the bedside this may be indistinguishable from post-infectious encephalitis, the pathology of which is perivenous demyelination thought to be caused by allergic or immune reactions triggered after a latent period by viral infection.[9 10] Viruses are far and away the commonest cause of encephalitis globally, but in certain locations and seasons other organisms such as malaria and other protozoans, rickettsiae, and fungi may induce an encephalitic syndrome.

As with meningitis, so with encephalitis, the virus reaches the brain by the bloodstream. Entry may be through the skin following an insect bite, as with arbovirus infection, or via the respiratory or gastrointestinal route. Local replication ensues, the inoculum spills into blood and so to the reticuloendothelial system whence, following further replication, viraemia increases, and spread takes place to other sites including the CNS. Modification of this process by host immune responses may occur, and if these are compromised, disease progression may be fulminant. Most cases of encephalitis are caused in this way. The virus may also ascend neurons centripetally to lodge in brain cells, as with herpes simplex encephalitis and rabies. Fortunately, encephalitis is a rare complication of common viral infections, and most patients with systemic viral infections do not develop neurological signs.

Certain viruses exhibit tropism towards specific cell types—the limbic system in rabies, temporal lobes in herpes simplex encephalitis—and this may produce clinical signs that are diagnostically useful. In most cases of encephalitis, however, signs and symptoms are common to most pathogens, and diagnostic clues must be sought elsewhere: is there evidence of infection elsewhere, such as the characteristic rash of varicella or measles, or the parotitis of mumps? Has there been travel to or from an area that harbours known vectors? Is there past or present evidence of an animal or insect bite? What is the season of the year? Diagnostic tests may help, yet in perhaps as many as a third of all cases, no specific aetiology can be established.

Viral encephalitis is not rare, and it occurs globally. In the United Kingdom and Europe, most cases are sporadic accompaniments of common infections such as mumps, measles, and herpes simplex (box 1). In the United States, sporadic and epidemic forms are caused by the arboviruses (*ar*thropod-*bor*ne), and Japanese B encephalitis causes most epidemic infections elsewhere. As many as 20 000 cases per annum may occur in the United States.[11]

Patients who develop viral encephalitis often have a prodrome lasting several days, which may include myalgia, fever, malaise, mild upper respiratory infection, rash, or parotitis. The development of headache, mental change, and drowsiness implies encephalitis, which is usually associated with meningitic features. As the disease progresses, disorientation and disturbance of behaviour and speech worsen, and drowsiness becomes coma. Epileptic seizures are common, and focal signs may appear appropriate to the area of the brain taking the brunt of the infection—hallucinations and memory upset from the temporal lobes, hemiparesis, spasticity, sensory loss and speech upset, and cerebellar deficits. There may also be signs of raised intracranial pressure. The very young, the very old, and those with compromised immune systems often have more severe disease. Signs should be sought in other organ systems, which may point to a particular virus. Some forms of encephalitis have specific features which are briefly discussed later.

Differential diagnosis

The list of other diseases that may cause a similar clinical picture is large, and includes all forms of bacterial meningitis, malaria and other protozoal and fungal infestations, intracranial suppuration, septicaemia and endocarditis, metastatic disease and collagenoses, and drug abuse.

Faced with a patient with rapid onset of pyrexia and stupor or coma, the above potentially remediable conditions need to be excluded quickly. Blood counts and biochemical tests are not diagnostic but may be abnormal as a result of inadequate hydration or inappropriate secretion of antidiuretic hormone. Blood films should be examined for malaria parasites, and blood cultures set up.

As these results are awaited, the intracranial contents should be imaged to determine if there is space-occupation, cerebral oedema, or focal areas of infarction such as may occur in the temporal lobes with herpes simplex encephalitis. Scans must be interpreted with close attention to their timing in the evolution of the disease: in the first two or three days no abnormality may be evident, and changes may not show for five or six days, so repeat scanning may be necessary. The EEG is abnormal, most often showing non-specific diffuse slow-wave activity, perhaps with seizure activity. Temporal lobe focal abnormality with high-voltage spike and slow-wave complexes is highly suggestive of herpes simplex encephalitis. CSF should be examined as soon as possible when deemed safe; unfortunately cranial scanning does not convey an accurate picture of intracranial pressure, and judgement of the potential safety of lumbar puncture requires not a little luck. CSF is often under pressure and the cell count is raised, from 10 to as many as several thousand white cells per mm^3, usually lymphocytes, but polymorphs may predominate in the early stages. Red cells may be found if there is a necrotising component, as in herpes simplex encephalitis. The glucose content is normal, protein is raised, and organisms are not seen.

Treatment

In the recent past, treatment of viral encephalitis was symptomatic, and no specific drug would influence the outcome. This has changed with the advent of acyclovir and other forms of antiviral chemotherapy, so it is now imperative to identify the organism as soon as possible, or at least to determine whether it is herpes simplex. Early reports of the application of PCR and other techniques to the rapid detection of viral antigen in CSF are encouraging.[12][13] In my view, brain biopsy no longer has a place in the diagnosis of viral encephalitis, except to determine if a lesion demonstrated by scan is an abscess, granuloma, or tumour. The complication rate is over 3%, and there is no guarantee that the area biopsied will contain virus. It is safer to begin treatment with acyclovir if clinical suspicion is high.

With the exception of that caused by herpes simplex, the treatment of viral encephalitis is symptomatic, and requires the maintenance of adequate nutrition, hydration, and oxygenation. Seizures are controlled with anticonvulsants, and secondary infections are treated as necessary. Intracranial hypertension and cerebral oedema may be a problem, and there is no consensus on the correct treatment. Intubation and hyperventilation, glycerol, mannitol, and dexamethasone have all been used, and I continue to use dexamethasone in severely ill patients, despite theoretical objections.

Specific encephalitides

Herpes simplex—This is the most common cause of sporadic encephalitis in Europe and North America, with an incidence of up to 0·5 per 100 000 population each year—almost certainly an underestimate because milder cases go unrecognised. It occurs throughout the year, and almost all cases are caused by herpes simplex virus type 1. It is no more common in those with compromised immune systems, and it affects patients of any age. A third are below 20, and half over 50.[14] The clinical presentation is enormously variable. Onset is usually insidious, with a prodrome of 4–10 days, with malaise, pyrexia, and irritability, followed by frontal and temporal lobe disturbance of personality change, hallucinations, psychiatric upset, and increasing focal signs, seizures, and deteriorating conscious level. In perhaps as many as 87%, focal signs appear.[15] In a few, the onset is cataclysmic, and the evolution is compressed into only a few days. Abscess, tumour, granuloma, vascular disease, and other forms of viral encephalitis are the other diagnoses that have been mistaken for herpes simplex encephalitis.[16] Focal changes on CT, MRI, and EEG, as already described, are helpful but not pathognomonic.

Treatment must be given quickly with acyclovir, 10 mg/kg by intravenous infusion over one hour, every eight hours for 10 days. This has been shown to diminish mortality rate to 30%.[17] Most people use dexamethasone despite objections that interferon synthesis may be inhibited.

Varicella zoster

Encephalitis accounts for 90% of the neurological complications of varicella, which are in themselves rare, affecting 0·1% of cases.[18] In half, the encephalitis is of cerebellar type, with ataxia, dysarthria, headache, and drowsiness coming on about a week after the rash begins,[9] but the neurological onset may precede the rash. Convulsions are common,[19] and progression to hemiplegia, cranial nerve palsies, aphasia, and coma may ensue. Patients with the cerebellar form usually recover completely, but 10% of those with the general form die.[9] Encephalitis may rarely follow shingles. Management is symptomatic, as already described.

Cytomegalovirus—This is not an important cause of encephalitis except in neonates and in immunocompromised patients, recipients of organ transplants, and patients with AIDS. Treatment with antiviral agents has, to date, been nugatory.

Epstein–Barr virus—Meningoencephalitis has been described as a rare complication of Epstein–Barr virus infection.[20] There are no specific features, and the prognosis is excellent.

Measles—Acute encephalitis occurring in the course of measles infection is usually caused by a postinfectious, perivenous, demyelinating, allergic phenomenon, although in some there may be direct virus-induced cellular damage, and virus has been isolated.[21] Clinically the manifestations are the same, and occur in up to one in 1000 cases above the age of two, the frequency increasing with age. Typically, as the exanthem begins to fade after seven or eight days, fever recurs and encephalitis develops rapidly, with convulsions, focal signs, myoclonus, and coma.[22][23] There are no specific features on investigation, and treatment is symptomatic. Mortality is high at 15%, and most are left with some disability.[23]

Mumps encephalitis—This complication is rare, occurring in less than 1% of cases, and has no specific features; it follows up to two weeks after development of parotitis, though this may be absent in up to half.[24][25] Treatment is symptomatic and prognosis is excellent.

Epidemic encephalitis

Arboviruses cause epidemic encephalitis in various parts of the world. They are not an important cause of encephalitis in Britain, but with the increasing ease and frequency of intercontinental travel, cases are now being recognised, and the likelihood is that the frequency will increase. It is imperative therefore that a full history of travel abroad be taken from anyone suspected of neurological infection, and arbovirus encephalitis should be suspected if there has been exposure to insect bites in countries known to harbour these viruses.

All of these arboviruses are perpetuated by zoonoses of insignificant infection in birds and smaller vertebrates. Transmission is by an arthropod vector, mosquito, or tick. Replication and viraemia develop after a bite. Most people suffer only a mild systemic illness, but some go on to develop encephalitis, the severity of which depends upon the strain of the virus. Clinical features are common to all, with some variation in incubation, progression, and severity, and they cannot be diagnosed on clinical grounds alone. There are no specific features to be found on imaging, on the EEG or in the CSF. Diagnosis is by demonstration of antibody rise in paired serum samples. Treatment is symptomatic.

Eastern equine encephalitis—Birds of the Atlantic and Gulf coasts of America are the reservoir of this rare condition. Epidemics may occur in horses. Cases occur at migration time, summer, and autumn, and children are most affected, with an acute encephalitis which may be abrupt and virulent, and a mortality rate of 70%.[26]

Western equine encephalitis—This is less severe, occurring in eastern, central, and western United States, Canada, and eastern South America.

St Louis encephalitis—This disease shares the same clinical features in the same areas and in central America. West of the Mississippi it is endemic, and cases occur in epidemics or sporadically from July to October. Most cases are benign and of short duration.

California and La Crosse viruses—These viruses are similar and cause the same disease in central and midwest United States. The reservoir is small rodents and the vector is the mosquito *Aedes* sp. Children are affected, with a peak in August and September. Clinical onset is sudden, and recovery takes place within 10 days.

Central European encephalitis—This encephalitis may be contracted from woodlands in Scandinavia through to northern

233

Greece and the former Yugoslavia, and more cases are being reported from Austria. The virus is maintained in small woodland mammals and transmitted to people who enter the forest for recreation or work and are bitten by the tick *Ixodes* sp. There is a biphasic course with an initial 'flu-like illness, followed within two weeks by mild meningitis or encephalitis, perhaps with muscle weakness. Management is symptomatic and recovery is usually complete. Diagnosis is serological.

Russian spring–summer encephalitis—Russian spring–summer encephalitis is a similar, more severe, condition.

Japanese encephalitis—This is the most common arbovirus infection worldwide, and is endemic in southeast Asia, Japan, China, Philippines, Borneo, and large areas of the Indian subcontinent. Birds and domestic animals are the reservoir, mosquitos the vector. Encephalitis is seen most commonly in those under 15 and in the aged. After an incubation period of 1–2 weeks there is abrupt onset of encephalitis, often with myalgia. Extrapyramidal features have been noted.[27][28] Convalescence may be prolonged and sequelae are common. Treatment is symptomatic and diagnosis is serological.[29]

Rabies

In Britain, recognition of a case of clinical rabies is exceptionally rare and, numerically, barely merits inclusion in a description of neurological emergencies. However, rabies is endemic throughout the world except for the UK, Ireland, Antarctica, Australasia, Japan, and islands of the Caribbean, Mediterranean, and Scandinavia. Most of the cases now seen in the United States have been contracted abroad and, where countries have introduced programmes to control domestic rabies in cats and dogs, the incidence in humans has dropped.[30]

Infection in humans results from transcutaneous inoculation through the bite of a rabid animal, although, rarely, aerosol inhalation of infected bat droppings has been implicated,[30a] and person-to-person contact by corneal transplantation has been documented.[30b] It is therefore necessary for all personnel who come in contact with such patients to exercise the strictest precautions, although no case has been reported to have been infected in

234

such circumstances. Once the skin has been broken, virus replicates at the site, then ascends peripheral nerves via acetylcholine receptors to the CNS. The weight of inoculum of virus and proximity of the bite to the brain are probably important because more severe bites nearer to the face result in a higher incidence of mortality—up to 60%—whereas more peripheral and less severe bites may not result in disease. Of bites from proven rabid beasts, 5–15% result in rabies in humans. If prompt attention can be given to local wound care and debridement, followed by the administration of human rabies immunoglobulin and active immunisation with human diploid fibroblast culture vaccine, clinical disease can be prevented.[30b]

The incubation period varies enormously, and may be as short as one week but is on average three weeks to three months, when the time of the bite can be established.[30c] In most cases history will reveal that there has been exposure to an animal bite,[30d] but if consciousness is impaired, or the child is young and fears chastisement, or, more worryingly, the original incident took place so long ago as to have been forgotten—six years in a recent report—this essential clue may be lacking. At first the symptoms may suggest 'flu—malaise, fever, headache, and myalgia—and may be associated with paraesthesiae at the site of the bite. Cerebral involvement declares itself within days, with apprehension, excitation, delirium, hallucinations, and seizures, and this progresses to the characteristic "hydrophobia" which results from laryngeal and pharyngeal spasms. These may be provoked by the smallest sensory stimulus, such as a draught of air, and become progressively worse and more severe, with opisthotonos and convulsions. Coma and death provide a merciful release within three weeks. Recovery has been recorded but, if it happens, it is exceptionally rare.

Diagnosis

Diagnosis is straightforward if an appropriate history can be obtained, but where that is lacking, the onset of hydrophobia provides the clue. Rabies should be considered in the differential diagnosis of all encephalitides contracted abroad, and it is important to remember that perhaps 15% of all cases present as a Guillain–Barré type of syndrome. Cranial imaging and EEG do not show specific features, and CSF may show a pleocytosis and raised protein. Rapid diagnosis can be reached by the demonstration of rabies antigen in neck skin biopsy,[31] which is said to be more accurate than corneal smears. Virus may be isolated from saliva and other fluids.

Treatment

Treatment does not alter the inevitably fatal outcome but does relieve distress to patients and relatives. Sedation may be necessary in the "furious" stage, anticonvulsants may prevent seizures, but it may be necessary to paralyse and ventilate the patient to prevent the severe generalised spasms of advanced hydrophobia. There is no evidence that steroids, immune suppression, antibiotics, or antiviral agents help. All secretions from the patient should be regarded as potentially hazardous, and any staff thought to have been inoculated by them should have a course of immunisation.

HIV

Cerebral infection is a frequent accompaniment of HIV infection. The virus itself affects the brain, and the systemic immune suppression which accompanies AIDS renders the sufferer liable to superadded and opportunistic infection which frequently attacks the brain. The manifestations of HIV infection of the brain coexist with opportunistic infection, and may result in a complex and confused syndrome constellation. Many of the features are chronic in evolution and some are acute. In practice, any change in neurological status in a patient with AIDS usually presents as an emergency because of the danger of opportunistic infection. Conversely, the finding of an unusual cerebral infection in a patient not known to be immune suppressed should raise the suspicion that he or she may have HIV infection. Many excellent accounts of the epidemiology and classification of the natural progression of HIV infection are available, and are not discussed further here.[32-34]

HIV is spread by inoculation of virus by homosexual or heterosexual intercourse, by contaminated blood or blood products, or vertically in utero, during birth or by breast milk. During the first eight weeks after infection, about 50% of patients will have a mild pyrexial illness like glandular fever, with a rash and lymphadenopathy, and seroconversion. At about this time the neurotropic HIV virus may infect the neuraxis and produce a self-limiting aseptic lymphocytic meningitis, or, less frequently, encephalitis.[34a] In 5–10% of patients, antibody tests at this stage are usually negative, but serum p24 antigen is found. HIVs are RNA retroviruses that encode for reverse transcriptase, which enables a DNA copy of viral RNA to be produced in an infected cell, where it becomes incorporated in the cell genome, conferring the property of persistent infection which lasts for life. It may remain latent or it may cause disease by producing virus. HIV attacks T helper lymphocytes via the CD4 molecule on the cell surface. Within a few weeks the cells die and the helper/suppressor ratio is disturbed, with resulting depression of cellular and humoral immunity and progression to full-blown AIDS.[34b 34c]

The severity of infection is determined by the strain and virulence of the virus, and the presence of concurrent viral infection with cytomegalovirus, Epstein–Barr virus, or herpes simplex virus. There may also be a genetic susceptibility. Mild prodromal symptoms of immuno-deficiency give rise to the syndromes of peristent generalised lymphadenopathy (PGL) and AIDS-related complex (ARC), which progress eventually to full-blown AIDS. Not all do so, however, perhaps 25% remaining healthy 12 years after infection. Because HIV can infect the neuraxis early, and persist in the CNS indefinitely, CSF studies cannot prove that HIV causes a particular neurological syndrome.[34d] Some 40% of all HIV patients have CSF abnormalities, and a large proportion are asymptomatic. There is a lymphocytic pleocytosis, raised protein, and normal glucose content, and as many as 20% may grow HIV in culture.[34e 34f] Antibodies, mainly immunoglobulin but also IgA and IgM, appear in CSF, and p24 antigen is often present in higher concentration than in serum. Unfortunately these levels do not correlate well with clinical status.[34g] Detection and quantification of viral load is now possible using PCR.[34h]

AIDS–dementia complex

AIDS–dementia complex occurs during established AIDS and, with more subtle neuropsychological and neurophysiological techniques, it is possible to demonstrate mild cognitive defects in early infection.[35] It is now recognised that 90% of AIDS patients will develop this complex before death. The usual course is for the subject to become withdrawn, apathetic, and mentally slow, and progress inexorably to become increasingly demented.[36] The course may, however, be interrupted by acute relapses with confusion and psychosis, when the patient may present as a neurological emergency, and it is necessary to exclude other CNS infections, neoplasia, and systemic illness as a cause.

In AIDS–dementia complex, CT is normal or shows cerebral atrophy, and MRI demonstrates diffuse white-matter abnormalities which correlate with neuropathological abnormalities of ADC.[36a] CSF examination is likely to be abnormal, as described, and is necessary to exclude complicating infection. In children, 50% develop a similar progressive encephalopathy which is usually fatal within a year.

Opportunistic infections

Infection and lymphoma can complicate and alter the progression of AIDS and precipitate a neurological emergency. Toxoplasma, cytomegalovirus, herpes simplex, herpes zoster, cryptococcus, histoplasma, and other fungi appropriate to geography, tuberculosis, and syphilis are all frequent pathogens. Progressive multifocal leucoencephalopathy may also complicate AIDS and, unfortunately, more than one syndrome may be present at any given time, so the clinical picture can be confused.

All patients with AIDS should be checked for syphilis with a specific antitreponemal test. A negative tuberculin skin test is likely in these patients even if they have tuberculosis.[37] If a focal lesion is seen on CT or MRI, it may be toxoplasmosis,[38 39] tuberculoma, lymphoma, or brain abscess. Lymphoma usually shows solid, multicentric lesions, but can show ring enhancement. Single or multiple, ring-enhancing, hyperdense or hypodense lesions may be caused by any of these pathologies: no appearance is specific. Because 10–40% of patients with AIDS will develop toxoplasmosis during the course of their illness, and serological tests are not sufficiently specific to confirm that toxoplasmosis is the cause of the lesion, biopsy must be considered. In such circumstances accepted practice (which I adopt) is to treat for toxoplasmosis with pyrimethamine and sulphadiazine, and with dexamethasone to reduce brain swelling. If the lesion is due to toxoplasmosis, improvement occurs within 10–14 days and can be monitored by serial scanning.[40]

If improvement does not occur, if there is clinical deterioration, or if diagnostic doubt remains, biopsy should take place, and treatment given as appropriate. Tuberculosis is an increasing problem due both to *Mycobacterium tuberculosis* and to *M avium* complex disease, and my threshold for deciding to perform a biopsy is diminishing, in order to make this diagnosis early: treatment of *M avium* complex disease responds better to regimens that incorporate clofazimine and amikacin.[41] At present there is no satisfactory regimen for the treatment of established HIV infection, but appropriate and prompt treatment of these infective complications can lead to prolonged remission.

Bacterial meningitis

Any bacterium is capable of causing meningitis, given favourable circumstances (boxes 2 and 3). Meningitis may come about as part of a generalised illness or as a complication of disease elsewhere. In practice, most cases are caused by organisms with properties of virulence which allow access to the CNS. With the exception of the neonatal period, *Haemophilus influenzae*, *Neisseria meningitidis*, and *Streptococcus pneumoniae* account for 70% of all cases. Neonatal meningitis may be caused by any organism, and the most frequently encountered pathogens are

---

Box 2—Bacterial meningitis: causal organisms

Neonates
    Gram-negative bacilli
    Streptococci (usually group B)
    Listeria sp.

Children
    Haemophilus sp.
    Meningococci
    Pneumococci

Adults
    Pneumococci
    Meningococci
    Staphylococci
    Listeria sp.
    Streptococci

Mycobacterium tuberculosis can affect children and adults

Box 3—Bacteria linked to underlying cause of
meningitis

Cause	Organism
Diabetes mellitus	Pneumococci
	Staphylococci
	Gram-negative bacilli
Alcohol	Pneumococci
Sickle cell disease	Pneumococci
Skull fracture	Gram-negative bacilli
	Staphylococci
Dural fistula/CSF leak	Pneumococci
	Gram-negative bacilli
CNS shunt	*Staphylococcus epidermidis*
Pregnancy/childbirth	*Listeria* sp.
	Streptococci
Cell-mediated immune defect	*Listeria* sp.
Humoral immune defect	Pneumocci
	Haemophilus sp.
	Meningococci
Neutropenia	*Pseudomonas* sp.

Gram-negative bacilli, particularly *E coli* K1, other enteric bacilli, *Pseudomonas* sp. and group B streptococci. Neonatal meningitis is not discussed further here.

The epidemiology of meningitis is complex, and varies with the age of the patient and geography. About 70% of cases are seen in children. *H influenzae* and *N meningitidis* are the main causes in this group; in adults, *S pneumoniae* and *N meningitidis* predominate, and there is an increasing number of cases caused by Gram-negative bacilli and *Listeria* sp., particularly in the elderly. Streptococci and staphylococci also cause sporadic cases—the meningococcus remains the only significant cause of epidemics. *H influenzae* is a more common pathogen in the United States than in the United Kingdom (48% v 29%) where the meningococcus and pneumococcus predominate (45% v 33%).[42 43] Gram-negative bacilli tend to occur in association with head injuries, following neurosurgery, in patients who have compromised immune systems, and in the elderly. One disturbing factor is the increase in the number of cases nosocomially acquired.[44] Streptococci infect puerperal women, the elderly, and those with immunosuppression, as does *Listeria* sp. Staphylococcal infection may complicate neurosurgical procedures and head trauma, and also affect those with immunosuppression or endocarditis. Anaerobic organisms cause less than 1% of cases. Infection with more than one organism also occurs in 1%, and in similar circumstances—paranasal sinus and ear infections, skull fractures, neurosurgery, and immunosuppression.[45 46] Tuberculosis remains a significant cause of meningitis in the United Kingdom and the United States. Many other organisms may also cause meningitis, commonly of a more chronic nature, which may rapidly develop into an acute emergency in patients with compromised immune systems.

Progress in diagnosis and treatment

Advances in the investigation and management of bacterial meningitis over the past 40 years or so, including the continuing development of antibiotics, the introduction of CT and MRI, the application of improved techniques of bacterial culture, and now the widespread use of molecular methods incorporating PCR,[47] have permitted treatment to be given on a more rational basis to a wider range of patients. It is disappointing therefore that mortality and morbidity from the main forms of bacterial meningitis have failed to diminish to any substantial degree over the same length of time. Fortunately, in recent years, new understanding of the pathophysiology of the changes that occur in bacterial meningitis has become available,[48-50] from which it will be possible to develop new strategies for treatment.

To cause bacterial meningitis, the infecting organisms must be able to overcome host defence mechanisms that protect the neuraxis, and their neurotropic properties derive from their ability to thwart these mechanisms. The upper respiratory tract is the favoured, but not the only, site for colonisation by these organisms, which must cross the mucosal epithelium which secretes IgA. They render IgA non-functional by secreting IgA protease, and attach to the epithelium by mechanisms that vary between species, and await full characterisation. To enter and survive in the bloodstream the bacterium must avoid circulating complement, and its ability to do this is attributed to capsular polysaccharide, the molecular basis of which varies between organisms and is a major factor determining virulence. Once established in

241

the bloodstream the blood–brain barrier must be penetrated to enter CSF: this is the least understood element of pathogenesis. The possession of pili to aid binding to surface molecules appears to influence virulence. Once within the CSF there is virtually no immunoglobulin and complement activity, and opsonic attack on bacteria cannot take place—low levels of CSF complement mediated opsonic activity have been associated with a poor outcome.[50a] Host reaction to this bacterial invasion determines the resulting clinical features of meningitis.

One of the major features of meningitis is a CSF neutrophil response. The exact mechanism by which white blood cells cross the blood–brain barrier is not yet known. The release of some bacterial cell wall components into the CSF stimulates the release of inflammatory cytokines, including interleukins 1 and 6, tumour necrosis factor, and prostaglandins into CSF, and there is strong evidence that their presence induces inflammation and disruption of the blood–brain barrier. By a complex series of interactions, as yet ill understood, cerebral blood flow increases, inducing vasogenic cerebral oedema and raised intracranial pressure. With the progression of inflammation, cytotoxic oedema develops, cerebral blood flow falls, vasculitis progresses, and intracranial pressure rises further. Interstitial oedema results from obstruction of CSF flow from subarachnoid space to blood. Cerebrovascular autoregulation is disrupted[51] and the brain becomes at risk from either hyper- or hypoperfusion. Evidence is accumulating that many of these changes occur early in the course of meningitis, and treatment regimens that reduce intracranial pressure while maintaining cerebral perfusion and blood flow may be useful.[50]

Diagnosis

The clinical features of a typical case of meningitis are easy to recognise—fever, malaise, headache, neck stiffness, irritability, and confusion. Usually these features appear over the space of a day or two but in some fulminant cases the signs may develop within hours. In as many as 20% of cases these typical features may be lacking: this is particularly so with the very young, the very old, the very ill, and those with compromised immune systems. The possibility of meningitis should be entertained in every child or adult in the above groups who has lethargy, altered mental status, drowsiness, or pyrexia, especially if neck stiffness is present. It is important to recognise that neck stiffness may *not* be present, and the physician must include meningitis in the differential diagnosis of a very wide range of diseases.

Epileptic convulsions occur with meningitis in any age group, are particularly common in young children, affecting up to 40% of cases, and may be the presenting feature.[52] Convulsions associated with pyrexia—"febrile convulsions"—commonly occur in the very young age group; each such patient may have meningitis, which poses the question, does each require lumbar puncture? Evidence suggests that the answer is "No". In one study,[53] four out of 328, and 15 of 304 in another,[54] had signs of meningitis on lumbar puncture. If the convulsion is brief and not associated with continuing neurological deficit or focal feature, if the child rapidly regains consciousness, and there are no other signs of meningitis, it is reasonable to observe the child closely for some hours rather than perform a lumbar puncture straight away.

Skin rashes are evident in about a third of patients, and their presence should be sought, because in some they may be sparse. A diffuse maculopapular eruption which progresses to include petechiae or frank purpura accompanies 50–60% of cases of meningococcal meningitis. Other bacteria—*Listeria* sp., staphylococci, pneumococci, *Haemophilus* sp., and viruses, particularly echo 9, may also cause rashes. Rarely, a rash may be due to a reaction to an antibiotic or other drug, but this seldom occurs early in the course of the disease. Shock may accompany any fulminant or overwhelming meningitis, and often complicates meningococcal infection. Focal neurological signs complicate meningitis in at least 15% of cases.[55] Hemiparesis implies arteritis or phlebitis and resulting infarction, or an evolving brain abscess. Cranial nerve palsies, commonly of the sixth and third nerves, are caused by basal exudation and inflammation. Sixth nerve palsies may indicate that intracranial pressure is rising dangerously. The level of consciousness must be closely observed and documented, because it correlates best of all with the likely clinical outcome. Mortality rate rises dramatically as consciousness decreases,[56 57] and approaches 55% for adults in coma. Cerebellar signs may be noted in some cases, and have no aetiological significance.

When assessing a case of meningitis, diligent search must be made for a non-neurological locus of infection, and cultures made from it, or for a pre-existing or contemporaneous illness that enables organisms to become more rapidly pathogenic.

There is some correlation between organism and condition.

Pneumococcal meningitis is associated with otitis media, skull fractures, alcoholism, and sickle cell disease, and up to 50% will have pneumonia. Haemophilus meningitis is uncommon after early childhood and its occurrence raises the possibility of a parameningeal focus of infection, including ear, nose, and basal skull fracture. Staphylococcal infection complicates the implantation of neurosurgical devices such as shunts. In those with immunosuppression, including AIDS, simultaneous infection with more than one organism can occur. Tuberculous meningitis may rarely be complicated by superadded infection. In the author's experience, diabetic patients are dangerously liable to misdiagnosis because their symptoms may be misinterpreted as being due to hypoglycaemia or to uncontrolled diabetes, and meningitis can exacerbate diabetes. If there is a history of meningitis in the past, there is probably a dural fistula from previous head injury or, much more rarely, the patient suffers from an inherited immunodeficiency state. In all cases, blood cultures should be taken before antibiotics are given.[55]

Once the possibility of meningitis is entertained the diagnosis must be confirmed straight away. Next to the conscious level on admission, the factor that has the most deleterious effect on prognosis is delay in beginning treatment. CSF examination is the only sure way to confirm the diagnosis, and this is almost always done by lumbar puncture. It may, in circumstances such as the existence of hydrocephalus, be necessary to puncture the ventricle to obtain a specimen. In established meningitis there is usually no difficulty in reaching a diagnosis. Very early in the evolution of the disease, however, or if antibiotics have already been administered, or if the organism is fastidious in its requirements for laboratory culture, it may not be possible to identify the causal bacterium. Discussion of the problem with the microbiological laboratory before taking CSF usually more than recoups the time spent, in order to ensure that appropriate culture media are available, and precautions taken to look for anaerobic organisms.

Lumbar puncture—Bacterial meningitis raises intracranial pressure. In most cases physiological mechanisms cope, and no long term, untoward effects result. It is now becoming recognised that the intracranial pressure can rise to potentially lethal levels, with cerebral oedema and brain herniation. In such circumstances, to do a lumbar puncture can lead to rapid deterioration and death.

To reconcile this with the necessity of reaching an early diagnosis is, in some cases, difficult; the correct decision depends on experience and a degree of luck. In my view, CT should be undertaken immediately if there is evidence of focal neurology on examination or historically, if the conscious level is reduced or the patient is confused, if headache is severe, or if there are frequent seizures. A recent report[57] suggested that CT had little influence on the management of bacterial meningitis in children, but did not address the problem of recognition of raised intracranial pressure and lumbar puncture. Cerebral herniation and death do occur as a result of injudicious CSF examination in cases of suspected meningitis,[58-60] and a normal CT scan does not always mean that it is safe to proceed to lumbar puncture: until better procedures to monitor intracranial pressure become routine, this decision must be left to clinical experience, reassured by brain imaging to exclude space occupation and cerebral oedema.

If there is a bleeding diathesis or coagulation defect, these should be corrected before lumbar puncture. If it is decided that lumbar puncture is too dangerous, or there will be a delay before scanning can be done, immediate treatment with antibiotics should be given, after blood cultures have been taken. The antibiotic regimen chosen will be a "best guess", based on the age, medical background, geographical location, and clinical findings of the patient. CSF may be examined later when it is considered to be safe, and evidence of bacterial infection can be found by demonstration of antigen with newer techniques.[61 62] Anxiety that infection may be introduced to CSF by lumbar puncture in patients with bacteraemia is largely unfounded.[63]

CSF findings are of a raised cell count with polymorphs predominating, at least 60%. There is no agreed value for the absolute count but usually this falls within the hundreds or more. The protein content is increased, and the glucose is reduced. A sample of blood should be taken at the time of lumbar puncture for comparison: a ratio of CSF:blood glucose of less than 0·3 is abnormal and is found in about three quarters of patients.[64] Unfortunately this is not specific and may be found in other chronic forms of meningitis.

Identification of the causal organism under the microscope or on culture should be possible in up to 80% of patients. A plethora of tests has been devised over the years to differentiate bacterial from other forms of meningitis: unfortunately they all suffer from

245

lack of specificity or sensitivity,[65] and are being superseded by newer, molecular techniques.[61]

CT and MRI scans need to be interpreted with due consideration given to the timing of the scan in relation to the evolution of meningitis: early in the disease the scan may be normal, but such a finding does not exclude meningitis. There may be meningeal and ventricular ependymal enhancement, basal purulent exudate, small ventricles with cerebral oedema, or large ventricles from CSF flow obstruction in the aqueduct or basal cisterns. Later in the disease, areas of infarction from vasculitis, and subdural collections may be seen, particularly in children with haemophilus infection.[66 67] Brain imaging also permits exclusion of other conditions that may present like meningitis—subarachnoid and intracerebral haemorrhage, infarction, tumour, and brain abscess. MRI is better at demonstrating more subtle changes than CT, but it is technically much more difficult to carry out MRI on a confused and uncooperative patient, or on one who requires artificial ventilation, than it is to perform CT.

A full blood count and sedimentation rate should be carried out. These are frequently abnormal but unfortunately do not point to a specific pathogen. Blood gases, electrolytes, and serum osmolality must be monitored carefully, especially in children. Inappropriate secretion of antidiuretic hormone can lead to a rapid fall in sodium, particularly but not exclusively with haemophilus infection.[68] Other tests should be carried out according to clinical need.

Treatment

Once the diagnosis of bacterial meningitis has been made, treatment must be begun immediately. Precedence is given to maintaining cardiorespiratory function, adequate oxygenation, and tissue perfusion while the causal organism is being identified and the appropriate antibiotic regimen determined. If no organism can be found, antibiotic treatment is given on a "best guess" basis (box 4).

As mentioned earlier, the release of bacterial cell wall products into CSF stimulates inflammation, mediated in part by cytokines. Studies to determine the efficacy of the anti-inflammatory action of corticosteroids in reducing this inflammation have produced encouraging results in children, and trials are proceeding with adults. There is now good evidence that dexamethasone in a dose of 0·15 mg/kg body weight every six hours for four days reduces the incidence of neurological sequelae,[69-72] and this should be begun just before antibiotics are given. I believe the evidence is sufficiently good to justify the adoption of a similar policy in adult bacterial meningitis until further trial results are available. Dexamethasone also helps to reduce raised intracranial pressure and, given for a short time, any side effects are minimal.

Other anti-inflammatory agents which act at different stages are currently undergoing trials. These include non-steroidal, anti-inflammatory drugs, pentoxifylline, and monoclonal antibodies targeted specifically against human β_2 integrin.[48 73] There is a complex inter-relationship between cerebral blood flow, cerebral blood volume, cerebral perfusion pressure, cerebral oedema, and intracranial pressure which becomes disturbed in bacterial meningitis. Decreased cerebral blood flow,[74] cerebral oedema,[58] and reduced cerebral perfusion pressure[75] all adversely affect the outcome. Intracranial pressure is raised maximally within the first 48 hours,[76 77] and it should be possible to anticipate this and ameliorate the effects. Patients whose conscious level deteriorates should be considered for intracranial pressure monitoring; if the level rises above 15 mm Hg, treatment to lower the pressure should be given. The head of the bed should be raised, hyperventilation induced, and dexamethasone and mannitol administered.[78]

Choice of antibiotic

To treat meningitis effectively, it is necessary to achieve adequate bactericidal levels of antibiotic in CSF 10–20 times higher than the minimal bactericidal concentration in vitro for the particular organism. Ideally the antibiotic should be lipid soluble to facilitate transfer across the blood–brain barrier but this is not

---

Box 4—Bacterial meningitis: empirical treatment

Children: ampicillin and chloramphenicol or third-generation cephalosporin
Adults: penicillin and third-generation cephalosporin
The obtunded infected patient with no history or diagnostic clues: acyclovir, penicillin, and chloramphenicol or third-generation cephalosporin, metronidazole; and consider tuberculosis as a cause.

usually a problem in practice because meningeal inflammation disrupts the barrier and allows sufficient penetration. The rate at which it is metabolised and cleared from CSF determines the frequency and amount which must be given, and it should be active within purulent and acidic CSF. The choice of antibiotic will be determined by the organism found on microscopy, culture, or antigen detection, and modified by knowledge of local and nosocomial drug resistance patterns.

As important as the choice of antibiotic is the identification and eradication of any parameningeal focus of suppuration.

For *H influenzae* type B infections, ampicillin and chloramphenicol have been the mainstay of treatment, but an increasing number of β-lactamase-producing strains are resistant to ampicillin, and a smaller number of chloramphenicol acetyltransferase-producing organisms are resistant to chloramphenicol.[79] Third-generation cephalosporins are to be preferred, and cefotaxime or ceftriaxone have been most widely used and demonstrated to be effective.[80][81] For meningococcal meningitis, penicillin remains the preferred drug. There have been reports of meningococci resistant to penicillin,[82] but to date this does not appear to cause problems if large doses are given. Chloramphenicol or a third-generation cephalosporin may be used in people with adverse reactions to penicillin. Pneumococcal meningitis is best treated with penicillin. Penicillin-resistant strains are being recognised[79] and, in these circumstances, a third-generation cephalosporin or vancomycin should be used. Cephalosporins have been shown to be more effective than aminoglycosides for the treatment of Gram-negative bacillary meningitis,[83] and third-generation antibiotics should now be used.

Group B streptococcal infection should be treated with penicillin or a combination of penicillin and ampicillin, which is said to be synergistic, and ampicillin covers those rare cases where the organism is penicillin-resistant. Listerial infection responds to ampicillin, and for those with penicillin allergies, trimethoprim–sulphamethoxazole (co-trimoxazole) is effective. Nafcillin, flucloxacillin, or oxacillin in high dose is the recommended treatment for *S aureus* meningitis, with vancomycin for those who cannot have penicillin.[84]

Shunt infections are commonly caused by coagulase-negative staphylococci, and vancomycin—perhaps with added rifampicin—is effective. In most cases it is necessary to remove the device to eradicate the infection completely. The combination of penicillin and chloramphenicol with metronidazole is recommended for anaerobic infections.

In cases where an organism cannot be identified, children should be treated with a combination of ampicillin and chloramphenicol, or a third-generation cephalosporin alone,[85] adults with penicillin or a third-generation cephalosporin, and the elderly with a third-generation cephalosporin and ampicillin. For empirical treatment of those with immunosuppression, the type of immunological abnormality governs the choice of antibiotic.[86] If the defect is of cell-mediated immunity, ampicillin should be included to treat *Listeria* sp.; if humoral immunity is depressed, penicillin and a third-generation cephalosporin are recommended; and for the patient with neutropenia, a third-generation cephalosporin, with ceftazidime and an aminoglycoside, are recommended if pseudomonas infection is likely.[49]

Parenteral treatment for all forms of bacterial meningitis is recommended, and dosage schedules and a description of the adverse effects of these drugs may be found in pharmacological texts. My policy is to discuss the treatment of any case which is at all complicated with a specialist in infectious diseases. The length of time for which treatment is given must be tailored to each case and should be at least 10 days. Failure to respond prompts a review of the diagnosis and treatment, search for a continuing source of infection, and repeat brain imaging to demonstrate abscess or subdural fluid accumulation. Repeat CSF examination should be considered in most cases where no explanation can be found.

Specific bacterial meningitides

Tuberculous meningitis—Tuberculous meningitis does not commonly present as a neurological emergency. The time course over which the clinical syndrome evolves is longer than purulent meningitis, up to three weeks in children, and rather longer in adults. In some cases, however, the onset may be acute and exactly similar to purulent meningitis, so tuberculosis must be considered in each case.

CT and MRI of the brain show changes of meningitis, and no specifically diagnostic features. Hydrocephalus is common, as is basal meningeal enhancement,[67 86a 86b] and tuberculomas may be seen. Low-density changes of infarction are common. CSF is typically under raised pressure and is clear or slightly turbid. Rarely it may look frankly purulent. There is moderate pleocytosis, often in the hundreds, with eventual lymphocytic predominance, but polymorphs may be in the majority at the onset. CSF protein is elevated, sometimes to very high levels, and the glucose content is reduced, on average not to the levels seen with pyogenic meningitis. If tubercle bacilli are seen, the diagnosis is confirmed, but several samples may be required for organisms to be identified,[86c] and even then, in as many as 30–50% of cases, none may be seen. In these it may now be possible to detect specific mycobacterial antigen or antibody in CSF, using modern techniques including polymerase chain reaction (PCR).[86d 86e] If tuberculous meningitis is suspected, treatment must be given straight away, as delay worsens morbidity and mortality.[86f]

Details of treatment regimens may be found in the literature.[87–89] Chemotherapy is given for between six months and a year, dependent upon the severity of disease and the response to treatment. Steroids are not given routinely. Dexamethasone in high dose for a short time is useful to reduce cerebral oedema. Hydrocephalus commonly develops, sometimes acutely, and should be treated early by surgical drainage.

Lyme disease—Lyme disease, caused by the spirochaete *Borrelia burgdorferi*, can present as meningitis, in most cases of chronic type but sometimes in an acute fulminant manner.

Meningitis may occur as part of the second stage of the disease, 1–6 months after a bite by the vector, a tick of the genus *Ixodes*, and because the original bite and the skin lesion of erythema chronicum migrans were not noticed or had been forgotten, presentation may rarely be with acute meningitis.[90–92]

Treatment should be given with parenteral third-generation cephalosporins[92] for a minimum of two weeks. Intravenous penicillin in high dose is also effective,[93] but may induce temporary worsening of symptoms akin to the Jarisch–Herxheimer reaction, which occurs when treating neurosyphilis; it would therefore be prudent to cover the first doses with steroids.

Syphilitic meningitis—Another spirochaete, *Treponema pallidum*, may also cause acute meningitis. Admittedly rare, such cases are occurring more frequently in association with HIV infection and clinical AIDS.[94 95] It occurs within two years of infection, and presents acutely with headache, vomiting, pyrexia, and neck stiffness. Cranial nerve palsies are not infrequent, nor are epileptic seizures.[96] CT scan appearances are of non-specific meningeal enhancement, and CSF contains a predominantly mononuclear pleocytosis, raised protein, and normal sugar. The diagnosis is made by finding a positive CSF or serum VDRL (Venereal Disease Reference Laboratory) test, and confirming it with the FTA-Abs (fluorescent treponemal antibody—absorbed) test. The results of PCR tests for treponemal DNA are awaited with interest, in the hope that it may be possible to differentiate active syphilis from an acute neurological syndrome occurring in a patient who has had yaws in the past.

Acute syphilitic meningitis is managed by the parenteral application of large doses of penicillin for 10 days, with steroids for the first 24 hours to diminish the possibility of inducing a Jarisch–Herxheimer reaction. It is necessary to follow up all cases closely to ensure that serological changes and CSF revert to normal, and to treat any re-infection rapidly.

Rickettsial meningitis—As a consequence of the proliferation of intercontinental travel by air, the person arriving from abroad may harbour an infection not usually seen in the UK and, as the incubation period of some of these infections may be 2–3 weeks, symptoms may not appear until some time has been spent in the country. It is therefore of the first importance to obtain a full history of recent travel, places visited, including stop-overs, and activities undertaken, from any patient who presents with an acute meningoencephalitis. Such an illness may be caused by rickettsial diseases, which are transmitted to humans by the bites of ticks or mites, and are prevalent in every continent except Antarctica. Rocky Mountain spotted fever caused by *R rickettsii* may be contracted in the Americas; Mediterranean spotted fever (*R conorii*) in Africa, Asia, and the Mediterranean basin; scrub typhus (*R tsutsugamushi*) in Asia, the Pacific, and Australia; typhus (*R prowazckii*) and Q fever (*Coxiella burnetii*) are ubiquitous. Rickettsiae invade small blood vessels throughout the body, multiply, causing endothelial wall proliferation, thrombosis, and perivascular inflammation and, when this affects the brain, meningoencephalitis results.

The incubation period, clinical features, and progression of the illness vary between organisms, but all share the triad of high

251

fever, skin rash, and headache, with meningoencephalitis developing during the second week of the illness in a significant proportion of cases. Rocky Mountain spotted fever may occur without a rash; Q fever is not usually accompanied by a rash; and Mediterranean spotted fever is characterised by a distinctive eschar at the site of the bite.

Neurological features are typically non-focal, with headache, neck stiffness, photophobia, and, in more severe cases, confusion and reduction in conscious level.[97][98] Convulsions may occur. CSF examination reveals no specific features: there may be a slight pleocytosis, the protein content may be raised, and glucose is normal. Diagnosis is confirmed by serological tests, but treatment must be started on the basis of clinical suspicion, and not delayed for test results to become available. Direct immunofluorescence of skin biopsies taken from a rash of Rocky Mountain spotted fever offered hope as a rapid method of diagnosis. Unfortunately it is not very specific, and is not widely available. The treatment of choice is tetracycline 500 mg four times per day for 10 days in adults. Chloramphenicol may also be used but it is thought that tetracycline is better and less likely to result in relapse.[99]

Malaria

Malaria is the most important parasitic disease in the world, affects as many as 300 million people, and is being imported to the United Kingdom more often—12 patients died of malaria in 1991, 10 in 1992.[100] Involvement of the brain occurs in patients infected with *Plasmodium falciparum* and results in cerebral malaria. For practical purposes, *P vivax*, *P ovale*, and *P malariae* do not cause cerebral malaria. Malaria is found in large parts of Asia, sub-Saharan Africa, parts of Greece, Turkey, and the Middle East, and Central and South America. People who live in endemic areas may acquire a degree of immunity which diminishes with time. Those most at risk of developing severe malaria are the traveller who has no immunity and is being exposed for the first time, the emigrant returning home from a long spell abroad, whose immunity has lapsed, pregnant women, and those who have immunosuppression.

Cerebral malaria is an acute diffuse encephalopathy with fever, which will kill within 72 hours if not recognised and treated, and even then carries a mortality rate of 25–50%.[101] Delay in making the diagnosis and initiating treatment is a major factor contributing to this.

Falciparum malaria is spread by female mosquitos of the genus *Anopheles*. When they feed on humans they inject falciparum sporozoites into the blood, which circulate and are rapidly cleared by the liver where they enter hepatocytes and reproduce asexually. One to three weeks later they rupture into the bloodstream as motile merozoites, which rapidly invade erythrocytes, where they can be seen on blood films under the microscope. There they feed on haemoglobin, and further asexual reproduction occurs (schizogeny). The progeny mature through the stage of trophozoite to merozoite, multiplying approximately 10-fold, to rupture out of the red cell and invade other uninfected red cells. This dispersal occurs every 48 hours and induces fever. A proportion of merozoites develop into the sexual, gametocyte stage of the parasite, and it is this which is ingested by a feeding mosquito to continue the cycle.

Pathogenesis

The clinical manifestations of cerebral malaria are the end result of a complex, and not fully understood, series of interactions within the cerebrovascular tree mediated by humoral, vascular, and haematological factors. There is evidence of an immune-mediated inflammatory reaction that releases vasoactive products which produce endothelial damage.[102 103] The presence of trophozoites within erythrocytes induces changes as they mature, which renders them capable of adhering to vascular endothelium, and these red cells packed with mature trophozoites are to be found sequestrated in small cerebral venules, resulting in microvascular congestion and tissue hypoxia.[104 105]

Other organ systems are vulnerable to similar changes. Acute tubular necrosis and the adult respiratory distress syndrome may need simultaneous treatment. Disseminated intravascular coagulation occurs in severe cases, but seems to be a complication and does not affect most patients. Whether cerebral oedema contributes significantly to the pathophysiology of cerebral malaria is debatable. It has been observed in pathological specimens and it is claimed that this may be an agonal event. CT studies do not support the presence of cerebral oedema,[106] yet CSF pressure has been found to be high at the time of lumbar puncture in a group

253

of African children.[107] Routine administration of dexamethasone does not improve the outcome.[108]

Hypoglycaemia is an important and frequent complication of cerebral malaria and undoubtedly contributes to depression of consciousness and the appearance of neurological signs. It results from a complex series of interactions which include malabsorption of glucose from the gut, hyperinsulinaemia which may be induced by treatment using intravenous quinine, the metabolic demands of infection, and increased metabolism of available glucose by a large biomass of parasites.[109 110] Pregnant women are particularly susceptible.

Diagnosis

Definitions of the clinical criteria required to justify a diagnosis of cerebral malaria have been drawn up to standardise parameters for research.[108] For the purposes of this discussion, any person from an endemic area, with cerebral symptoms or signs, should be suspected of suffering from cerebral malaria, and demands immediate monitoring, investigation, and treatment. Such a patient will usually have been ill for days and have a temperature. Exceptions occur: the onset of neurological symptoms may be abrupt, and very ill patients can be hypothermic. Commonly there are convulsions, more so in the young and in 45% of adults; coma follows the convulsion. Young children have febrile convulsions associated with many varieties of infection, and with these, consciousness is rapidly regained. Coma lasting more than an hour or two in such circumstances should raise the suspicion of cerebral malaria.

Symptoms before the onset of the cerebral state are diverse and non-specific, and the most common misdiagnosis is of 'flu. The level of consciousness is invariably impaired, and there is evidence of an organic brain syndrome which manifests as confusion, hallucinations, delirium, and psychosis, complicated in some by motor signs and movement disorders. Meningism and opisthotonos may be found, and it is important to remember that bacterial and other forms of meningitis may coexist with malaria. Furthermore, severely ill patients are susceptible to Gram-negative septicaemia. There may be signs of damage to other organ systems—anaemia is common and may be severe, jaundice complicates severe infection in adults, hepatosplenomegaly of mild to moderate degree is frequent, and haemorrhages may be found in the retina.

Prolonged coma and frequent convulsions should trigger a search for hypoglycaemia and pyogenic meningitis.

Treatment

Confirmation of the diagnosis of a case of suspected cerebral malaria must be obtained forthwith, but if this cannot be done, and suspicion is high, treatment should be given straight away. The best way to confirm the diagnosis is to have thick and thin smears of blood examined by an experienced microscopist after appropriate staining. Should no parasites be seen, and the diagnosis seems likely, treatment should be given and the blood re-examined every 6–8 hours for the next 48 hours. Blood sugar should be estimated and monitored frequently, and hypoglycaemia corrected if found. A full blood count, urea, electrolytes, and blood gases must be checked and monitored as treatment progresses. It is necessary to examine the CSF to exclude pyogenic or other forms of meningitis as a cause of coma: CSF examination is not otherwise helpful in the diagnosis of malaria. In the United Kingdom it should be possible to obtain an urgent CT brain scan, to give some estimate of intracranial pressure before lumbar puncture and, if the brain looks swollen, it may be better to treat for meningitis empirically, with cover for Gram-negative organisms, and to consider giving mannitol. Blood cultures should be taken. All such patients should be nursed in intensive care.

Because of widespread resistance of *P falciparum* to chloroquine, this should not be used: quinine is the drug of choice. In the United States quinine is not available, and quinidine gluconate is used instead.[111][112] Quinine is given by slow, intravenous infusion after an initial loading dose (provided none has been given in the preceding two days). Dosage schedules vary but approximate to 5 mg/kg by intravenous infusion over two hours every 8–12 hours. In patients from southeast Asia, it may be necessary to double the loading dose. Quinine should not be given by bolus injection. When the patient regains consciousness, oral treatment can be given. Plasma concentrations should be monitored, as should the ECG. It is recommended that an antifolate metabolite, either pyrimethamine–sulfadoxine (three tablets) or doxycycline, be given during the course of quinine. If the parasite load is very high and the patient very ill, exchange transfusion is useful. Anticonvulsants are given to counter any tendency to seizures. Intravenous glucose is given for hypoglycaemia, anaemia is corrected by blood transfusion, and renal failure by dialysis. Mechanical ventilation is necessary for the adult respiratory distress syndrome. Gram-negative septicaemia causing septic shock can be a life-threatening complication which should be anticipated and treated. Chloroquine is just as effective as quinine provided that the organism is not resistant.

Features that adversely affect the outcome are failure to make the diagnosis, delay in starting treatment, not recognising concurrent infection, deep and prolonged coma, and continuing seizures.

Primary amoebic meningoencephalitis

This condition is caused by free living amoebae of the species *Naegleria fowleri*. *Acanthamoeba* sp. tends to cause a subacute granulomatous meningoencephalitis. They live in moist soil, and most cases have been reported in children who have been swimming or playing in stagnant water.[113] Amoebae enter the nasal cavity, cross the nasal epithelium, and ascend to the brain along olfactory nerves and blood vessels to frontal and basal meninges, and spread, causing a florid necrotising inflammation.

Clinically the presentation is of sudden onset, with a severe meningitis indistinguishable from bacterial meningitis—the clue to diagnosis is the history of exposure to warm, stagnant water. CSF examination reveals pleocytosis in which polymorphs predominate, raised protein, and reduced glucose. No organisms are seen on the Gram stain, and special examination of fresh, warm specimens of CSF will show motile trophozoites. Most patients die rapidly despite treatment, but survival following therapy with amphotericin B has been described,[114] and this should be given in the highest tolerated dose parenterally, reinforced by intracisternal injection, and by rifampicin and tetracycline, which have some activity against naegleriae.

Brain abscess

Parenchymal brain abscess remains a diagnostic and therapeutic challenge to the physician and surgeon, notwithstanding the considerable advances that have taken place in the last decades in imaging techniques, neurosurgical practice, bacteriological isolation of causal organisms, and the introduction of more potent antibiotics. Patterns of infection are changing but the number of cases seen is not diminishing, and the result of treatment is little better than it was years ago. Brain abscesses frequently present as emergencies, and as with other forms of cerebral infection, delay in diagnosis and implementation of treatment, and inappropriate investigation, adversely affect the end result.

The incidence of brain abscess has remained at one in 10 000 of general hospital admissions, approximating to a prevalence of 4–5 per million population,[115] which is almost certainly an underestimate.

Pathogenesis

Bacteria reach brain parenchyma via the bloodstream, by direct extension from an adjacent focus of infection or by implantation through wounds as a result of trauma or neurosurgery. In as many as 20% of cases the source of infection cannot be identified. Experimental data indicate that bacteria cannot set up a nidus of infection in normal, undamaged brain, and it may be that thrombophlebitis spreads from contiguous infection, or microinfarction occurs from emboli or hypoxaemia to produce a microscopic area of necrosis where infection can become established. Thereafter the evolution of an abscess passes through four main stages, which have been documented experimentally and correlate well with both clinical and CT findings.

The first stage is of cerebritis, with surrounding oedema of white matter; next the centre of cerebritis becomes necrotic, enlarges, capsule formation begins with the appearance of fibroblasts and neovascular change at the periphery, reactive astrocytosis, and surrounding oedema. The third stage is of capsular development; the fourth is of capsular maturity as it thickens and reactive astrocytosis increases.[116 117] The time course is variable and probably related to the virulence of the organism and to the immune status of the host, and may be as short as three weeks to encapsulation and fibrosis, and the capsule may thicken by 1 mm per month.

The range of primary foci from which bacteria spread to produce an abscess is large. There is a relationship between the primary focus and the bacterial composition of the abscess. Otogenic infection from otitis media or a cholesteatoma spawns abscesses in the temporal lobe or cerebellum. Paranasal sinusitis leads to abscess formation in the frontal lobes and the deeper parts of the temporal lobes. Metastatic abscesses, borne by blood, have a

257

predilection for grey–white matter junctions where the blood supply is relatively reduced, and they are often multiple. The primary source may be lung, heart, or teeth, but a source of infection such as osteomyelitis may be implicated. Chronic pulmonary sepsis, congenital heart disease (fig 1), particularly cyanotic, and pulmonary arteriovenous fistulae are all fruitful sources, as are dental sepsis and dental manipulation. Those abscesses that are caused by direct implantation occur in proximity to the site of injury or surgery, commonly a depressed fracture or gunshot wound. Bacterial meningitis may be complicated by brain abscess but it is difficult to know how often this happens.

Depression of the immune system from drugs or a disease such as AIDS renders the neuraxis vulnerable to attack by a wide range of organisms, including those that would not normally be pathogenic. The relative frequency with which these predisposing factors occur changes with time, age of the patient, population studied, and geographical location. In any single patient, all

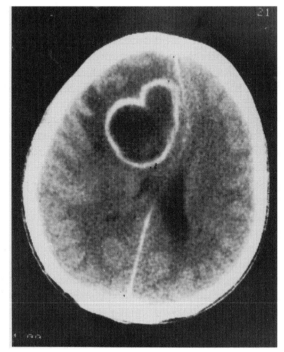

Figure 1—CT brain scan of a man of 20 years with surgically corrected Fallot's tetralogy and bacterial endocarditis, showing a large frontal abscess with ring enhancement caused by an anaerobic streptococcus and *Eikonella corrodens*.

potential sources should be considered and excluded in turn by appropriate investigation.

Causative organisms—A very wide spectrum of organisms has been isolated from brain abscesses, and is set to widen further as immune suppression and AIDS spread. The ability to identify an organism from pus is dependent on several factors: have antibiotics already been administered? Has there been a delay between collection and culture? Is the organism fastidious, and have the correct methods of culture been used? When proper attention has been given to those details it has become evident that anaerobic bacteria play a larger role in brain abscess than had been appreciated, and the yield of positive cultures can be significantly increased.[118]

Otogenic brain abscesses commonly have a mixed flora, which include Enterobacteriaceae, streptococci, and *Bacillus fragilis*. Those caused by sinus infection grow *Streptococcus milleri* and *Bacteroides* sp. Dental sepsis causes mixed infection with streptococci, *Bacteroides,* and *Fusobacterium* spp.; pulmonary disease results in a very mixed bag including fusobacteria, other anaerobes, streptococci, and actinomycetes. Patients with congenital heart disease are likely to have *S viridans,* anaerobic, and microaerophilic streptococci. Staphylococci are found with penetrating head trauma, as are streptococci and *Clostridium* sp. In patients who are immune compromised, *Nocardia* sp. and a wide range of fungi may be implicated.

Published reports abound of single cases of abscesses from which unusual organisms have been grown. It therefore behoves the attending physician to alert the bacteriological laboratory to the relevant circumstances of the case under investigation so that appropriate techniques can be employed to identify the causal organism.

Diagnosis

The clinical features of brain abscess are many and varied. Typically there is a combination of raised intracranial pressure, focal neurological signs, signs of infection—either focal or systemic—and rapid progression. Unfortunately such a combination exists in only half of all patients, with the result that many other disease states may be mimicked: "Any neurologist or neurosurgeon who can claim never to have made an error in the clinical diagnosis of a brain abscess either has a conveniently short memory span or has not been in practice long enough."[119]

Headache is common and may be diffuse, localised, and intermittent.

Emergency presentation may be with focal signs pointing to the site of the lesion, with convulsions, which are usually generalised but may be focal, with raised intracranial pressure even to the point of coning, and with neck stiffness to suggest meningitis. There may be a pyrexia in 50% of patients and, in some, symptoms relating to the source of infection, such as otitis, may predominate.[120-124] In young children, the presentation may be even more confusing—an enlarging head associated with vomiting and seizures can be mistaken for tumour or congenital anomaly. Cerebral abscess therefore must be included in the differential diagnosis of those who present acutely with raised intracranial pressure, epileptic seizures, strokes, meningitis and encephalitis, and primary and secondary intracranial malignancy.

Faced with a patient in whom intracranial abscess is a possible diagnosis, the priority is to confirm the diagnosis, identify the source of infection and the responsible organism or organisms, once vital functions have been stabilised. A full examination should be made for a locus of infection, such as otitis media or pelvic sepsis, and if found, cultures should be made and steps taken to eradicate the source. Blood cultures should be set up. Baseline haematological and biochemical parameters should be established: they are seldom useful for diagnosis but may change rapidly in the course of the disease. CT of the head should be done as soon as possible. In addition to visualising the intracranial contents, note should be made of the state of the paranasal sinuses and the mastoid air cells. Skull fractures and cranial defects should be looked for.

Interpretation of the CT scan should always be made with reference to timing in the evolution of the abscess. In the earliest stages of cerebritis, a low-density area may be evident, perhaps with surrounding oedema, and no enhancement after contrast injection. Later there may be patchy enhancement which, with maturity, adopts a "ring" appearance as encapsulation takes place. Later still this becomes more evident and the centre of the lesion or lesions becomes increasingly hypodense. Adjacent white matter is swollen with cerebral oedema. Location and multiplicity of abscesses, hydrocephalus, and cerebral mass effect are readily identified.[125 126] Unfortunately such appearances are not specific and may be seen with brain tumours, granulomas, necrotising encephalitis, and infarction. If ventriculitis is demonstrated by ependymal enhancement, then infection is likely.

MRI is likely to prove more sensitive than CT in demonstrating early cerebritis, cerebral oedema, and the contents of abscess cavities.[127 128] As an emergency investigation it is not widely available in the United Kingdom, however, and there are problems accommodating severely ill patients within the machine. Lumbar puncture should *never* be carried out on patients suspected of harbouring a brain abscess. If the urgency of the patient's condition allows, a chest radiograph should be carried out.

Treatment

When the diagnosis of brain abscess is confirmed, the therapeutic strategy will be influenced by several factors, and there is no overall agreement on when surgery should be undertaken, and if it is, which technique should be used. Indications for surgery are relief of space occupation, confirmation of the diagnosis, and obtaining specimens of pus for culture. If the abscess is a consequence of head trauma, then surgery is mandatory for appropriate toilet, debridement, removal of fragments, and closure of dural defects. If lesions are multiple or deeply situated, it is best to treat with antibiotics on the basis of organism identification from other sources, or if that is not possible, on a "best guess" principle governed by the likely source of infection. Close monitoring of the lesions with serial CT or MRI is necessary; if they do not diminish in size, aspiration should be undertaken. In people with immunosuppression, including those with AIDS, the threshold for aspiration of pus to identify the offending organism is substantially lowered. It is seldom necessary to resort to complete surgical excision of an abscess: simple aspiration of the contents of an abscess is the most frequently advocated technique—when carried out under CT stereotactic control, diagnostic material may be obtained in as many as 95% of cases.[129–131] There is an increasing trend towards treating multiple abscesses, or those that are deeply situated, with antibiotics alone.[124 132 133] Results seem to justify this course of action.

Choice of antibiotics—The choice of antibiotic to be used is influenced by its capacity to penetrate not only into CSF but through the capsule wall and into the pus, and to be active in the presence of pus. Little information is available on the penetration of newer antibiotics into brain. Currently the favoured regimen for empirical treatment, while awaiting the results of culture studies, is a combination of penicillin 24 mega units per day intravenously, chloramphenicol 1 g intravenously every six hours, and metronidazole. If staphylococci are suspected, nafcillin or flucoxacillin, vancomycin, or fusidic acid should be used. The length of time for which treatment should be given must be determined for each case by clinical response and improvement of CT scan appearances, and is usually no less than six weeks, often longer. In patients with AIDS, toxoplasmosis is the likeliest cause of a focal brain lesion, particularly if multiple. The range of possible pathogens is very wide, however, and biopsy should be considered for every patient who has a negative toxoplasma serology test or in whom CT scans are atypical. In others, treatment should be given with pyrimethamine and sulphadiazine, and progress monitored. Clinical and CT improvement should take place within 14 days.

Dexamethasone is commonly used to treat cerebral oedema, and in practice the benefit obtained in reducing intracranial pressure outweighs the potential hazard of diminishing the host inflammatory response. Mannitol and hyperventilation may be necessary in addition. The risk of developing epileptic seizures is not insubstantial, and prophylactic anticonvulsants are recommended.

Subdural empyema

This potentially lethal infection of the space between the dura and arachnoid mater is most often due to spread of infection from ear or nose,[134 135] and less commonly osteomyelitis (fig 2). Rarely it may be caused by haematogenous spread from a distant focus, and it may follow penetrating head trauma. In children, subdural effusions that complicate meningitis become infected.[136] Because the subdural space is extensive, pus can readily track over the brain surface from one side to another, and may accumulate along the falx, or it may remain localised and become encapsulated in proximity to the primary focus. The organisms that are found reflect the underlying cause. In adults organisms from otitis and sinusitis predominate—aerobic and anaerobic streptococci, staphylococci, and Gram-negative organisms including *Proteus*

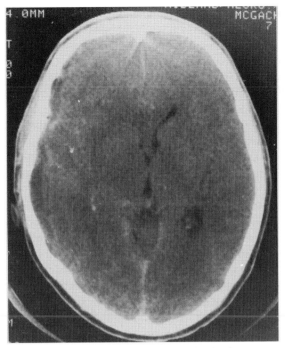

Figure 2—CT brain scan showing subdural empyema caused by an α-haemolytic streptococcus in a man of 19 years who presented six weeks following a head injury causing a fracture of the cribriform plate.

and *Pseudomonas* spp. In infants and young children *H influenzae*, Gram-negative bacteria, and pneumococci are common. In as many as a quarter of all cases no organism can be cultured from pus.[134]

Diagnosis

Subdural empyema affects the young—more than half of all cases are aged less than 20, and it is more common in boys. Presentation is frequently acute, as an emergency with rapid deterioration. There is usually evidence of general infection: fever, tachycardia, malaise and rigors; there may be signs of local infection: face ache, and tenderness over the sinuses or over the mastoid process. Headache and signs of meningeal irritation are common, vomiting, papilloedema, and diminution of conscious level imply raised intracranial pressure. Focal signs of hemiparesis, dysphasia, and, less frequently, cerebellar disturbance may

263

occur. Epileptic seizures are very common and are often focal.[137] A parafalcine collection may herald its presence with signs of a paraparesis, sphincter disturbance, or weakness of one leg.[138] The diagnosis should be considered in any patient who presents acutely with neurological dysfunction on a background of infection, especially if there are focal seizures and if there is evidence of infection in the ear or paranasal sinuses.

To confirm the diagnosis, CT of the head with contrast enhancement should be undertaken as an emergency. MRI may be more sensitive,[139] but the same strictures apply as for brain abscess. CT appearances may be subtle in the early stages of development. The classical appearance is of an extracerebral collection of lower density than brain over the surface of the hemispheres and in the parafalcine region. A rim of enhancement follows contrast injection. If large enough, adjacent structures will be displaced, but bilateral effusions may not cause evident shift. There may be adjacent infarction and brain oedema.[140] Pus or fluid may be seen in the paranasal sinuses or in the ear, and there may be evidence of osteomyelitis. A blood count should be taken: it often shows a polymorphonuclear leucocytosis and raised ESR. Lumbar puncture should *not* be carried out even if meningitis is suspected.

Treatment

Most authorities agree that once the diagnosis is established, treatment should be started immediately with a combination of systemic chemotherapy together with surgical exploration and removal of pus, and the eradication of the primary source of infection. Unless culture sensitivities indicate otherwise, a combination of penicillin, chloramphenicol, and metronidazole is given, as for brain abscess. Prophylactic anticonvulsants should be prescribed and measures taken to combat raised intracranial pressure.

There are considerable differences of opinion concerning the relative merits of burrhole aspiration and craniotomy in the treatment of subdural empyema, and which method is employed depends upon the prejudices and experience of the neurosurgeon on call. Whichever technique is used it is important to ensure that all loculi of pus are removed. Working in an institution where there are vociferous proponents of each method, I consider that craniotomy produces better results.

264

Management of cerebral infection

- Cerebral infection occurs clinically as meningitis, encephalitis, or localised suppuration in the form of parenchymal abscess or subdural empyema, or a combination of these.

- Most cases of *meningitis* are caused by viruses, are benign and self-limiting, and require symptomatic treatment only. Bacterial meningitis attacks any age, most commonly infants, children, and young adults in whom *Haemophilus* sp., the meningococcus, and pneumococcus predominate as pathogens. Other organisms should be sought according to circumstances. Successful management demands immediate diagnosis by CSF examination incorporating appropriate precautions to manage intracranial hypertension, followed by the parenteral administration of suitable antibiotics, and the maintenance of cerebral perfusion and nutrition.

- Encephalitis is almost always of viral origin, and is treated symptomatically, care being taken to manage intracranial pressure. Because of the relative lack of toxicity of acyclovir, this is given to most cases whether the diagnosis of herpes simplex encephalitis has been confirmed or not. Less common causes, such as rickettsiae, must not be overlooked, and falciparum malaria should always be suspected if there has been travel abroad, and should be treated promptly with quinine.

- Intracranial suppuration is of bacterial origin, and is diagnosed by cranial imaging. Treatment combines the administration of antibiotics, control of intracranial hypertension, relief of space-occupation by surgery, and the eradication of foci of infection.

- Subdural empyema is best treated by craniotomy and evacuation of pus.

1 Wallgren A. Une nouvelle maladie infectieuse du système nerveux central? (Meningite septique aigue). *Acta Paediatr Scand* 1925;4:158–82.
2 Johnson RT, Mims CA. Pathogenesis of viral infections of the nervous system. *N Engl J Med* 1968;278:23–30, 84–92.
3 Dropulic B, Masters GL. Entry of neurotropic arboviruses into the central nervous system: an *in vitro* study using mouse brain epithelium. *J Infect Dis* 1990;161:685–91.
4 Ponka A, Pettersson T. The incidence and aetiology of central nervous system infections in Helsinki in 1980. *Acta Neurol Scand* 1982;66:529–35.
5 Beghi E, Nicolosi A, Kurland LT, Mulder DW, Hauser WA, Shuster L. Encephalitis and

aseptic meningitis, Olmsted County, Minnesota 1950–1981. 1. Epidemiology. *Ann Neurol* 1984;**16**:283–94.

6 Centers for Disease Control. Summary of notifiable diseases, United States 1988. *MMWR* 1989;**37**:1–57.

7 Feigin RD, Shackelford PG. Value of repeat lumbar puncture in the differential diagnosis of meningitis. *N Engl J Med* 1973;**289**:571–4.

8 Birkenmayer LG, Mushahwar IK. DNA probe amplification methods. *J Virol Methods* 1991;**35**:117–26.

9 Miller HG, Stanton JB, Gibbons JL. Parainfectious encephalomyelitis and related syndromes: a critical review of the neurological complications of specific fevers. *Q J Med* 1956;**25**:427–505.

10 Johnson RT. The pathogenesis of acute viral encephalitis and post-infectious encephalomyelitis. *J Infect Dis* 1987;**155**:539–64.

11 Whitley RJ. Viral encephalitis. *N Engl J Med* 1990;**323**:242–9.

12 Klapper PE, Cleator GM, Dennett C, Lewis A. Diagnosis of herpes encephalitis via Southern blotting of cerebrospinal fluid DNA amplified by polymerase chain reaction. *J Med Virol*, 1990;**32**:261–4.

13 Rowley AH, Whitley RJ, Lakeman FD, Wolinsky SM. Rapid detection of herpes simplex virus DNA in cerebrospinal fluid of patients with herpes simplex encephalitis. *Lancet* 1990;**335**:440–1.

14 Whitley RJ, Tilles J, Linneman C, *et al*. Herpes simplex encephalitis: clinical assessment. *JAMA* 1982;**247**:317–20.

15 Barza M, Pauker SG. The decision to biopsy, treat or wait in suspected herpes encephalitis. *Ann Intern Med* 1980;**92**:641–9.

16 Whitley RJ, Cobbs CG, Alford CA, *et al*. Diseases which mimic herpes simplex encephalitis: diagnosis, presentation and outcome. *JAMA* 1989;**262**:234–9.

17 Whitley RJ, Alford CA, Hirsch MS, *et al*. Vidarabine versus acyclovir therapy of herpes simplex encephalitis. *N Engl J Med* 1986;**314**:144–9.

18 Kennedy PGE. Neurological complications of varicella zoster virus. In: PGE Kennedy, RT Johnson, eds, *Infections of the nervous system*. London: Butterworths, 1987:177–208.

19 Johnson R, Milbourn PE. Central nervous system manifestations of chicken pox. *Can Med Assoc J* 1970;**102**:831–4.

20 Gautier-Smith PC. Neurological complications of glandular fever (infectious mononucleosis). *Brain* 1965;**88**:323–34.

21 Ter Meulen V, Muller D, Kackell Y, Katz M. Isolation of infectious measles virus in measles encephalitis. *Lancet* 1972;**2**:1172–5.

22 Johnson RT, Griffin DE, Hirsch RL, *et al*. Measles encephalomyelitis—clinical and immunologic studies. *N Engl J Med* 1984;**310**:137–41.

23 Aarli JA. Nervous complications of measles: clinical manifestations and prognosis. *Eur Neurol* 1974;**12**:79–93.

24 Koskiniemi M, Donner M, Pettay O. Clinical appearance and outcome in mumps encephalitis in children. *Acta Paediatr Scand* 1983;**72**:603–9.

25 Azimi PH, Cramblett HG, Haynes RE. Mumps meningoencephalitis in children. *JAMA* 1969;**207**:509–12.

26 Goldfield M, Sussman O. The 1959 outbreak of Eastern encephalitis in New Jersey. 1. Introduction and description of outbreak. *Am J Epidemiol* 1968;**87**:1–10.

27 Dickerson RB, Newton JR, Hausen JE. Diagnosis and immediate prognosis of Japanese B encephalitis. *Am J Med* 1952;**12**:277–90.

28 Lincoln AF, Siverston SE. Acute phase of Japanese B encephalitis. Two hundred and one cases in American soldiers, Korea. *JAMA* 1950;**150**:268–73.

29 Burke DS, Nisalak A, Ussery MA, Laorakpogese T, Chantavibul S. Kinetics of IgM and IgG responses to Japanese encephalitis virus in human serum and cerebrospinal fluid. *J Infect Dis* 1985;**151**:1093–9.

30 Acha PN. A review of rabies prevention and control status in the Americas 1970–1980: overall status of rabies. *Bull World Health Organ Int Epiz*, 1981;**93**:9–52.

30a Constantine DG. Rabies transmission by non-bite route. *Public Health Rep* 1962;**77**:287–9.

30b Centers for Disease Control. Rabies prevention, United States, 1984. Recommendations of the Immunization Practices Advisory Committee (ACIP). *MMWR* 1984;**33**:393–402.

30c Warrell DA. The clinical picture of rabies in man. *Trans R Soc Trop Med Hyg* 1976;**70**:188–95.

30d Lakhanpal U, Sharma RC. An epidemiological study of 177 cases of human rabies. *Int J Epidemiol* 1985;**14**:614–7

30e Smith JS, Fishbein DB, Rupprecht CE, Clark K. Unexplained rabies in three immigrants in the United States. A virological investigation. *N Engl J Med* 1991;**324**:205–11.

31 Blenden DC, Creech W, Torres-Anjel MJ. Use of immunofluorescence examination to detect rabies virus antigen in skin of humans with clinical encephalitis. *J Infect Dis* 1986;**154**:698–701.

32 Heyward WL, Curran JW. The epidemiology of AIDS in the US. *Sci Am* 1988;**259**:72–81.

33 Selik RM, Jaffe HW, Solomon SL, Curran JW. CDC's definition of AIDS. *N Engl J Med* 1986;**315**:761.

34 Redfield RR, Wright DC, Tramont EC. The Walter Reed staging classification for HTLV-III/LAV infection. *N Engl J Med* 1986;**314**:131–2.

34a Carne CA, Tedder RS, Smith A, Sutherland S, Elkington SG, Daly HM, Preston FE, Craske J. Acute encephalopathy coincident with seroconversion for anti-HTLV-III. *Lancet* 1985;**ii**:1206–8.

34b Dalgleish A, Beverley PCL, Clapham PR, Crawford DH, Greaves MF, Weiss RA. The CD_4 (T_4) antigen is an essential componentt of the receptor for the AIDS retrovirus. *Nature* 1984;**312**:763–7.

34c Seligmann M, Chess L. Fahey JL, *et al.* AIDS—an immunologic re-evaluation. *N Engl J Med* 1984;**311**:1286–92.

34d Hollander H. Cerebrospinal fluid normalities and abnormalities in individuals infected with human immunodeficiency virus. *J Infect Dis* 1988;**158**:855–8.

34e Levy JA, Shimabukuro J. Hollander H, Mills J, Kaminsky L. Isolation of AIDS associated retroviruses from cerebrospinal fluid and brain of patients with neurological symptoms. *Lancet* 1985;ii:586–8.

34f Hollander H, Levy JA. Neurologic abnormalities and recovery of human immuno-deficiency virus from cerebrospinal fluid. *Ann Intern Med* 1987;**106**:692–5.

34g Portegies P, Epstein LG, Hung ST, de Gans J, and Goudsmit J. Human immuno-deficiency virus type 1 antigen in cerebrospinal fluid: correlation with clinical neurologic status. *Arch Neurol* 1989;**465**:261–4.

34h Levy JA. Changing concepts in HIV infection: challenges for the 1990s. *AIDS* 1990;**40**: 1051–8.

35 Goodin DS, Aminoff MJ, Chernoff DN, Hollander H. Long latency event related potentials in patients infected with Human Immunodeficiency Virus. *Ann Neurol* 1990;**27**:414.

36 Navia BA, Jordan BD, Price RW. The AIDS dementia complex. I. Clinical features. *Ann Neurol* 1986;**19**:517–24.

36a Navia BA, Cho E-S, Petito CK, Price RW. The AIDS dementia complex. II. Neuropathology. *Ann Neurol* 1986;**19**:525–35.

37 Barnes PF, Bloch AB, Davidson PT, Snider DE. Tuberculosis in patients with human immunodeficiency virus infection. *N Engl J Med* 1991;**324**:1644–50.

38 Navia BA, Petito CK, Gold JWM, Cho E, Hordan BD, Price RW. Cerebral toxoplasmo-sis complicating the acquired immune deficiency syndrome: clinical and neuropathologi-cal findings in 27 patients. *Ann Neurol* 1986;**19**:224–38.

39 Porter SB, Sande MA. Toxoplasmosis of the central nervous system in the acquired immunodeficiency syndrome. *N Engl J Med* 1992;**327**:1643–8.

40 Cohn JA, McMeeking A, Cohen W, Jacobs J, Holzman RS. Evaluation of the policy of empiric treatment of suspected Toxoplasma encephalitis in patients with the acquired immunodeficiency syndrome. *Am J Med* 1989;**86**:521–7.

41 Young LS. Mycobacterium avium complex infection. *J Infect Dis* 1988;**157**:863–7.

42 Noah ND. Epidemiology of bacterial meningitis: UK and USA. In: Williams JD, Burnie J, eds, *Bacterial meningitis*, London: Academic Press, 1987;93–115.

43 Roos KL, Tunkel AR, Scheld WM. Acute bacterial meningitis in children and adults. In: Scheld WM, Whitley RJ, Durack DT, eds, *Infections of the central nervous system*, New York: Raven Press, 1991:335–409.

44 Durand ML, Calderwood SB, Weber DJ, *et al.* Acute bacterial meningitis in adults. A review of 493 episodes. *N Engl J Med* 1993;**328**:21–8.

45 Downs NJ, Hodges GR, Taylor SA. Mixed bacterial meningitis. *Rev Infect Dis* 1987;**9**:693–703.

46 Heerema MS, Ein ME, Musher DM, Bradshaw MW, Williams TW. Anaerobic bacterial meningitis. *Am J Med* 1979;**67**:219–27.

47 Tompkins LS. The use of molecular methods in infectious diseases. *N Engl J Med* 1992;**327**:1290–7.

48 Quagliarello V, Scheld WM. Bacterial meningitis: pathogenesis, pathophysiology and progress. *N Engl J Med* 1992;**327**:864–72.

49 Tunkel AR, Wispelwey B, Scheld WM. Bacterial meningitis: recent advances in pathophysiology and treatment. *Ann Intern Med* 1990;**112**:610–23.

50 Ashwal S, Tomasi L, Schneider S, Perkin R, Thompson J. Bacterial meningitis in children: pathophysiology and treatment. *Neurology* 1992;**42**:739–48.

50a Simberkoff MS, Moldover NH, Ranal J. Absence of detectable bacterial and opsonic activities in normal and infected human cerebrospinal fluids: a regional host defense deficiency. *J Lab Clin Med* 1980;**95**:362–72.

51 Tureen JH, Dworkin RJ, Kennedy SL, Sachdeva M, Sande MA. Loss of cerebral autoregulation in experimental meningitis in rabbits. *J Clin Invest* 1990;**85**:577–81.

52 Hambleton G, Davies PA. Bacterial meningitis. Some aspects of diagnosis and treatment. *Arch Dis Child* 1975;**50**:674–84.

53 Rutter N, Smales OR. Role of routine investigations in children presenting with their first febrile convulsion. *Arch Dis Child* 1977;**52**:188–91.

54 Lorber J, Sunderland R. Lumbar puncture in children with convulsions associated with fever. *Lancet* 1980;**i**:785–6.

55 Klein JO, Feigin RD, McCracken GH. Report on the task force on diagnosis and management of meningitis. *Pediatrics* 1986;**78S**:959–82.

56 Geiseler PJ, Nelson KE, Levin S, Reddy KT, Moses VK. Community acquired purulent meningitis: a review of 1316 cases during the antibiotic era, 1954–1976. *Rev Infect Dis* 1980;**2**:725–45.

57 Friedland IR, Paris MM, Rinderknecht S, McCracken GH. Cranial computed tomographic scans have little impact on management of bacterial meningitis. *Am J Dis Child* 1992;**146**:1484–7.

58 Horwitz SJ, Boxerbaum B, O'Bell J. Cerebral herniation in bacterial meningitis in childhood. *Ann Neurol* 1980;**7**:524–8.

59 Addy DP. When not to do a lumbar puncture. *Arch Dis Child* 1987;**62**:873–5.

60 Rennick G, Shann F, de Campo J. Cerebral herniation during bacterial meningitis in children. *BMJ* 1993;**306**:953–5.

61 Darnell RB. The polymerase chain reaction: application to nervous system disease. *Ann Neurol* 1993;**34**:513–23.

62 Eisenstein BI. The polymerase chain reaction: a new method of using molecular genetics for medical diagnosis. *N Engl J Med* 1990;**322**:178–83.

63 Eng RHK, Seligman SJ. Lumbar puncture induced meningitis. *JAMA* 1981;**245**:1456–9.

64 Marton KI, Gean AD. The spinal tap: a new look at an old test. *Ann Intern Med* 1986;**104**:840–8.

65 Anderson M. Bacterial meningitis. In: Matthews WB, Glaser GH, eds, *Recent advances in clinical neurology 4*. Edinburgh: Churchill Livingstone, 1984:87–121.

66 Cabral DA, Flodmark O, Farrell K, Speert DP. Prospective study of computed tomography in acute bacterial meningitis. *J Pediatr* 1987;**111**:201–5.

67 Sze G, Zimmerman RD. The magnetic resonance imaging of infections and inflammatory diseases. *Radiol Clin North Am* 1988;**26**:839–59.

68 Kaplan SL, Feigin RD. The syndrome of inappropriate secretion of antidiuretic hormone in children with bacterial meningitis. *J Paediatr* 1978;**92**:758–61.

69 Lebel MH, Freij BJ, Syrogiannopoulos GA, *et al*. Dexamethasone therapy for bacterial meningitis. *N Engl J Med* 1988;**319**:964–71.

70 Lebel MH, Hoyt MJ, Waagner DC, Rollins NK, Finitzo T, McCracken GH. Magnetic resonance imaging and dexamethasone for bacterial meningitis. *Am J Dis Child* 1989;**143**:301–6.

71 Havens PL, Wenderberger KJ, Hoffman GM, Lee MB, Chusid MJ. Corticosteroids as adjunctive therapy in bacterial meningitis. A meta analysis of clinical trials. *Am J Dis Child* 1989;**143**:1051–5.

72 Odio CM, Faingezicht I, Paris M, *et al*. The beneficial effects of early dexamethasone administration in infants and children with bacterial meningitis. *N Engl J Med* 1991;**324**:1525–31.

73 Schattner A. Should we add corticosteroids to the treatment of acute bacterial meningitis? *Q J Med* 1992;**82**:181–3.

74 Ashwal S, Stringer W, Tomasi L, Schneider S, Thompson J, Perkin R. Cerebral blood

flow and carbon dioxide reactively in children with bacterial meningitis. *J Paediatr* 1990; **117**:523–30.

75 Rebaud P, Berthier JC, Hartemann E, Floret D. Intracranial pressure in childhood central nervous system infections. *Intensive Care Med* 1988;**14**:522–5.

76 Minns RA, Engleman HM, Stirling H. Cerebrospinal fluid pressure in pyogenic meningitis. *Arch Dis Child* 1989;**64**:814–20.

77 McMenamin JB, Volpe JJ. Bacterial meningitis in infancy: effects on intracranial pressure and cerebral blood flow velocity. *Neurology* 1984;**34**:500–4.

78 Pickard JD, Czosnyka M. Management of raised intracranial pressure. *J Neurol Neurosurg Psychiatry* 1993;**56**:845–58.

79 Kaplan SL, Fishman MA. Update on bacterial meningitis. *Child Neurol* 1988;**3**:82–93.

80 Peltola H, Anttila M, Renkonen O-V, Finnish Study Group. Randomised comparison of chloramphenicol, ampicillin, cefotaxime and ceftriaxone for childhood bacterial meningitis. *Lancet* 1989;**1**:1281–7.

81 Lebel MH, Hoyt MJ, McCracken GH. Comparative efficacy of ceftriaxone and cefuroxime for treatment of bacterial meningitis. *J Pediatr* 1989;**114**:1049–54.

82 Sutcliffe EM, Jones DM, El-Sheikh S, Percival A. Penicillin-insensitive meningococci in the UK. *Lancet* 1988;**i**:657–8.

83 Landesman SH, Corrado ML, Shah PM, Armengaud M, Barza M, Cherubin CE. Past and current roles for cephalosporin antibiotics in the treatment of meningitis: emphasis on use in gram negative bacillary meningitis. *Am J Med* 1981;**71**:693–703.

84 Schlesinger LS, Ross SC, Schaberg DR. Staphylococcus aureus meningitis: a broad based epidemiological study. *Medicine (Baltimore)*, 1987;**66**:148–56.

85 Klein NJ, Heyderman RS, Levin M. Antibiotic choices for meningitis beyond the neonatal period. *Arch Dis Child* 1992;**67**:157–61.

86 Rubin RH, Hooper DC. Central nervous system infections in the compromised host. *Med Clin North Am* 1985;**69**:281–93.

86a Bullock MRR, Welchman JM. Diagnostic and prognostic features of tuberculous meningitis on CT scanning. *J Neurol Neurosurg Psychiatry* 1982;**45**:1098–1101.

86b Chu N. Tuberculous meningitis: computerised tomographic manifestations. *Arch Neurol* 1980;**37**:458–60.

86c Kennedy DH, Fallon RJ. Tuberculous meningitis. *JAMA* 1979;**241**:264–8.

86d Chandramuki A. Rapid diagnosis of tuberculous meningitis by ELISA to detect mycobacterial antigen and antibody in the cerebrospinal fluid. *J Infect Dis* 1989;**160**:343–4.

86e Kaneko K, Onodera O, Miyatake T, Tsuji S. Rapid diagnosis of tuberculous meningitis by polymerase chain reaction (PCR). *Neurology* 1990;**40**:1617–18.

86f Fallon RJ, Kennedy DH. Treatment and prognosis in tuberculous meningitis. *J Infect Suppl* 1981:39–44.

87 Wood M, Anderson M. CNS tuberculosis. In: Walton J, ed. *Neurological infections*, London: Saunders, 1988:172–96.

88 Sheller JR, Des Prez RM. CNS tuberculosis. *Neurol Clin* 1986;**4**:143–58.

89 American Thoracic Society. Treatment of tuberculosis and tuberculosis infections in adults and children. *Am Rev Respir Dis* 1986;**134**:355–63.

90 Reik L, Steere AC, Bartenhagen NH, Shope RE, Malawista SE. Neurologic abnormalities of Lyme disease. *Medicine (Baltimore)*, 1979;**58**:281–94.

91 Pachner AR, Steere AC. The triad of neurologic manifestations of Lyme disease: meningitis, cranial neuritis and radiculoneuritis. *Neurology* 1985;**35**:47–53.

92 Finkel MJ, Halperin JJ. Nervous system Lyme borreliosis—revisited. *Arch Neurol* 1992; **49**:102–7.

93 Steere AC, Pachner AR, Malawista SE. Neurologic abnormalities of Lyme disease: successful treatment with high dose intravenous penicillin. *Ann Intern Med* 1983;**99**:767–72.

94 Katz DA, Berger JR. Neurosyphilis in acquired immunodeficiency syndrome. *Arch Neurol* 1989;**46**:895–8.

95 Katz DA, Berger JR, Duncan RC. Neurosyphilis. A comparative study of the effects of infection with human immunodeficiency virus. *Arch Neurol* 1993;**50**:243–9.

96 Merritt HH, Moore M. Acute syphilitic meningitis. *Medicine* 1935;**14**:119–83.

97 Kirk LJ, Fine PD, Sexton JD, Muchmore G. Rocky mountain spotted fever: a clinical review based on 48 confirmed cases 1943–1986. *Medicine* 1990;**69**:35–45.

98 Raoult D, Zuchelli P, Weiller PJ, *et al*. Incidence, clinical observations and risk factors in the severe form of Mediterranean spotted fever among patients admitted to hospital in Marseilles 1983–1984. *J Infect* 1986;**12**:111–16.

99 Shaked Y. Rickettsial infection of the central nervous system: the role of prompt antimicrobial therapy. *Q J Med*, 1991;**79**:301–6.

100 Molyneux M, Fox R. Diagnosis and treatment of malaria in Britain. *Br Med J* 1993; **306**:1175–80.

101 Romans GC. Cerebral malaria: the unsolved riddle. *J Neurol Sci* 1991;**101**:1–6.

102 Maegraith B, Fletcher A. The pathogenesis of mammalian malaria. *Adv Parasitol* 1972;**10**:49–75.

103 Molyneux M. Cerebral malaria in children; clinical implications of cytoadherence. *Am J Trop Med Hyg* 1990;**43**:38–41.

104 MacPherson GG, Warrell MJ, White NJ, Looareesuwan S, Warrell DA. Human cerebral malaria: a quantitative ultrastructural analysis of parasitized erythrocyte sequestration. *Am J Pathol* 1985;**119**:385–401.

105 Warrell DA, White N, Veall S, *et al.* Cerebral anaerobic glycolysis and reduced cerebral oxygen transport in human cerebral malaria. *Lancet* 1988;**2**:534–4.

106 Looareesuwan S, Warrell DA, White NJ, *et al.* Do patients with cerebral malaria have cerebral oedema? A computed tomography study. *Lancet* 1983;**1**:434–7.

107 Newton CRJC, Kirkham FJ, Winstanley PA, *et al.* Intracranial pressure in African children with cerebral malaria. *Lancet* 1991;**337**:573–6.

108 Warrell DA, Looareesuwan S, Warrell MJ, *et al.* Dexamethasone proves deleterious in cerebral malaria. A double blind trial in 100 consecutive patients. *N Engl J Med* 1982; **306**:313–19.

109 White NJ, Looareesuwan S. Cerebral malaria. In: Kennedy PGE, Johnson RT, eds. *Infections of the nervous system*, London: Butterworths, 1987:118–44.

110 Phillips RE. Hypoglycaemia is an important complication of Falciparum malaria. *Q J Med* 1989;**71**:477–83.

111 Miller KD, Greenberg AE, Campbell CC. Treatment of severe malaria in the United States with a continuous infusion of quinidine gluconate and exchange transfusion. *N Engl J Med* 1989;**321**:65–70.

112 Wyler DJ. Malaria: overview and update. *Clin Infect Dis* 1993;**16**:449–58.

113 Carter RF. Primary amoebic meningoencephalitis: clinical, pathological and epidemiological features of six cases. *J Pathol Bacteriol* 1968;**96**:1–25.

114 Seidel JS, Harmatz P, Visvesvara GS, Cohen A, Edwards J, Turner J. Successful treatment of primary amoebic meningo-encephalitis. *N Engl J Med* 1982;**306**:346–8.

115 McLelland CJ, Craig BF, Crockard HA. Brain abscesses in Northern Ireland: a 30-year community review. *J Neurol Neurosurg Psychiatry* 1978;**41**:1043–7.

116 Britt RH, Enzmann DR, Yeagar AS. Neuropathological and computerized tomographic findings in experimental brain abscess. *J Neurosurg* 1981;**55**:590–603.

117 Britt RH, Enzmann DR. Clinical stages of brain abscesses on serial CT scans after contrast infusion. Computerized tomographic, neuropathological and clinical correlations. *J Neurosurg* 1983;**59**:972–89.

118 de Louvois J, Gortvai P, Hurley R. Bacteriology of abscesses of the central nervous system: a multicentre prospective study. *BMJ* 1977;**ii**:981–4.

119 Ingham HR, Sisson PR, Mendelow AD, Kalbag RM, McAllister VL. Brain abscess—clinical features. In: *Pyogenic neurosurgical infections.* London: Edward Arnold, 1991:39–50.

120 Chun CH, Johnson JD, Hofstetter M, Raff MJ. Brain abscess. A study of 45 consecutive cases. *Medicine* 1986;**65**:415–31.

121 Nielsen H, Gyldensted C, Harmsen A. Cerebral abscess: etiology and pathogenesis, symptoms, diagnosis and treatment. *Acta Neurol Scand* 1982;**65**:609–22.

122 Shaw MDM, Russell JA. Cerebellar abscess—a review of 47 cases. *J Neurol Neurosurg Psychiatry* 1975;**38**:429–35.

123 Saez-Llorens XJ, Umann MA, Odio CM, McCracken GH, Nelson JD. Brain abscess in infants and children. *Pediatr Infect Dis J* 1989;**8**:449–58.

124 Mampalam TJ, Rosenblum ML. Trends in the management of bacterial brain abscess; a review of 102 cases over 17 years. *Neurosurgery* 1988;**23**:451–8.

125 New PFJ, Davis KR, Ballantine HT. Computed tomography in cerebral abscess. *Radiology* 1976;**121**:641–6.

126 Miller ES, Psrilal SD, Uttley D. CT scanning in the management of intracranial abscess: a review of 100 cases. *Br J Neurosurg* 1988;**2**:439–46.

127 Davidson HD, Steiner RE. Magnetic resonance imaging in infections of the central nervous system. *Am J Neuroradiol* 1985;**6**:499–504.

128 Schroth G, Kretzschmar K, Gawehn J, Voigt K. Advantage of magnetic resonance imaging in the diagnosis of cerebral infections. *Neuroradiology* 1987;**29**:120–6.

129 Apuzzo ML, Chandrasoma PR, Cohen D, Zee CS, Zelman V. Computed imaging stereotaxy: experience and perspective related to 500 procedures applied to brain masses. *Neurosurgery* 1987;**20**:930–7.

130 Dyste GN, Hitchon PW, Menezes AH, Vangilder JA, Greene GM. Stereotaxic surgery in the treatment of multiple brain abscesses. *J Neurosurg* 1988;**69**:188–94.

131 Young B. Role of stereotactic biopsy in the management of transplant patients with intracranial lesions. *Neurol Clin* 1988;**6**:639–44.

132 Boom WH, Tuazon CV. Successful treatment of multiple brain abscesses with antibiotics alone. *Rev Infect Dis* 1985;**7**:189–99.

133 Rousseaux M, Lesoin F, Destee A, Jomin M, Petit H. Developments in the treatment and prognosis of multiple brain abscesses. *Neurosurgery* 1985;**16**:304–8.

134 Bannister G, Williams B, Smith S. Treatment of subdural empyema. *J Neurosurg* 1981;**55**:82–8.

135 Kaufman DM, Miller MH, Steigbigel NH. Subdural empyema. Analysis of 17 recent cases and review of the literature. *Medicine* 1975;**54**:485–98.

136 Smith HP, Hendrick EB. Subdural empyema and epidural abscess in children. *J Neurosurg* 1983;**58**:392–7.

137 Cowie R, Williams B. Late seizures and morbidity after subdural empyema. *J Neurosurg* 1983;**58**:569–73.

138 Hitchcock E, Andreadis A. Subdural empyema: a review of 29 cases. *J Neurol Neurosurg Psychiatry* 1964;**27**:422–34.

139 Weingarten K, Zimmerman RD, Becker RD, Heier LA, Haimes AB, Deck MDF. Subdural and epidural empyemas: MR imaging. *Am J Neuroradiol* 1987;**10**:81–7.

140 Zimmerman RD, Leeds NG, Danziger A. Subdural empyema CT findings. *Radiology* 1984;**150**:417–22.

10 Acute spinal cord compression

ROBIN A JOHNSTON

A wide variety of pathological lesions causes spinal cord compression. The clinical presentation may indicate the nature of the lesion although with modern imaging techniques the importance of making a clinical diagnosis of pathology has diminished. The important diagnostic aspect of acute spinal cord compression is that it should be recognised as early as possible and the patient referred with the urgency that each particular case merits. The over-riding reason for this is to enhance the chances of reversing the neurological damage by appropriate decompression surgery. Prognosis for recovery depends mainly on two factors: (a) the severity of the neurological deficit and (b) the duration of the deficit before decompression. There will be other factors taken into consideration when planning surgical management including general fitness, life expectancy, tumour pathology, and the extent of any metastatic spread. Successful spinal cord decompression means return of normal function in affected limbs and a stable, painless spine. Generally this means restoring independent walking although both patient and surgeon may have to settle for lesser degrees of functional recovery.

Spinal cord compression implies a "structural" lesion of the vertebral column compromising the spinal canal and producing a myelopathy. The signs and symptoms of spinal cord compression are those of motor and sensory deficit, but the common feature of "structural" lesions is pain. Spine pain or nerve root pain, occurring in the presence of myelopathic symptoms, strongly implies a surgically remediable aetiology. Most patients presenting with spinal cord compression reach hospital by referral through their general practitioner or through an accident and emergency department, and are usually admitted to general medical or surgical wards. In the early stages it may be difficult to detect abnormal neurological signs, especially if these are subtle and the pain component is large. For a variety of reasons, including late self-referral to any medical practitioner, delays can and do occur in the referral of such a patient to a specialist spinal unit. This was the subject of a candid and disturbing report by Maurice-Williams and Richardson in which they illustrate the diverse causes for delayed referral and the consequences of this.[1] Any neurosurgeon or orthopaedic surgeon who carries out spinal decompression, will have experience of patients who are referred having been paraplegic for several days, well beyond the time of useful surgical treatment. Recognition of signs and symptoms of spinal cord compression may be difficult outside a neuroscience environment and it is important that both neurosurgeons and neurologists take the trouble to facilitate referral from physicians and general surgeons at an early stage. This includes an ongoing educational element of which a most important aspect is to encourage colleagues to recognise the early signs of myelopathy. Easier access to spinal imaging should help.

Trauma

The most acute form of spinal cord compression is caused by trauma of which 50% occurs in the cervical spine and most of the remainder in the thoracolumbar junction and lumbar spine. Patients are usually young males involved in road traffic accidents, falls, and occasionally sport related activities.[2] The forces involved can be resolved into flexion, extension, compression, and rotation, although usually more than one is involved to produce the variety of different fracture patterns and subluxations seen in the cervical spine. In about 10% of cases, two non-contiguous levels of the cervical spine are damaged, separated by several normal segments.[3]

The management of acute spinal cord injury is the subject of many text books and publications and may be intimidating to those unfamiliar with this clinical problem. In fact the major components of management of spine trauma are analogous to the

273

management of a fracture of a long bone. The management steps involved are recognition, immobilisation, investigation, reduction, fixation, and rehabilitation. The cervical fracture should be recognised for what it is and in most cases the combination of neurological deficit, plus a painful and tender cervical region will indicate at least the possibility of cervical spine damage. Situations do occur where a patient is unable to provide a history because of decreased consciousness and in these it is better to make the assumption that cervical damage is present until proved otherwise. The cervical spine can be immobilised simply by holding the head firmly between two hands and maintaining the cervical spine in a neutral position until better facilities are available. Depending on the circumstances the patient may be fitted with an appropriate sized Philadelphia style collar, or be placed in cervical traction. The frequently used soft, spongy, cervical collars are particularly ineffective in restricting cervical movements. One study indicates that this type of collar prevents only 25% of flexion and extension movements. A Philadelphia style collar rises to the occiput, spreads over the shoulders, rises over the chin, and provides more effective immobilisation. Cervical tongs may be applied in the casualty department within a matter of seconds if the Gardner–Wells variety are used. These require only a little local anaesthetic and are placed 4 cm above the external auditory meatus. They are simply hand-screwed through the anaesthetised scalp into the outer skull cortex to a pre-set tension. The doctor then has full control of the patient's cervical spine. Definitive investigations at an early stage must include a lateral plain radiograph of all cervical vertebrae. So many cases of missed fracture in the cervical spine are the result of inadequate radiographs which omit the lower vertebrae. Flexion/extension views can be particularly revealing. If carried out carefully the patient will come to no harm and the films may show abnormal movement. Cervical spine radiographs are difficult to read, especially for inexperienced junior staff, and recourse should be had to experienced staff before management decisions are made on these patients. More definitive investigation is carried out by CT, which almost always reveals more damage than was initially expected from plain radiographs. If C7 is invisible with ordinary radiographs it is always accessible through CT. MRI is beginning to be made available to patients with acute spinal injuries.[4] It is particularly helpful in recognising damage to ligaments, discs, and pre-vertebral tissues which have clearly altered signals with this form of scanning, but which may not be recognised using radiographs (fig 1).

At or about this stage in management, referral should be made to a specialised spinal unit, preferably an acute spinal cord injury unit. The newly opened National Spinal Cord Injuries Unit for Scotland now receives patients with spine trauma, with and without cord injury, within hours of injury in some cases. The pathophysiological consequences of acute spinal cord injury on the cardiovascular and respiratory symptoms and the intensive nursing requirements make early referral of these patients to an appropriate unit imperative. Spinal cord damage results in loss of sympathetic neural control causing hypotension and bradycardia. These are normal for the patient who has cord transection and should not be the subject of volume loading in misplaced attempts

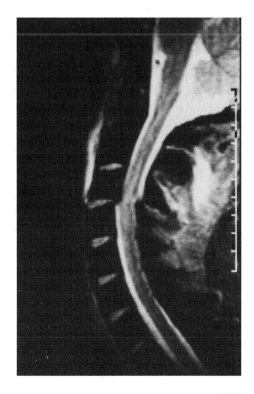

Figure 1—MRI (1·5 T Siemens Magnetom, T2-weighted scan) 24 hours after acute spinal trauma. The altered signal from the anterior longitudinal ligament opposite C2 and C3 is clearly seen. This cervical spine has lost a substantial degree of stability.

275

to restore "normal" blood pressure. Loss of intercostal innervation due to cranial cord trauma produces ventilatory insufficiency which is best managed in specialised units.[5]

Fractures, subluxations, or dislocations require reduction into normal alignment. This may be relatively easily brought about using simple cervical traction. In the 1970s there was a vogue for using high loads of cervical traction, but this carries the risk of damage by traction on the spinal cord itself. Depending on the type and displacement of the injury, the position of the cervical spine can be altered using a rolled up sheet to exaggerate the lordotic curve. The vector of traction may be varied to enhance the likelihood of reducing the spine back to normal alignment. These techniques require frequent radiographic assessment and management experience. Should appropriate cervical traction be unsuccessful in reducing the fracture/dislocation, the options are for manipulation under anaesthesia, which should only be carried out by experienced staff or, more commonly now, by open reduction and internal fixation. These latter decisions should be made by those experienced in dealing with spine trauma. Those patients who have vertebral damage but no spinal cord injury are to some extent vulnerable to secondary injury through inadvertent or accidental mishandling of the spine and in some ways have considerably more to lose than those patients who already have major spinal cord damage.

Fixation of the cervical spine may be carried out using external orthotic supports such as the halo fixator which is particularly useful for high cervical fractures. Even in this device a small degree of flexion and extension can still occur. Methods of internal fixation have evolved and improved, especially in recent years. In the cervical spine these involve plate and screw, wire or laminar clamp devices and do provide the patient with the ability to begin mobilisation and rehabilitation at an earlier stage.[6] For thoracic and lumbar fractures the use of pedicle screw fixation reduces the number of vertebral levels permanently immobilised and allows intraoperative fracture reduction and restoration of alignment in some cases.[7] Malalignment of vertebrae is reduced using internal fixation, but long term stability only comes through bony union. There is, and will continue to be, great debate among specialists in the management of patients with spinal cord injury concerning the merits and demerits of surgical intervention. What is clear is that in selected circumstances internal fixation and fusion does have a role to play and does impart advantages to patients, their rehabilitation, and their spines. What surgical intervention does not do, however, is improve neurological outcome. Although there have been spurious and isolated reports of this, there is no generally recognised association between surgical decompression and fixation, and neurological recovery in patients with acute spinal trauma.

The use of high doses of methylprednisolone has become standard practice in North America for patients with acute spinal trauma. This follows the results of studies that showed statistical improvement in limb function where these steroids were administered.[8] This statistical improvement, however, may not be reflected in any significant functional or clinical gain by the patient. Although the use of high dose methylprednisolone has, for reasons other than those which are entirely medical, gained widespread use in America this practice has not become established in the United Kingdom.

In patients who incur a severe head injury, the primary traumatic event is followed by a series of microvascular and biochemical changes which are recognised as the means by which secondary damage can compound the original injury. The same is true of spinal cord injury and it is possible that similar mechanisms are involved. The effect of the excitotoxic glutamate which is released following trauma to central neural tissue can be modified using N-methyl-D-aspartate receptor blockade. Considerable attention currently focuses on biochemical methods of preventing or modifying the secondary damage produced following brain and spinal cord injury.[9]

Inflammatory conditions

The most common, surgically relevant, inflammatory spinal condition is rheumatoid disease which affects approximately 1% of the population in western Europe. The cervical spine is involved in a substantial percentage of those patients who have rheumatoid disease, with the incidence and severity increasing with the duration of the disease. The most common site of involvement is at the occipito-C1/C2 level, although all levels of the cervical spine may be involved.[10]

The fibrous inflammatory tissue mass is generally referred to as pannus although by strict definition pannus refers to the exudate overlying the synovial membrane. The fluctuating progress of the condition gradually destroys the joint tissues and articular surfaces which will lead to subluxation or even dislocation. This is frequently seen in the fingers and wrist joints of patients with rheumatoid disease, but does also occur at the occipito-C1/C2 level. The most common form of dislocation is anterior subluxation of C1 on C2 and this may be fixed or mobile depending on the activity of the inflammatory process.[11–13] Eventually the condition will "burn out" and the joints may become ankylosed in an abnormal position. Loss of height of the lateral masses of C1 will result in vertical translocation of the odontoid process and this occurs in about 10% of the affected population. Less frequently occurring abnormalities include posterior subluxation of C1 on C2 where the odontoid is totally eroded and the atlas can move posteriorly relative to the body of C2. Asymmetrical involvement of the lateral mass joints may lead to rotational deformities or lateral subluxations.[14] The demonstration of these different types of atlantoaxial abnormalities has been enormously enhanced through the use of CT myelography including sagittal plane reconstruction, and with magnetic resonance scanning, both carried out with the patient flexing and extending the neck.[15 16]

With any subluxation in this region, or in the subaxial region, the spinal canal will be compromised and the patient may develop a myelopathy. One of the burning issues of epidemiological investigation into rheumatoid disease addresses the question of which patients with cervical spine involvement will go on to develop spinal cord compression. Unfortunately despite considerable effort there is no firm method of predicting which patients will deteriorate neurologically and which patients, with perhaps relatively severe radiological involvement, will never develop neurological signs or symptoms. Clinical markers have proved to be of little value, but more recent work involving measurement of cord diameter may prove to be of more value in predicting those patients who will require surgical intervention.[17]

Acute spinal cord compression is not common in rheumatoid disease although there are anecdotal cases of patients suddenly collapsing with paralysis and succumbing due to gross odontoid subluxation. Usually neurological symptoms develop over a period of weeks or even months, but a few patients do develop neurological signs and deteriorate with progressive myelopathy over a short period of days. They present with deterioration in gait quality and complain of sensory alteration or sensory loss, including loss of manual dexterity in the upper limbs. A clear clinical history is of paramount importance in confirming a myelopathy, since severe and widespread synovial joint involvement frequently precludes accurate assessment of deep tendon reflexes and muscle power. Patients will often be able to distinguish between new symptoms such as loss of strength or paraesthesia or significant gait deterioration, and identify these separately from the symptoms of multiple joint involvement with which they are already very familiar. Isolated tendon reflexes may be elicited although plantar responses are almost never obtainable because of local joint involvement or previous surgery. Vertical subluxation of the odontoid process makes it possible that patients will develop lower cranial nerve signs. In the past, speech difficulty, dysphonia, and nystagmus have been attributed to high spinal cord or low medullary compression by pannus around the odontoid process. Although this may be so in some cases, rheumatoid disease in the temporomandibular and cricoarytenoid joints may provide a more pragmatic cause.[18 19] In one of the largest series of rheumatoid patients that have been studied, Crockard found that nystagmus only occurred in those patients with pre-existing Chiari I malformation.[17]

When an acute cervical myelopathy is confirmed in a patient with rheumatoid disease, the most likely cause will be anterior atlantoaxial subluxation. This can easily and rapidly be confirmed by a plain lateral radiograph of the cervical spine taken in flexion and extension. This will confirm only bone movement and position whereas soft tissue involvement will require the use of CT myelography or MRI. The purpose of management in this situation is to reduce the compression on the cervical cord and in most cases this will be achieved by extending the upper cervical spine and bringing into more normal alignment the C1 and C2 vertebrae. It cannot be assumed, however, that because vertebral alignment has been restored spinal cord compression has been reduced. This will become apparent once scanning of the region has been carried out. Restoration of normal vertebral alignment is achieved using light cervical traction, preferably with titanium or carbon fibre tongs so there is no interference with subsequent scanning. The simplest and easiest type of cervical tong to apply is the Gardner–Wells version. As the patient will most frequently be female and small, the weight required will rarely exceed 3 or

4 kg. Over the next 24–48 hours the patient will experience any neurological improvement that is likely to occur if reduction of cord compression has been achieved. It is at this time that the interest of a spine surgeon must be engaged and appropriate imaging of the region carried out. It is also important to recall that patients with multiple joint involvement due to rheumatoid disease do not tolerate prolonged cervical traction. If neurological improvement is not obvious within 72 hours it is probably unlikely to occur and traction should be discontinued. Once appropriate scanning has been carried out the surgical decision concerning continued immobilisation or interventional decompression, fixation, and fusion will be made.

There are a variety of surgical procedures from which the surgeon may select those most appropriate to individual patients. The odontoid region can be approached directly by the transpharyngeal route in order to directly decompress the cervicomedullary region. It is recommended that this should be followed by a posterior stabilising operation which will generate fusion of C1 and C2 or occipital bone to C2.[20-22] Subaxial cranial compression is less common than at C1–C2 and usually also requires a combination of anterior and posterior surgery. At all levels the aim is to directly decompress the spinal cord, to restore vertebral alignment and to prevent further malalignment. For many patients a posterior C1–C2 fixation and fusion will be sufficient but in others the surgical procedure may be more complex.[23-28]

The postoperative mortality and morbidity rates are greatest in those patients who are severely neurologically affected, that is, quadriparetic and unable to walk. The systemic effects of rhematoid disease, especially interstitial pulmonary involvement, may adversely affect postsurgical recovery. In those patients in whom the myelopathy is recognised and treated in the early stages the outlook for recovery is good and postoperative mortality is low.[11]

Infective lesions

Infections of the spine are uncommon, but can usefully be classified as either vertebral osteomyelitis or intraspinal infection. Vertebral osteomyelitis is the more common variety of infection and can lead to intraspinal infection, whereas "pure" intraspinal infection comprises extradural, subdural, or intramedullary abscess in descending order of frequency and without concomitant infection of the vertebral column.[29][30] Intraspinal infections occur at a frequency of approximately one per million per year in United Kingdom neurosurgical units and are predominantly caused by pyogenic organisms, usually *Staphylococcus* sp., whereas in Asia or Africa *Mycobacterium tuberculosis* is the common infecting organism.[31]

Extradural spinal abscess may be found anywhere within the spinal extradural space but this does not communicate with the intracranial extradural space because the two are separated at the foramen magnum where the outer, endosteal layer of the intracranial dura adheres to bone. The spinal dura is a single layer with the extradural space most prominent posteriorly and it is here that most extradural abscesses are found, most being in the thoracic or lumbar spine. Cervical extradural abscess is uncommon and is usually associated with vertebral osteomyelitis. The abscess may extend over a few or many vertebral levels and it is well recognised that non-contiguous abscesses may occur.[32][33]

A spinal extradural abscess is a neurosurgical emergency and is one of the few instances where the history and clinical examination may provide an instant pathological diagnosis. The patient may, or may not, present with systemic signal illness, but as the abscess enlarges and compression of the spinal cord occurs then myelopathic symptoms gradually develop, usually over the course of a small number of days.[34-36] The outstanding clinical feature is spinal pain and the marked local tenderness of the spine at the level of abscess formation. Tapping the spinous processes lightly with a tendon hammer may elicit this and indicate the pathological diagnosis. Several studies have reported the high frequency of misdiagnosis of this condition in its early stages. The complaint of spinal pain, particularly in younger patients, and of thoracic pain in all patients should be regarded seriously enough to make a definitive pathological diagnosis rather than to assume the symptom is due to minor "mechanical dysfunction". By the time neurological symptoms are present, even in the absence of neurological signs, the probability of some form of surgically remediable structural spinal lesion increases considerably. Should the patient present with a paraplegia this should be regarded as a failure of diagnosis, as symptoms are frequently present for several days before this end stage.

The most valuable diagnostic exercise is high grade MRI.[37] This will confirm the diagnosis of extradural abscess, indicate its upper and lower limits, demonstrate whether or not there is an associated primary osteomyelitis and in most cases differentiate between extradural abscess and subdural abscess. Myelography with CT is the next best diagnostic investigation although the distinction between abscess, haematoma, or even in some cases metastatic tumour is not possible.

Investigations should be carried out without delay and management is by immediate surgical decompression. As the abscesses are very commonly located in the posterior extradural space, albeit extending laterally on either side, this is one occasion where a decompressive laminectomy is the operation of choice. Attention should be paid to the upper and lower limits of the abscess although the laminectomy may not require to be taken to these extremes should the pus be of a liquid nature. On other occasions the laminectomy may need to be taken to the limits if the compressive material is semi-solid infected granulation tissue.

The results of surgery tell their own story and indicate that when patients are severely affected or paraplegic the likelihood of neurological recovery is poor. The mortality rate for this condition has diminished over the years with improving diagnosis, but is nevertheless substantial for a spinal condition and is variously reported at between 17% and 36%.[31 38]

Vertebral osteomyelitis is a relatively uncommon condition, but familiar to spine surgeons in the United Kingdom. The commonest causes are staphylococci, streptococci, *E coli* and occasionally unusual organisms such as salmonellae or *Brucella* sp. For the most part the spinal cord is not affected and the problem is one of structural integrity of the vertebral column.[39] Both pyogenic and tuberculous osteomyelitis may lead to the formation of an extradural abscess lying anterior to the spinal cord, which may cause acute spinal cord compression in a fashion not dissimilar to a "pure" extradural abscess. The gradual progressive nature of bone infection will produce a more protracted preceding history, including spinal pain, aches, malaise, discomfort, and system signs of infection culminating in an acute neurological deterioration.

Plain radiographs of the spine may give the diagnosis by revealing erosion and loss of height in contiguous vertebrae with destruction of the intervertebral disc. The coexistence of an extradural abscess is made by MRI or by CT myelography and is done as a matter of some urgency. It requires only a few millilitres of localised liquefied pus in the anterior cervical spinal canal to cause substantial tetraparesis, recovery from which is entirely possible with expeditious decompression. Scanning also reveals the extent of vertebral and paravertebral infection and can usually be distinguished from metastatic disease.[40]

For pyogenic osteomyelitis, which predominates in the United Kingdom, direct ventral spinal canal decompression is often required. In the cervical spine this will involve an anterior cervical decompression procedure which can be carried out through an intervertebral disc space by a medial vertebrectomy. Division of the posterior longitudinal ligament usually results in the egress of a small volume of liquefied pus which is sometimes less than impressive considering the degree of paralysis which it has produced. In these acute situations the surgeon is best advised not to incorporate spinal reconstruction, but rather to return the patient to a period of external spinal stabilisation, usually by cervical traction, accompanied by appropriate intravenous antibiotic therapy. Once the infection has been treated in such a way for a period of several days, then more definitive means of stabilising the spine can be employed. In these situations where the pyogenic infection is under control, bone grafting almost always results in a solid fusion and in selected cases it is becoming accepted practice to use one or more of the forms of internal metal fixation while continuing antibiotic treatment.

In the thoracic and lumbar spine surgical decompression involves more difficult access, either by costotransversectomy or posterior thoracotomy in the thoracic region and by the extraperitoneal route in the lumbar region. In tuberculous osteomyelitis a limited posterolateral decompression by costotransversectomy to release indolent purulent material is a satisfactory means of decompression with reconstruction and stabilising surgery reserved for later if necessary.[41]

Degenerative pathology

Degenerative change within the spine only causes acute spinal cord compression in a small group, but usually has a more prolonged course involving progressive neurological symptoms.[42] Protrusion of intervertebral disc into the spinal canal, whether this be in the presence of existing osteophyte or not, can produce a rapidly developing myelopathy. Acute disc protrusions most commonly occur in the lumbar spine with 80% being located either at L4–L5 or L5–S1. Central compression of the spinal theca at this level causes an acute cauda equina syndrome which is a spinal emergency. Isolated or "pure" cervical intervertebral disc protrusion is much less common than compression due to osteophyte formation although it is common to find a combination of both. "Pure" cervical disc prolapse can occur at any age and it may be that a pre-existing and relatively mild myelopathy rapidly becomes much worse because of protrusion of cervical disc a few millimetres further into the spinal canal. Acute myelopathy will present in older patients who have degenerative changes superimposed on a developmentally narrow cervical spinal canal (<10 mm anteroposterior diameter). In these patients the usual mechanism is violent hyperextension of the neck.[43] "Pure" thoracic disc protrusion is uncommon and these patients present to neurosurgical units at a frequency of one per million per year.[44] It is common to find that the so called thoracic "disc" is in fact a combination of osteophyte and calcified disc material, rather than degenerate nucleus pulposus which has prolapsed into the spinal canal.

In cases of acute disc protrusion, whichever the level, spinal pain usually accompanied by root pain is a common clinical symptom. The level of root pain provides a good indication of which intervertebral disc is the culprit. When the disc protrudes sufficiently into the spinal canal to cause spinal (or cauda equina) compression then neurological symptoms and signs accompany the pain. In the cervical and thoracic region these will lead to a myelopathy commensurate with the level of compression. Clinical determination of the sensory level gives a good indication of the level of thoracic disc prolapse. The distribution of pain, numbness, or "dropped" reflexes in the upper limbs provides a good clinical indicator as to the level of cervical disc disease. When the patient produces symptoms which illustrate loss of manual dexterity it is often the case that compression is at the level of the C3–C4 intervertebral disc. In the lumbar spine, compression of the cauda equina produces loss of sensation across the sacral dermatomes, either unilaterally or bilaterally, associated with root pain in both legs and loss of bladder sphincter function. The clinical diagnosis of an acute disc prolapse in the cervical and lumbar spine is relatively straightforward, but misdiagnosis often occurs in the thoracic region. There may be a background history of thoracic spine pain and several studies have confirmed that, probably because of the rarity of thoracic disc disease, other pathological diagnoses are given prior consideration.[44]

The diagnosis is of disc prolapse confirmed radiologically by MRI of the appropriate spinal region. The alternative is CT myelography but with modern CT scanners contrast is usually not required to confirm lumbar disc prolapse, although it is still required in the thoracic and cervical spine.[45]

The management of acute myelopathy or an acute cauda equina syndrome due to intervertebral disc prolapse involves urgent surgical decompression. In the lumbar spine this is carried out through a micro-discectomy approach and in most cases this gives adequate access to the disc prolapse on both sides. Occasionally the access has to be increased by either a hemi-laminectomy or on occasions by a full laminectomy. For those patients with coexisting lumbar canal stenosis, it is recommended by some that a laminectomy is used to reduce the risk of a post-surgical cauda equina syndrome which occurs at a frequency of one in 500 lumbar disc operations.[46]

In the cervical spine, disc prolapse causing myelopathy is removed through an anterior access route between the carotid sheath laterally and the pharynx/larynx medially. This is an approach to the subaxial spine and when the compression is due to disc prolapse alone a simple disc excision is satisfactory. This is carried out using an operating microscope with excision of the disc material and the cartilaginous end plates down to the level of the posterior longitudinal ligament and laterally to the medial part of the uncovertebral joints. It is necessary to open the posterior longitudinal ligament to directly visualise and explore the extra-dural space as disc material can find its way through the longitudinally orientated fibres of this ligament into the extradural space. It is not necessary to carry out a fusion procedure although this can be carried out either by the Smith–Robinson or Cloward technique if preferred. The use of a bone fusion does not confer additional neurological recovery, although it may be required (or preferred) if spinal stability is significantly degraded. Those patients in whom a fusion procedure is not carried out may be more susceptible to cervical pain for the first few weeks following the decompression and the use of a cervical collar is recommended. Laminectomy is not indicated for a patient with myelopathy due to acute cervical disc prolapse as this would involve unacceptable cord retraction to remove the disc.

For those patients who develop an acute myelopathy due to hyperextension forces superimposed on a narrow spinal canal, there is little, if any, convincing evidence that surgical decompression improves neurological recovery. In those few patients who have a narrow cervical spinal canal and who develop an acute non-traumatic myelopathy, a laminectomy or a multiple level anterior decompression and fusion are the surgical alternatives although the presumed ischaemic pathogenesis does not incline to the favourable outcome associated with slowly developing spondylitic myelopathy.[42]

For a thoracic disc protrusion the surgical access must be either lateral or anterior or a combination of both. The approaches to the thoracic spinal canal are those which give access to the disc prolapse without requiring any retraction of the thoracic spinal cord and are such that the disc material may be removed in a direction away from the spinal theca. The recommended approaches are pediculectomy, costotransversectomy, or transthoracic partial vertebrectomy.[44 47 48] A laminectomy is *only* indicated for thoracic disc prolapse if the disc material is entirely free and is located in a position lateral to the spinal cord. This does happen, but not commonly. A laminectomy for an anteriorly placed thoracic disc prolapse invites major neurological deterioration.

For patients who present with an acute disc prolapse causing cauda equina syndrome, prognosis for recovery is based on the severity of the pre-decompression neurological deficit rather than the duration of neurological symptoms, although it is difficult to entirely separate these two components.[49] The same is likely to apply to prognosis for recovery following cervical and thoracic disc induced myelopathy. Full recovery for expeditiously diagnosed and optimally managed patients is to be expected.

Neoplastic cord compression

By far the commonest type of neoplastic spinal cord compression is that caused by secondary tumour deposits and up to one third of patients with malignant disease have deposits in the spine.[50 51] These are most commonly found in the vertebral body and pedicles with direct spread into the spinal canal. In about 5% of cases, metastatic tumour is confined to the spinal extradural space.[52] The usual and most common primary tumours are bronchus, breast, gastrointestinal tract, prostate, kidney, myeloma, and lymphoma. Most secondary deposits are found in the thoracic spine and multiple lesions may be non-contiguous. The reasons for this are likely to be related to the venous drainage of affected primary organs being routed through the spinal extradural venous plexus. The relative size of the thoracic spine clearly also has an effect. Secondary deposits are less common in the lumbar and cervical spine. They are uncommon or even rare in the sacral spine.

As the tumour enlarges and encroaches on the spinal cord the signs and symptoms of myelopathy progressively develop. This is associated with spinal pain in over 90% of patients and in retrospect these patients are often found to have complained of pain in the affected region for many weeks before the development of clinical myelopathy.[53] In most cases the myelopathy progresses gradually, usually over a period of days or weeks. As the compression increases the ability of the spinal canal to accommodate the extra volume is exhausted and the rate of neurological deterioration increases rapidly. The typical patient will have complained of thoracic spinal pain for perhaps 4–6 weeks with gradual development of fatigue in the lower limbs followed by decreased gait quality, and finally with rapid development of weakness and loss of sensation. The apparent acute presentation is therefore usually only the final stage of a more gradual process.[54]

Acute spinal cord compression due to secondary tumour does occur when the tumour enlarges very rapidly as a result of haemorrhage or where a vertebral body suddenly collapses because its structure has been extensively infiltrated by the neoplastic process.

The clinical features of presentation are not sufficiently characteristic to permit an accurate pathological diagnosis. Other causes of acute cord compression may present in a similar clinical fashion. The diagnosis must be confirmed by appropriate spinal imaging, initially by plain radiograph of the relevant spinal region although the whole spine needs to be managed as up to 17% of patients have multiple lesions.[53] The typical features of metastatic involvement include loss of vertebral height, an irregular lucent appearance within the fine architecture of the bone, preservation of the intervertebral disc space, and the possibility of multiple lesions. Spinal radiographs should be taken in combination with chest radiographs and the clinical examination, either or both of which may reveal evidence of a primary lesion. The optimal form

287

of spinal imaging is by MRI or CT myelography.[55] All the relevant information can be obtained from MRI including the number of levels affected, the extent of any local extravertebral infiltration and soft tissue involvement. CT gives a clear indication of the extent of bone involvement and makes surgical planning of the route of access and the achievable extent of excision easier.

It may be that the pathological nature of the secondary tumour is circumstantially identified by locating the primary tumour. When no primary can be found it is important to identify the histopathological type of the tumour by biopsy. In the spine between T5 and L5 this can be achieved through percutaneous vertebral body biopsy carried out under biplanar image intensifier control.[56] An alternative method is to use CT guided needle biopsy at almost any level, although this technique does not as readily provide samples of bone tissue, but rather of infiltrated soft tissue immediately adjacent to the vertebra. Either technique is safe in experienced hands and yields a high rate of positive diagnosis.

The subsequent management usually takes account of a number of factors, each with a varying influence on the management in different circumstances.[57] The histopathology of the tumour must be taken into account with the overall tumour load, that is, the number of secondary deposits and the best estimate of the patient's life expectancy. The severity of the neurological deficit probably has the major influence on the neurological recovery following decompression surgery. The most severely affected patients and those who are paraplegic have the lowest chance of regaining the ability to walk independently. Lesser levels of recovery, which do not permit the patient to either transfer, stand or walk, are of little practical benefit although return of sensation is of great importance to someone who is confined to a wheelchair.

The first surgical decision to be made is whether or not a surgical procedure is indicated. Surgery will provide the most rapid means of cord decompression, in contrast to radiotherapy which may take several days to have its optimum effect as a decompressing agent. Even patients with highly radiosensitive tumours such as myeloma or lymphoma occasionally require urgent surgical management where the compression is due to a collapsed vertebra rather than to tumour tissue surrounding the spinal cord.

The route of access should then be decided and at all spinal

288

levels the surgeon has a choice of posterior, lateral, or anterior routes. In general where the compression and major disease lie anterior to the spinal cord this should be the preferred route to decompression. This may be transoral, transcervical, transthoracic, or retroperitoneal depending on the level of the spine affected. Lateral access can be achieved through a laminectomy extended laterally to include the pedicle and facet joint, a true costotransversectomy or a lateral extra-cavity approach which is in effect an extended multiple level costotransversectomy. Where the spinal cord is primarily compressed posteriorly then a laminectomy still has a role to play. The days of simply carrying out a laminectomy for any form of neoplastic spinal cord compression are long since past. Studies from the late 1970s and early 1980s clearly showed how ineffective a laminectomy is in the presence of vertebral body disease. In this situation 20% of patients are made neurologically worse and a similar number are made unstable. The decompression process may entail removal of considerable amounts of bone from the spine and require replacement using internal metallic fixation, bone graft, or in some cases methyl methacrylate in combination with metal fixation.

Surgical decision making in these situations is complex and preparing contingency plans for every clinical situation is not a practical proposition. The over-riding aims are to provide the most effective form of decompression of the spinal cord to leave the patient with a pain-free stable spine, with return of function of the spinal cord. In some situations, such as a patient with widespread metastatic bronchogenic tumour, it is entirely inappropriate to carry out a transthoracic spinal decompression. In a patient who has multiple non-contiguous spinal lesions, major surgery on any one of these is likely to be followed by further cord compression at a different level. In selected patients, however, even relatively major surgery to access and decompress the spinal cord is indicated before further treatment with radiotherapy or chemotherapy.

Haematogenous spinal cord compression

Epidural and subdural haematomas are common and well known conditions in cranial neurosurgery, but are distinctly uncommon in the spine. Subdural haematomas in particular are rare, with few cases being reported.[58] Epidural haematomas,

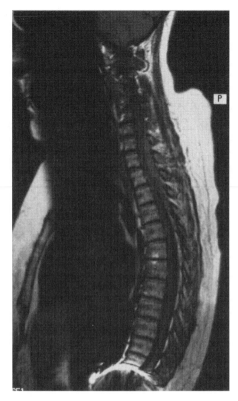

Figure 2—MRI (1·5 T Siemens Magnetom) showing a cervicothoracic extradural haematoma of spontaneous onset and unknown cause. The haematoma lies posterior to the spinal cord.

although uncommon, are a recognised cause of cord compression and about a third are associated with patients receiving anticoagulant therapy. Lumbar puncture in this group of patients may lead to the formation of a spinal epidural haematoma. A substantial proportion occur for no particular reason although in the literature they are associated with, or even causally related to, what might otherwise be described as minor traumas of everyday living.[59][60] It seems more likely that these are coincidental factors rather than causal. There is little evidence that arteriovenous abnormalities in the vertebra or other form of angiomatous malformation are causally related to more than a small number of spinal epidural haematomas.[61][62]

Their clinical presentation is similar to several other forms of structural spinal cord compression. Haematomas produce a combination of spinal pain and root pain, followed by a progressive myelopathy, whose features will depend on the level of compression. Occasionally the process develops over several days and there are documented cases in whom the myelopathy has developed over several weeks.[63] Most present relatively rapidly, within one or two days, and the diagnosis is confirmed by MRI or CT myelography.[64] (fig 2). The appearances are those of an extradural compressive lesion although with MRI it is possible to distinguish haematoma from pus or extradural tumour in some cases. Treatment is by laminectomy at the level of compression.[65]

Management of acute spinal cord compression

● The symptoms of patients who have acute spinal cord compression comprise motor loss, sensory loss and pain, although the combination and severity of these will vary according to the degree of compression and the level affected. Whatever the cause, pain is very common and may be midline and spinal, or radiating along a nerve root distribution. Careful examination will reveal that reflexes are depressed at the level of compression and exaggerated below.

● The causes of acute spinal cord compression fall into the general categories of traumatic, inflammatory, infective, degenerative, neoplastic, and haemorrhagic. A few of these have clinical features which indicate the pathological diagnosis. However, diagnosis usually awaits definitive radiological investigation.

● When the history and clinical examination suggest spinal cord compression it is reasonable and sometimes very useful to carry out relevant plain radiography of the appropriate spinal region. This may indicate the pathological diagnosis. The decision to proceed to further imaging will depend on the availability of appropriate equipment and the urgency of the clinical situation. This should be clarified by urgent discussion of the case with a spine specialist.

Management of acute spinal cord compression (cont)

● It is important to make a clinical diagnosis of spinal cord compression at the earliest opportunity, to provide the patient with the best prognosis for neurological recovery. Unfortunately, and all too frequently, the diagnosis is not made at an optimum time and the patient is presented to a specialist spine unit in a more advanced stage of myelopathy than is necessary. With the stakes for the patient being so high, it is better to err on the side of "false alarm" than to make a late diagnosis. Patients with thoracic spinal pain are more likely to have an organic lesion and they should not be diagnosed to have non-specific, degenerative, or soft tissue pain, but rather a definitive diagnosis should be sought. This also applies to patients below the age of about 25 who present with any form of spinal pain. The diagnosis of "hysterical paralysis" should not be made or assumed, especially by junior staff and those inexperienced in diagnosing spinal conditions. When junior staff are in doubt, recourse must be made to senior colleagues or to a specialist spine unit (neurosurgical or orthopaedic). I strongly encourage junior staff to be aware of the clinical advice contained in this paragraph.

1 Maurice-Williams RS, Richardson PL. Spinal cord compression: delay in the diagnosis and referral of a common neurosurgical emergency. *Br J Neurosurg* 1988;**2**:55–60.
2 Meyer PR. Acute injury retrieval and splinting techniques. In: Meyer PR, ed. *Surgery of spine trauma*. New York: Churchill Livingstone, 1989:1–21.
3 Vaccaro AR, An HS, Lin S, *et al*. Noncontiguous injuries of the spine. *J Spinal Dis* 1992;**5**:320–9.
4 Schaefer DM, Flanders AE, Osterholm JL, Northrup B. Prognostic significance of magnetic resonance imaging in the acute phase of cervical spine injury. *J Neurosurg* 1992;**76**:218–23.
5 Cane RD, Shapiro BA. Pulmonary effects of acute spinal cord injury: assessment and management. In: Meyer PR, ed. *Surgery of spine trauma*. New York: Churchill Livingstone, 1989:173–83.
6 Aldrich EF, Weber PB, Crow WN. Halifax interlaminar clamp for posterior cervical fusion: a long term follow up review. *J Neurosurg* 1993;**78**:702–8.
7 McNamara MJ, Stephens GC, Spengler DM. Transpedicular short segment fusions for treatment of lumbar burst fractures. *J Spinal Dis* 1992;**5**:183–7.
8 Bracken MB, Shephard MJ, Collins WF, *et al*. Methylprednisolone or naloxone treatment after acute spinal cord injury: 1 year follow up data. Results of the second national acute spinal cord injury study. *J Neurosurg* 1992;**76**:23–31.
9 Tator CH, Fehlings MG. Review of the secondary injury theory of acute spinal cord trauma with emphasis on vascular mechanisms. *J Neurosurg* 1991;**75**:15–26.
10 Johnston RA, Kelly IG. Surgery of the rheumatoid cervical spine. *Ann Rheum Dis* 1990;**49**:845–50.

292

11 Santavirta S, Kottinen YT, Laasonen E, Honkanen V, Antti-Poika I, Kauppi M. Ten year results of operation for rheumatoid cervical spine disorders. *J Bone Joint Surg* 1991;**73-B**:116–20.
12 Mathews JA. Atlanto-axial subluxation in rheumatoid arthritis. *Ann Rheum Dis* 1974;**33**: 526–31.
13 Pellicci PM, Ranawat CS, Tsairis P, Bryan WJ. A prospective study of the progression of rheumatoid arthritis of the cervical spine. *J Bone Joint Surg* 1981;**63-A**:342–50.
14 Santavirta S, Kankaanpaa U, Sandelin J, Laasonen E, Kottinen Y, Slatis P. Evaluation of patients with rheumatoid cervical spine. *Scand J Rheumatol* 1987;**16**:9–16.
15 Bell GR, Stearns KL. Flexion-extension MRI of the upper rheumatoid cervical spine. *Orthopaedics* 1991;**14**:969–74.
16 Krodel A, Refior HJ, Westermann S. The importance of functional magnetic resonance imaging in the planning of stabilizing operations on the cervical spine in rheumatoid patients. *Arch Orthop Trauma Surg* 1989;**109**:30–3.
17 Dvorak J, Grob D, Baumgartner H. Gschwent N, Graver W, Larsson S. Functional evaluation of the spinal cord by magnetic resonance imaging in patients with rheumatoid arthritis and instability of the upper cervical spine. *Spine* 1989;**14**:1057–64.
18 Rogers MA, Crockard HA. Nystagmus and joint position sensation; their importance in posterior occipito-cervical fusion in rheumatoid arthritis. Presented in part, *19th Annual Meeting, Cervical Spine Research Society*, December 1991, Philadelphia PA.
19 Toolaner G. Cutaneous, sensory impairment in rheumatoid atlanto-axial subluxation assessed quantitatively by electrical stimulation. *Scand J Rheumatol* 1987;**16**:27–32.
20 Dickman CA, Locantro J, Fessler RG. The influence of transoral odontoid resection on stability of the craniovertebral junction. *J Neurosurg* 1992;**77**:525–30.
21 Crockard HA, Calder I, Ransford AO. One stage transoral decompression and posterior fixation in rheumatoid atlanto-axial subluxation. *J Bone Joint Surg* 1990;**72-B**:682–5.
22 Hadley MN, Spetzler RF, Sonntag, VKH. The transoral approach to the superior cervical spine. *J Neurosurg* 1989;**71**:16–23.
23 Wertheim SB, Bohlman HH. Occipitocervical fusion. *J Bone Joint Surg* 1987;**69-A**:833–6.
24 Ranawat CS, O'Leary P, Pellicci P, Tsairis P, Marchisello P, Dorr L. Cervical spine fusion in rheumatoid arthritis. *J Bone Joint Surg* 1979;**61-A**:1003–10.
25 Chan CP, Ngian KS, Cohen L. Posterior upper cervical fusion in rheumatoid arthritis. *Spine* 1992;**17**:268–72.
26 Ferlic DC, Clayton, ML, Leidholt JD, Gamble WE. Surgical treatment of the symptomatic unstable cervical spine in rheumatoid arthritis. *J Bone Joint Surg* 1975; **57-A**: 349–54.
27 Brattström H, Granholm L. Atlanto-axial fusion in rheumatoid arthritis. *Acta Orthop Scand* 1976;**47**:619–28.
28 Grob D, Dvorak J, Gschwend N, Froehlich M. Posterior occipito-cervical fusion in rheumatoid arthritis. *Arch Orthop Trauma Surg* 1990;**110**:38–44.
29 Dutton JEM, Alexander GL. Intramedullary spinal abscess. *J Neurol Neurosurg Psychiatry* 1954;**17**:303–7.
30 Fraser RAR, Ratzan K, Wolpert SM, *et al*. Spinal subdural empyema. *Arch Neurol* 1973;**28**:235–8.
31 Johnston RA. Intraspinal infection. In: Findlay G, Owen R, eds. *Surgery of the spine*. London: Blackwell, 1992:621–8.
32 Dandy WE. Abscesses and inflammatory tumors in the spinal epidural space (so called pachymeningitis externa). *Arch Surg Chicago* 1926;**13**:477–94.
33 Heusner AP. Non tuberculous spinal epidural infections. *N Engl J Med* 1948;**239**:845–54.
34 Statham P, Gentleman D. Importance of early diagnosis of acute spinal extradural abscess. *J R Soc Med* 1989;**82**:584–7.
35 Baker AS, Ojemann RG, Swartz MN, *et al*. Spinal epidural abscess. *N Engl J Med* 1975;**293**:463–8.
36 Hakin RN, Burt AA, Cook JB. Acute epidural abscess. *Paraplegia* 1979;**17**:330–6.
37 Ross J. Inflammatory disease. In: Modic M, Masaryk T, Ross J, eds. *Magnetic resonance imaging of the spine*. Chicago: Year Book Medical, 1989:167–82.
38 Holme A, Dott NM. Spinal epidural abscess. *BMJ* 1954;**64**:64–8.
39 Ho EKW, Leong JCY. Spinal osteomyelitis. In: Findlay G, Owen R, eds. *Surgery of the spine*. London: Blackwell Scientific, 1992:621–8.
40 Modic MT, Feiglin DH, Piraino DW, *et al*. Vertebral osteomyelitis; assessment using MR. *Radiology* 1985;**157**:157–63.

41 Johnston RA, Hadley DM. Tuberculous infection of the thoracic spine. In: Tarlov EC, ed. *Neurosurgical treatment of disorders of the thoracic spine*. Illinois: American Association of Neurological Surgeons, 1991:95–109.

42 Ferguson RJL, Kaplan LR. Cervical spondylitic myelopathy. *Neurol Clin* 1985;**3**:373–82.

43 Epstein N, Epstein J. Benjamin V, *et al*. Traumatic myelopathy in patients with cervical spinal stenosis without fracture or dislocation. *Spine* 1980;**5**:489–96.

44 Russell T. Thoracic intervertebral disc protrusion: experience of 67 cases and review of the literature. *Br J Neurosurg* 1989;**3**:153–60.

45 Wesolowski DP, Wang AM. Radiologic evaluation. In: Rothman RH, Simeone FA, eds. *The Spine*. Philadelphia: WB Saunders, 1992:570–6.

46 McLaren AC, Bailey SI. Cauda equina syndrome: a complication of lumbar discectomy. *Clin Orthop* 1986;**204**:143–9.

47 Fidler MW, Goedhart ZD. Excision of prolapse of thoracic intervertebral disc. *J Bone Joint Surg* 1984;**66–B**:518–22.

48 Russell T. Thoracic intervertebral disc protrusion. In: Findlay G, Owen R, eds. *Surgery of the spine*. London: Blackwell Scientific, 1992:813–20.

49 O'Laoire SA, Crockard HA, Thomas DG. Prognosis for sphincter recovery after operation for cauda equina compression owing to lumbar disc prolapse. *BMJ* 1981;**282**:1852–4.

50 Schaberg J, Gainor B. A profile of metastatic carcinoma of the spine. *Spine* 1985;**10**:19–20.

51 Wong D, Fornasier V, MacNab I. Spinal metastases: The obvious, the occult and the imposters. *Spine* 1990;**15**:1–4.

52 Constans J, de Divitus E, Donzelli R, *et al*. Spinal metastases with neurological manifestations: review of 600 cases. *J Neurosurg* 1983;**59**:111–18.

53 Gilbert R, Kim J, Posner J. Epidural spinal cord compression from metastatic tumor: diagnosis and treatment. *Ann Neurol* 1978;**3**:40–51.

54 Shapiro W, Posner J. Medical versus surgical treatment of metastatic spinal cord tumour. In: Thompson R, Green J, eds. *Controversies in Neurology*. New York: Raven Press, 1983:57–65.

55 Godersky J, Smoker W, Knutzon R. Use of magnetic resonance imaging in the evaluation of metastatic spinal disease. *Neurosurgery* 1987;**21**:676–80.

56 Findlay G, Sandeman D, Buxton P. The role of needle biopsy in the management of malignant spinal compression. *Br J Neurosurg* 1988;**2**:479–84.

57 Findlay GFG. Metastatic spinal disease. In: Findlay G, Owen R, eds. *Surgery of the spine*. London: Blackwell Scientific, 1992:557–72.

58 Reinsel TE, Goldberg E, Granato DB, *et al*. Spinal subdural haematoma: A rare cause of recurrent postoperative radiculopathy. *J Spinal Dis* 1993;**6**:62–7.

59 Cowie RA. Acute spinal haematoma. In: Findlay G, Owen R, eds. *Surgery of the spine*. London: Blackwell Scientific, 1992:621–8.

60 Bruyn GW, Bosma NJ. Spinal extradural haematoma. In: Vinken PJ, Bruyn GW, eds. *Handbook of clinical neurology*. Amsterdam: Elsevier, 1976;1–30.

61 Harris DJ, Fornasier VL, Livingstone KE. Haemangiopericytoma of the spinal canal. Report of three cases. *J Neurosurg* 1978;**49**:914–20.

62 Stuart Lee K, McWhorter JM, Angelo IV. Spinal epidural haematoma associated with Pagets disease. *Surg Neurol* 1988;**30**:131–4.

63 Boyd HR, Pear BL. Chronic spontaneous spinal epidural haematoma: report of two cases. *J Neurosurg* 1972;**36**:239–42.

64 Larsson EM, Holtas S, Cronqvist S. Emergency magnetic resonance examination of patients with spinal cord symptoms. *Acta Radiol* 1988;**29**:69–75.

65 Johnston RA, Bailey IC. Spinal extradural haematoma; report of two cases. *Ulster Med J* 1983;**52**:157–61.

11 Acute neuromuscular respiratory paralysis

R A C HUGHES, D BIHARI

This chapter reviews the recognition, diagnosis, and management of respiratory failure in acute neuromuscular disease. Respiratory failure requiring artificial ventilation occurs in about 14% of patients with Guillain–Barré syndrome (GBS),[1] a small percentage of patients with myasthenia gravis and polymyositis, and also in acute rhabdomyolysis and a wide range of other less common disorders (box 1, tables I–III). Neuromuscular disorders are responsible for only a tiny proportion of admissions to most intensive care units, 23 (1·1%) of 2097 consecutive admissions to our own unit in the last two years. Of those cases, 15 (60%) required mechanical ventilation and two (8·7%) died in hospital. The APACHE III study in North America[2] documented neuromuscular disease as the cause of intensive care unit admission in only 45 patients (0·26%) of the cohort of 17 440 patients with a 15·6% unadjusted hospital mortality rate. These figures exclude those patients who were admitted to the intensive care unit because of operation or systemic disease and then developed neuromuscular disease which caused respiratory failure or delayed weaning off the ventilator. Respiratory failure occurring in the setting of chronic progressive neuromuscular disease, such as Duchenne muscular dystrophy and motor neuron disease, presents a challenging management problem which is outside the scope of this chapter.

TABLE II—Disorders of neuromuscular transmission that cause respiratory failure

Condition	Specific test	Specific treatment
Myasthenia gravis[27]	Edrophonium test	PE, S, IVIg
	Anti AChR antibody	
Anticholinesterase overdose	Negative edrophonium test	Drug withdrawal
Antibiotic-induced paralysis[30]	—	Drug withdrawal
Hypermagnesaemia[29]	Plasma Mg	Intravenous
	EMG increment on 50 Hz stimulation	calcium
Botulism[32]	Injection of serum into mice	Antitoxin
Snake, scorpions and spider bite[32]	Identifying the snake	Antitoxin
Fish, shellfish, crab poisoning[32 33 86]	Identifying the fish	Varies
Tick paralysis[32 34]	Finding the tick	Removal
Eaton–Lambert syndrome[27]	EMG increment on repetitive stimulation	PE, S

PE = plasma exchange; S = steroids; AChR = acetylcholine esterase receptor; EMG = electromyogram.

TABLE III—Disorders of muscle that cause acute respiratory failure

Condition	Specific test	Specific treatment
Hypokalaemia[38]	Plasma K$^+$	K$^+$
Polymyositis[40]	Plasma CK	S
	EMG	
	Muscle biopsy	
Acute rhabdomyolysis[40]	EMG	Urine alkalinisation
	Muscle biopsy	
Hypophosphataemia[39]	Plasma phosphate	Phosphate
Acid maltase deficiency[37]	PAS stain of blood film	—
Combined neuromuscular blockade and steroids[28]	Muscle biopsy	Withdrawal
Barium intoxication[88]	Plasma K$^+$	Intravenous K$^+$
		Oral magnesium sulphate
		haemodialysis

CK = creatinine kinase; PAS = periodic acid-Schiff reagent.

sleep nearly all the work of breathing is performed by the diaphragm.

When the diaphragm is paralysed, expansion of the ribcage is performed by the accessory muscles of respiration. When the ribcage expands, the fall in intrapleural pressure moves the flaccid diaphragm cephalad into the thorax and the anterior abdominal wall, being coupled to the diaphragm movement through the abdominal contents, moves passively inwards during inspiration. This "paradoxical abdominal movement" is most marked in the supine posture as gravity assists the cephalad movement of the abdominal contents. The change in volume of the ribcage is partly absorbed by the cephalad movement of the abdominal contents and the volume of air inspired is reduced. In the upright posture gravity partially counteracts the upward movement of the abdominal contents and improves the efficiency of the accessory muscles producing inspiration. Consequently, in diaphragmatic paralysis, patients use the accessory muscles of respiration, become distressed when supine, and have smaller supine than erect vital capacities. Furthermore, the majority of neural drive to the respiratory muscles during sleep is directed to the phrenic nerves, so that patients with diaphragm paralysis are particularly prone to hypoventilation during sleep.

Patients with intact diaphragms but impaired intercostal and abdominal muscle function show paradoxical ribcage movement. As the diaphragm lowers intrapleural pressure during inspiration the intercostal spaces and the upper ribcage move inwards because of the lack of intercostal muscle tone. In the upright posture, gravity pulls the abdominal contents caudally and the flaccid anterior abdominal wall bulges anteriorly. The diaphragm is thus flattened and shortened and is inefficient in lifting the ribcage and elongating the thorax. In this situation respiratory distress may be experienced in the upright position. The resultant poor vital capacity and inability to cough contribute to ventilatory failure.

Clinical diagnosis of neuromuscular respiratory failure

The danger of respiratory failure should be considered in every patient with progressive weakness, especially if the upper limbs and bulbar muscles are involved. The patient complains of weakness and fatigue but, unlike a patient with parenchymal lung disease or airway obstruction, does not appear wheezy or cyanosed. Instead, the patient prefers to sit or lie still in bed, becomes breathless on talking or swallowing, and uses the accessory muscles of respiration (pectoral, scalene, sternocleidomastoid, and levators of the nostrils). Diaphragm weakness may be detected by indrawing of the abdominal wall, that is, paradoxical abdominal movement. Although the respiratory rate may be rapid and shallow, and the observation chart may show an increase in heart and

299

respiratory rate over the previous few hours, this is not invariable and some patients present with ventilatory failure and a normal or reduced respiratory rate. All such patients should be monitored from the outset, especially during sleep, by pulse oximetry for the early detection of arterial desaturation. Clinical assessment, however, is better than blood gas analysis in assessing the need for ventilatory support. As respiratory failure worsens, the patient becomes increasingly anxious and, though exhausted, may be unable to sleep. Additional bulbar weakness or insensitivity with the attendant danger of inhalation is particularly hazardous.

Although the decision to intubate and start artificial ventilation depends primarily on the overall clinical assessment, quantitative assessment and monitoring of respiratory muscle function are helpful. The most convenient method is the measurement of vital capacity. A common error is to measure peak expiratory flow because devices for its measurement have always been more readily available on a general medical ward. Fortunately, small portable electronic devices are now available for monitoring respiratory frequency, tidal volume, and vital capacity at the bedside in the spontaneously breathing patient. Care is needed to educate the patient to obtain a meaningful measurement since facial weakness may prevent an adequate lip seal around a mouth piece. In such cases, a padded, tightly fitting face mask attached to the measuring device may help. As a rule of thumb ventilatory support of some form should be considered when the vital capacity in an adult falls to less than one litre. The exact figure depends upon the predicted normal vital capacity for the weight and age of the individual concerned.

Maximal static respiratory pressures (maximum inspiratory pressure, PI_{max}, measured at residual volume; maximum expiratory pressure, PE_{max}, measured at total lung capacity) obtained while breathing against an occluded mouthpiece are said to be more sensitive indicators of respiratory muscle weakness.[5] A PE_{max} of less than 40 cm H_2O (adult normal = 100 cm H_2O) has been associated with an inability to cough and clear secretions adequately whereas a PI_{max} of more than -20 cmH_2O (adult normal of more than -70 cmH_2O) precludes effective ventilation with the maintenance of a normal arterial carbon dioxide tension. Nevertheless, a falling vital capacity approximates these changes with impaired clearance of secretions occurring at around a vital capacity of less than 30 ml/kg and frank ventilatory failure at less than

10 ml/kg. Further assessment can be obtained by the measurement of transdiaphragmatic pressure during tidal breathing and on maximal inspiration. Such studies may be coupled with the measurement of the diaphragm EMG, but this is not routinely performed outside research centres.

Diagnosis of the cause

Central nervous system causes

Diseases of the nervous system can cause respiratory failure by damaging the respiratory centre in the medulla or its connections with the cervical and thoracic spinal cord. In practice the commonest causes are the secondary consequences of CNS depression by drugs or metabolic abnormalities or of primary cerebral or brainstem disease. These are important in differential diagnosis but this review is confined to disorders affecting the lower motor neuron, peripheral nerves, neuromuscular junction, and muscles. The localisation of the disease process to the brainstem or spinal cord does not usually present the neurologist with any difficulty because of the presence of symptoms and signs at the level of the lesion and involvement of the long tracts.

Poliomyelitis remains a common problem in eastern Europe, the Middle East, and the Indian subcontinent. It should still be considered in the differential diagnosis of acute flaccid paralysis throughout the world, especially when sensory deficit is absent, the onset is asymmetrical, and the CSF shows a pleocytosis.[6 7] The diagnosis may be confirmed by culturing the stool, and sometimes a throat swab or CSF, and by finding a rising titre of neutralising antibody in the serum.

Peripheral neuropathy

Peripheral neuropathy causing respiratory failure can usually be diagnosed clinically from the gradual evolution of ascending or sometimes descending weakness associated with paraesthesiae and sensory deficit and reduced or absent tendon reflexes. Difficulties in diagnosis arise in rapidly evolving pure motor neuropathies, especially in the earliest stages when the tendon reflexes may be preserved. Also paraesthesiae occur in occasional cases of toxic neuromuscular conduction block, including botulism.[8]

Guillain–Barré syndrome is so much more common than any of the other causes of neuromuscular respiratory failure that there is a danger that other causes and particularly other causes of neuropathy will be overlooked.[19] The diagnosis of GBS cannot be made by any diagnostic test but requires the exclusion of other causes. These are listed in table I. In most cases the pathological process is inflammatory, demyelinating, and probably auto-immune.[1] The presence of demyelination can be confirmed by the neurophysiological demonstration of multifocal conduction block.[10] GBS is a heterogeneous condition, however, whose pathological substrate also includes an acute axonal form which may have an explosively rapid onset and be associated with a particularly slow and incomplete recovery.[11] The neurophysiological diagnosis of the axonal form of GBS requires the demonstration of reduction in evoked muscle and nerve action potentials without marked slowing or conduction block. If the nerves are already inexcitable by the time of the first neurophysiological study, the distinction between demyelination and axonal degeneration may need to be made by biopsy, preferably of a motor nerve.[12 13]

The other causes of neuropathy (table I) can be ruled out by a careful history. Critical illness polyneuropathy occurs in the setting of an extremely ill patient who is being ventilated, has had sepsis and multiorgan failure, and cannot be weaned from the ventilator. It is due to an axonal neuropathy and its distinction from the axonal form of GBS may be merely semantic. The aetiology of critical illness polyneuropathy is not known but may be multifactorial.[14 15] Careful enquiry about possible toxin exposure as a cause of polyneuropathy is always necessary. Poisoning with organophosphates or heavy metals severe enough to cause a neuropathy with respiratory failure has usually been preceded by an acute illness with vomiting and an altered level of consciousness. Prominent cutaneous and muscular pain, especially in the feet, and preservation of the reflexes in the early stages should raise the suspicion of thallium poisoning.[16] Painful tingling and weakness begin within 1–5 days from ingestion of thallium, before the characteristic hairfall. In arsenic poisoning the early clinical picture sometimes closely resembles GBS and neurophysiological changes may initially show partial conduction block and slowing of conduction before giving way to changes suggestive of axonal degeneration.[17] Diphtheria is extremely rare in developed countries but cases were recently reported from Sweden,[18] and the diagnosis should be considered in patients with a recent upper respiratory infection, especially if there is prominent palatal involvement.[19] Buckthorn neuropathy need only be suspected in those who have consumed berries in Mexico.[20] Drugs usually cause an insidiously progressive distal axonopathy without respiratory involvement, but acute paralysis with respiratory failure occurred in a patient being treated with vincristine, possibly due to coincidental GBS.[21] Both T and B cell lymphomas may cause acute neoplastic infiltration of the peripheral nervous system which closely resembles GBS.[22-24] Sometimes acute neuropathy is the presenting feature of the lymphoma. Vasculitic neuropathy rarely causes respiratory failure and usually only does so in the setting of a systemic illness with cutaneous, renal, and lung involvement. Acute neuropathy occurs in acute intermittent porphyria, usually after abdominal pain and vomiting, but sometimes as the presenting feature.[25] It may be diagnosed during attacks by detecting increased urine porphobilinogen excretion, a test which should be undertaken in every case of undiagnosed acute neuromuscular paralysis. Recurrent neuropathy in infants is a feature of hereditary tyrosinaemia.[26]

Neuromuscular junction disorders

Respiratory failure can herald disorders of the neuromuscular junction, which can be distinguished from neuropathic causes by the absence of sensory deficit and preservation of tendon reflexes. In myasthenia gravis respiratory failure usually occurs in the setting of established disease which has failed to respond to conventional treatment. Even in an acute case the diagnosis is usually evident because of ptosis, facial weakness, and bulbar palsy with muscle fatigue. The diagnosis can be confirmed by the injection of intravenous edrophonium, neurophysiogical tests, and a positive test for acetylcholine receptor antibodies in a reliable laboratory.[27] In treated myasthenia, weakness can be caused by overdosage of anticholinesterase drugs causing depolarisation cholinergic block. This will be accompanied by diarrhoea, colic, excessive salivation, and small pupils and will be worsened rather than improved by intravenous edrophonium.

Other causes of neuromuscular junction blockade are rare and the diagnosis is usually obvious from the clinical setting. Botulism should be suspected when acute descending paralysis has been heralded by autonomic features, dry mouth, constipation, poorly reactive pupils, and ptosis and bulbar palsy. These symptoms have usually been immediately preceded by nausea, vomiting,

303

abdominal pain, and diarrhoea from eating foul smelling food contaminated by *Clostridium botulinum*.[28] Severe hypermagnesaemia can be produced by magnesium-containing antacids and aperients in patients with impaired renal function. The increased magnesium interferes with the release of acetylcholine so as to cause weakness which may develop into respiratory failure.[29] The aminoglycoside and polymyxin antibiotics and some other drugs also cause neuromuscular blockade by interfering with the release of acetylcholine.[30] This is usually only significant when weaning infected patients off ventilation.[31] Physicians practising in the tropics have to cope with a much wider range of toxic causes of neuromuscular conduction blockade whose diagnosis will be obvious from the history (table II).[32] Fish or shellfish toxin poisoning (usually Caribbean or Pacific fish) causes a gastrointestinal upset before the development of weakness.[32 33] In North America paralysis is sometimes caused by the bite of a female tick whose saliva contains an unidentified toxin which probably also interferes with neuromuscular conduction.[32 34] The tick may be difficult to find but its removal is reported to be curative. Respiratory failure occurs in the Lambert-Eaton myasthenic syndrome, but only rarely and then usually in the setting of gradually progressive weakness. The diagnosis may be suggested clinically by autonomic symptoms, including a dry mouth, the finding of depressed reflexes which are enhanced after exercise, and confirmed by electrophysiological tests showing an increment in muscle action potential amplitude following repetitive nerve stimulation.[27] It may be associated with a small cell lung carcinoma or autoimmune disease.

Myopathy

Respiratory failure in muscle disease usually occurs insidiously following progressive proximal weakness, which has evolved over months or years, and presents with nocturnal hypoventilation causing morning headache and daytime sleepiness. This form of respiratory failure may develop in the advanced stages of severe muscular dystrophy and also in polymyositis. Sometimes, especially in myotonic dystrophy, the respiratory failure is worsened by depression of central respiratory drive. When the ventilatory reserve has fallen so far that the vital capacity is less than 55% of its predicted normal, there is a grave danger that an intercurrent lung infection will precipitate respiratory failure.[35] In acid maltase deficiency the diaphragm is particularly severely affected and the patient may present with respiratory failure before consulting a neurologist about weakness.[36] Acid maltase deficiency should be suspected if there is proximal upper limb weakness and marked wasting of the paraspinal muscles, and confirmed by seeking glycogen-containing granules in the lymphocytes which stain red with periodic acid–Schiff reagent applied to a blood film.[37]

When a patient presents with flaccid paralysis and respiratory failure over a few hours or days, a correctable electrolyte disturbance should be sought immediately. The feature that distinguishes muscle disease from neuropathy is the preservation of the reflexes and the absence of sensory symptoms or signs. Hypokalaemia induced by potassium loss from the gut or kidneys is the commonest cause and is probably responsible for the muscle fibre necrosis in acute rhabdomyolysis which occurs following some drugs, such as carbenoxolone.[38] Severe hypophosphataemia can also cause paralysis requiring respiratory failure. It is usually precipitated by parenteral glucose infusions in alcoholic patients.[39]

Acute rhabdomyolysis is a rare condition in which acute muscle necrosis causes the very rapid onset of muscle pain, tenderness, swelling, and weakness, sometimes severe enough to cause respiratory failure. The muscle enzyme concentrations, including creatinine kinase, are markedly increased in the plasma, and the electromyograph (EMG) shows myopathic changes and spontaneous fibrillation. A muscle biopsy is necessary to confirm the diagnosis and will show massive muscle fibre necrosis and often numerous regenerating fibres but relatively little inflammation. The neurological picture is overshadowed by the development of myoglobinuria and acute renal failure. Causes of acute rhabdomyolysis are alcohol abuse, viruses (influenza, coxsackie B5, echo 9, adenovirus 21, Epstein–Barr), mycoplasmae,[40] and a wide variety of drugs, especially potassium-lowering drugs, amphetamine-like agents, barbiturates, and the combination of the muscle relaxant pancuronium and corticosteroids.[30 41] If the causative agent is withdrawn and the patient can be nursed through the period of respiratory and renal failure, regeneration of the necrotic muscle and full recovery are usual.

Respiratory muscle involvement was a presenting feature in 4% of 118 patients with polymyositis. More commonly it developed later, contributing to death in 14%.[42] Neuromuscular respiratory failure may be worsened by simultaneous interstitial infiltration and fibrosis of the lungs.[40] Inflammatory changes in muscle are usually so extensive that the diagnosis can be readily confirmed by the increased plasma creatinine kinase concentration, myopathic EMG with additional spontaneous discharges, and inflammatory changes in a muscle biopsy.

Institution of mechanical ventilation

The decision to institute respiratory support depends much more on the clinical state of the patient than on any physiological measurement. Arterial blood gas analysis is not particularly helpful. Intervention is required to prevent the development of arterial hypoxaemia and carbon dioxide retention before they become life threatening. Continuous positive airway pressure administered by face mask may be useful in the temporary correction of arterial hypoxaemia but is uncomfortable and poorly tolerated for prolonged periods of time. It has little effect on carbon dioxide retention although it may reduce the work of breathing by correcting any reduction in functional residual capacity in patients with sputum retention and atelectasis. Nevertheless, it is only a "stop-gap" measure used to avoid tracheal intubation in a small minority of cases in whom some basic treatment, for example, drug therapy or plasma exchange, will reverse the primary disease process. On the whole, it is safer to proceed rapidly to tracheal intubation to ensure control of the airway, adequate oxygenation, ventilation and tracheal toilet (especially in patients with an inadequate cough reflex), and the prevention of pulmonary aspiration.

Intubation is best performed by a skilled operator in the setting of an intensive care unit. This requires referral and involvement of the intensive care medical staff at an early stage to prevent any emergency intervention on a general medical ward. Intubation is best achieved by the oral route following adequate intravenous sedation in combination with muscle relaxation. Although it is often said that nasotracheal tubes are a well tolerated alternative, we have found them to be unsuitable because they carry a high risk of sinusitis,[43] and their extra length with the narrow internal diameter makes them more difficult to aspirate adequately and increases the resistance of the ventilatory circuit. Any increase in work of breathing associated with nasotracheal intubation is especially harmful during the weaning period when a weak patient is asked to make some effort while receiving graded reductions in ventilatory support. Following pre-oxygenation, etomidate, propofol, or a benzodiazepine (midazolam) may be used to render the patient unconscious and this on its own—in the presence of cricoid pressure—may be sufficient for the experienced operator to perform the necessary laryngoscopy and intubation. A non-depolarising muscle relaxant (atracurium, vecuronium) in adequate doses will abolish all remaining muscular tone and can improve the inexperienced operator's ability to visualise the larynx. Suxamethonium should never be used in this setting because of reports of ventricular tachycardia and asystole caused by a sudden rise in serum potassium in patients with denervated muscles.[44 45] Cricoid pressure should always be used because, although patients may not have eaten for some time before the induction of anaesthesia, gastric stasis and ileus are common particularly in the early stages of GBS. Following successful tracheal intubation, a nasogastric tube (if not already present) should be placed to facilitate the initiation of enteral nutrition.

Management during mechanical ventilation

General principles

The principles that govern management during mechanical ventilation centre upon three primary concerns—access to the airway with the provision of adequate pulmonary gas exchange, the maintenance of nutrition, and the prevention of nosocomial infection. Other issues, very often taken for granted but which require special attention, include the need for scrupulous nursing care to avoid nerve compression syndromes and bed sores; physiotherapy with the provision of splints to prevent irreversible contractures and joint immobilisation; subcutaneous heparin for the prophylaxis of deep venous thrombosis; prevention of deep vein thrombosis; and finally, extensive psychological support throughout the period of their illness when individual patients with neuromuscular disease are entirely dependent upon their attendants and the mechanical ventilator. Keeping a paralysed but conscious patient comfortable requires careful positioning and frequent gentle repositioning: sitting up, especially out of bed, may help and is good for morale. A particular problem in patients with GBS is the management of autonomic dysfunction which can result in wide fluctuations in pulse and blood pressure as well as a wide variety of atrial and ventricular arrhythmias.[1 45]

Airway access and mechanical ventilation

Most patients who develop respiratory failure as a consequence of neuromuscular dysfunction will require a tracheotomy. Although mechanical ventilation via an orotracheal tube can be performed for a limited period of time (usually for 5–7 days in our unit), a tracheotomy simplifies management considerably and allows the withdrawal of all sedation.[46] The tracheostomy tube is well tolerated, gives excellent access for tracheal toilet and chest physiotherapy, and, as the patient can be placed on and off different forms of respiratory support at will, permits easier "weaning". Tracheotomy can now be performed at the bedside, using a percutaneous Seldinger technique, and this appears to be the preferred technique.[47] Nevertheless, tracheotomy by whatever method is not without risk (infection of the stoma; primary and secondary haemorrhage).

In the absence of severe pulmonary aspiration or infection, it is not difficult to achieve adequate pulmonary gas exchange in these patients. Initially, most patients are too weak to generate an adequate negative pressure to "trigger" the ventilator and so require "controlled ventilation". More modern ventilators, for example, the Siemens Servo 300, have a different method of triggering which requires the patient to change a baseline flow within the machine rather than to reduce a pressure. These machines are much more sensitive to the respiratory efforts of a patient and should theoretically be beneficial in management. In fact, no particular kind of ventilation or ventilator has been shown to be superior in supporting these patients and most intensivists rely on pressure support or some combination of intermittent mandatory ventilation with pressure support to provide an adequate tidal volume and minute ventilation. Positive end expiratory pressure (with a pressure of 3–6 cm H_2O) together with physiotherapy is used in the often vain attempt to prevent atelectasis.

Provision of nutrition

Every effort should be made to feed these patients early via the enteral route.[48] Although it is impossible to prevent muscle wasting related to denervation, loss of muscle bulk will only be more exaggerated if an external source of calories and nitrogen is not forthcoming.[49] Muscle wasting is particularly marked in those cases who develop nosocomial sepsis and may contribute to a prolongation of the period of dependence on mechanical ventilation.[50] Use of the enteral route ensures that the gastrointestinal mucosa does not atrophy and the integrity of gut barrier is maintained. Theoretically this should contribute to the prevention of nosocomial infection by reducing the likelihood of translocation of bacteria and endotoxin from the lumen of the gut into the portal venous circulation and lymphatic system.[51] Parenteral nutrition on the other hand, especially that containing large amounts of intravenous fat, may contribute to an increased risk of sepsis and is best avoided.[52 53] It may be difficult to establish enteral nutrition in occasional patients with an ileus. A distended abdomen and large nasogastric aspirates with the absence of bowel sounds are the usual features of ileus. In our experience these features have usually been related to the excessive use of sedatives, especially opiates. Early tracheotomy and the subsequent withdrawal of all sedation (other than simple night sedation to ensure an appropriate sleep pattern) will reduce the incidence of ileus. Diarrhoea usually reflects the administration of broad spectrum antimicrobials rather than any effect of enteral nutrition. It should be treated symptomatically and every effort made to withdraw the offending antibiotics.

Prevention of nosocomial infection

The prevention of hospital acquired infection is at the heart of good intensive care practice.[54] It is especially important in patients requiring prolonged mechanical ventilation, as uncontrolled nosocomial sepsis is likely to be an important cause of death in those cases who die in the intensive care unit. Several studies have demonstrated an association between the likelihood of developing a nosocomial pneumonia and the number of days of mechanical ventilation.[55] Prevalence rates vary enormously from unit to unit and reflect local practices and resources. Every intensive care unit should have a written infection control policy developed in conjunction with local microbiological experts. Central issues are local practices of handwashing, nursing numbers, strict intravenous line/urinary catheter and antimicrobial policies, the avoidance of gastric alkalinisation with H_2 receptor antagonists and antacids, and an infection surveillance programme. These aspects concerning the organisation of intensive care are fundamental in the prevention of infection in individual cases.

Recently, the practice of "selective decontamination of the digestive tract" has been proposed as another means of reducing

309

the incidence of unit-acquired Gram-negative infections.[56] This method requires the application of a paste of non-absorbable antimicrobials (most commonly the combination of tobramycin, polymyxin, and amphotericin) to the oropharynx and, via the nasogastric tube, to the stomach. It has been best studied in patients following multiple trauma and major surgery. Although several studies have demonstrated reductions in the incidence of infection using this technique, no influence on survival has been observed. Many believe that selective decontamination only works well in the setting of a high nosocomial infection rate and we do not use it.

Autonomic dysfunction

In respiratory paralysis due to acute neuropathy, and especially in GBS, autonomic dysfunction is common.[1 45 57–59] Tachycardia and loss of sinus arrhythmia are usual. Rapid fluctuations of pulse and blood pressure and sweating may occur and are sometimes the harbingers of asystole. In particular tracheal suction may cause bradycardia and asystole. This can usually be prevented by hyperoxygenation beforehand but if it persists it may be necessary to use atropine and even an endocardial pacemaker. Serious arrhythmias usually only occur in patients who need ventilation but we have had a patient with early GBS who developed asystole before needing ventilation. We monitor the ECG from the time of admission in all patients with GBS who have any sign of respiratory or bulbar involvement. Although the bladder is spared in the early stages of GBS, it may be affected in severe cases and bladder catheterisation is often needed as part of the intensive care of the ventilated patient. Postural hypotension is common when the patient is being mobilised so that the blood pressure should be monitored. This is best done with the aid of a tilt table.

Specific interventions

Guillain–Barré syndrome

In two large randomised trials, patients with GBS who received plasma exchange (PE) recovered more quickly than those not so treated.[60–62] It is valuable during the first week, and its use after the second week is doubtful, although so long as the disease is still progressing it would be worth using PE. In the North American trial continuous flow PE appeared more effective than intermittent flow although intermittent flow was better than none.[62] There is no information concerning the relative merits of filtration compared with centrifugation systems. Albumin is the preferred exchange fluid since fresh frozen plasma caused more reactions and was no more effective.[61] The North American trial exchanged 200–250 ml/kg body weight (4–5 plasma volumes) over 7–14 days, and the French trial two plasma volumes on alternate days for a total of four exchanges. It is not known whether more exchanges would be more effective, but 10–25% of patients show a limited relapse after 1–6 weeks and usually respond to a further PE.[63 64] We used to space five 50 ml/kg PEs over 14 days and add further exchanges if there was a subsequent relapse.

Although steroids might have been expected to be beneficial in GBS, neither a small trial of oral prednisolone nor a large double-masked trial of intravenous methylprednisolone 500 mg daily for five days demonstrated any benefit.[65 66]

(Intravenous immunoglobulin (IVIg) has now replaced PE as the preferred treatment for GBS.) A Dutch trial showed that the rate of recovery was similar or possibly slightly faster in patients treated with IVIg 0·4 g/kg daily for five days compared with those treated with PE. The median time to walk unaided was 55 days in 75 patients treated with IVIg and 69 days in the same number treated with PE (p = 0·07 two-tailed). Lung and circulatory complications were more common in the PE treated group than the IVIg group.[67] Although IVIg is expensive, it is not usually more expensive than PE and it is more widely available and simpler to give. A large international trial compared PE alone with IVIg alone and PE followed by IVIg. There was no significant difference in outcome between the treatments. Although there was a trend towards more rapid recovery in the patients who received combined treatment, this was not significant, and not sufficient to justify the extra inconvenience, risk, and cost.[68]

Myasthenia gravis

After establishing with an edrophonium test that a patient has respiratory failure due to myasthenia gravis the dose of anticholinesterase drugs should be optimised. The vital capacity should be monitored before and after small (2 mg) doses of intravenous edrophonium. Swallowing is usually impaired and a nasogastric tube is often needed. Pyridostigmine should be given orally or via the nasogastric tube, but when enteral fluids cannot be absorbed, neostigmine should be given intramuscularly, substituting each 60 mg of pyridostigmine with 1 mg of neostigmine.

Patients with myasthenia gravis respond so dramatically in the short term to PE that a controlled trial has never been undertaken. We use 50 ml/kg exchanges on alternate days until an adequate response has been achieved, usually after 2–5 exchanges. Improvement is usually noticeable after the second exchange and lasts for about 4–6 weeks. Similar clinical benefit and falls in anti-acetylcholine receptor antibody titre have been reported following IVIg. The largest published experience is that of Cosi et al [69] who reported clinical improvement 12 days after a standard course of 0·4 g/kg in 70% of 37 patients treated which lasted for 60 days in 57%. Arsura et al [70] reported improvement in 11 of 12 patients beginning 3·6 days after IVIg treatment began, reaching a maximum after 8·6 days and lasting an average of 52 days. Sustained improvement has been maintained with repeated courses in a small number of cases.[71] Judgement of the relative merits of PE and IVIg must await comparative trials. In the meantime it would be reasonable to try IVIg to treat a myasthenic crisis if PE is not available.

As PE provides only temporary relief, immunosuppressive treatment should be started, or increased, at the same time. We follow the practice of Newsom-Davis[27] and use prednisolone 120 mg on alternate days. In patients with early respiratory failure steroids should be introduced slowly and cautiously because of the danger of a transient worsening during the first week or two of the course. In patients with established respiratory failure on artificial ventilation, this cautious approach is superfluous and a full dose of steroids can be started immediately. Very large doses of steroids, including boluses of intravenous methylprednisolone, should be avoided because of the danger of inducing necrotic myopathy.[72] For patients who are inadequately controlled with steroids we add azathioprine. If azathioprine is not tolerated, other immunosuppressive agents, such as cyclophosphamide or methotrexate, and as a last resort, low dose total body irradiation can be tried. When the respiratory failure due to myasthenic crisis has been controlled, younger patients and those with thymoma should be assessed for thymectomy.

Polymyositis

Treatment of polymyositis with large doses of steroids is universally recommended and so clearly helpful, at least in the short term, that a controlled trial has never been considered necessary. A typical regimen, recommended by Mastaglia and Ojeda,[40] is prednisone 60–80 mg/kg daily for 6–8 weeks followed by gradual withdrawal at the rate of 5 mg of the daily dose per week. After the dose has reached 30 mg daily further reductions should be made at 2·5 mg per week. A wide range of doses are used however; some prefer an alternate day dose but others feel that this is not so effective.[40] It is important to bring the disease under control before beginning the reduction and then to monitor the course of the disease closely with serial measurements of muscle strength and plasma creatinine kinase concentrations. Although PE combined with cyclophosphamide has been reported beneficial in polymyositis,[73] the usefulness of PE alone was not confirmed in a controlled trial in which three groups of 13 patients were treated with leucopheresis, PE, or sham PE.[74] The authors of that trial claim an 80% power of detecting a minimal improvement in functional capacity. The trial did not answer the question whether PE followed by immunosuppression would provide a more rapid response than immunosuppression alone. Further exploration of this possibility would be worthwhile as the PE group had a highly significant fall in plasma creatinine kinase concentration compared with the sham PE group. Intravenous immunoglobulin was dramatically effective in two cases resistant to steroids and immunosuppressive drugs,[75] but its usefulness requires more study. Immunosuppressive treatment with azathioprine, cyclophosphamide, or methotrexate has often been tried when steroids have failed,[40] but probably does not have the rapid effect necessary to prevent or reverse the acute onset of respiratory failure. In desperation, total body low dose irradiation has sometimes been used and remissions have occurred in those cases that have been published.[40]

Withdrawal of mechanical ventilation

The course of respiratory failure related to neuromuscular disease is extremely variable. Various factors such as the primary diagnosis, chronic health status, treatment, and the presence or absence of supervening complications dictate the rate of recovery. It eventually becomes evident that an individual patient has regained adequate neuromuscular function to be placed on a spontaneous mode of ventilation. At this stage, lung compliance and spontaneous minute ventilation should be relatively normal with a stable cardiovascular system. We prefer pressure support as a weaning mode and it is our practice to reduce gradually the amount of pressure support while monitoring the clinical appearance of the patient, respiratory rate, tidal volume, and arterial saturation by pulse oximetry. Daily measurements of vital capacity are also performed but it is not clear how helpful these are in the assessment of the recovery of respiratory muscle function. One study has clearly demonstrated that tidal volume rather than vital capacity is more closely related to recovering diaphragm function.[76] We have not found the more complex assessments of diaphragmatic performance such as maximum transdiaphragmatic pressure (P_{Dimax}) or inspiratory time fraction (T_i/T_{tot}) useful in the withdrawal of ventilatory support in these cases.

As respiratory muscle strength increases, it is possible to ask the patient to breathe for longer periods off the ventilator, either on continuous positive airway pressure or a T piece. A relatively low level of pressure support (10 cm H_2O) is usually maintained overnight to allow a patient to rest and to prevent nocturnal hypoxaemia. Many patients find that this period of ventilator withdrawal provokes extreme anxiety because of psychological dependence on the presence and the sound of the ventilator. Careful assessment of respiratory function and extensive psychological support are required to meet the physical and emotional needs of the patient.

Aftermath

Prevention of death from respiratory failure is merely the first stage in treatment of an illness such as GBS. Maintenance of morale and recognition and treatment of depression are important and difficult tasks which call on all the resources of the intensive care team. For some conditions, patient support groups exist which offer counselling services (for example, Guillain–Barré Syndrome Support Group International, PO Box 262, Wynnewood, Pa 19096, United States; Guillain–Barré Syndrome Support Group, Foxley, Holdingham, Sleaford, Lincs NG34 8NR, United Kingdom). There are no easy guidelines. The patient and the family need clear information about what is happening and what may be expected. Over-optimistic prognoses may be greeted eagerly at first but reap a grim harvest of dashed hopes later. Above all, a conscious patient festooned with monitoring equipment in a modern intensive care unit needs a sympathetic caring approach tailored to his or her own needs.

We thank our colleagues and the nursing staff of Russell Brock and Starling Wards for their help, Dr L Loh, Radcliffe Infirmary, Oxford, Dr D F Moore, Guy's Hospital Poisons Information Service, and Professor C M Wiles, University of Wales, Cardiff for advice, and the Medical Research Council and Guillain–Barré Syndrome Support Group for financial support.

Management of acute neuromuscular paralysis

● Respiratory paralysis occurs in a small percentage of patients with acute neuromuscular disease and accounts for less than 1% of admissions to intensive care units. Its development may be insidious so that patients with acute neuromuscular disease should have their vital capacity monitored. Orotracheal intubation and ventilatory support should be instituted prophylactically when the vital capacity is falling towards 1000 ml or 10 ml/kg. Earlier intervention is necessary in the presence of bulbar palsy.

● The cause of the respiratory paralysis can usually be deduced from the clinical history and examination. It is necessary to distinguish diseases affecting the respiratory centre and its CNS connections to the cervical and thoracic spinal cord (see box 1), peripheral neuropathy, disorders of neuromuscular conduction, and muscle disease. In practice the commonest cause is Guillain–Barré syndrome but the possibility of porphyria, vasculitis, and toxic neuropathies should not be ignored (table II). If the reflexes are preserved and there is no sensory deficit, the possibility of myasthenia, botulism, other rare causes of neuromuscular conduction block (table III), and muscle disease (table III) should be considered.

● If artificial ventilation is likely to be required for more than about seven days, a tracheotomy should be performed and is much more comfortable for the patient. Nutrition should be provided early via a nasogastric tube. Strenuous efforts should be made to reduce the incidence of nosocomial infection. In patients with neuropathy, in particular, autonomic function causing cardiac arrhythmia and fluctuating blood pressure should be sought and if necessary treated. Deep vein thrombosis should be avoided by regular passive limb movements and low dose subcutaneous heparin.

> ## Management of acute neuromuscular paralysis (cont)
>
> ● Specific interventions to shorten the duration of artificial ventilation should be applied appropriate to the nature of the underlying condition. Metabolic disturbances such as hypokalaemia or hypermagnesaemia should always be sought and corrected first. In Guillain–Barré syndrome we recommend intravenous immunoglobulin. In myasthenia gravis we recommend plasma exchange followed by thymectomy or, where thymectomy is inappropriate or has been unsuccessful, plasma exchange combined with steroids. In polymyositis steroids are the mainstay of treatment.

1 Hughes RAC. *Guillain-Barré syndrome*. Heidelberg: Springer-Verlag, 1990.
2 Knaus WA. The APACHE III Prognostic System—risk prediction of hospital mortality for critically ill hospitalized adults. *Chest* 1991;**100**:1619–36.
3 Kelly BJ. The diagnosis and management of neuromuscular diseases causing respiratory failure. *Chest* 1991;**99**:1485–94.
4 Roussos C. The respiratory muscles. *New Engl J Med* 1982;**307**:786–97.
5 Black LF. Maximal static respiratory pressures in generalized neuromuscular disease. *Am Rev Respir Dis* 1971;**103**:641–7.
6 Hall AJ. Polio eradication as 2000 approaches. *BMJ* 1992;**305**:69–70.
7 Joce R, Wood D, Brown D, Begg N. Paralytic poliomyelitis in England and Wales. *BMJ* 1992;**305**:79–82.
8 Goode GB, Shearn DL. Botulism. A case with associated sensory abnormalities. *Arch Neurol* 1982;**34**:55.
9 Ropper AH, Wijdicks EFM, Truax BT. *Guillain-Barré syndrome*. Philadelphia: FA Davis, 1991.
10 Albers JW, Kelly JJ. Acquired inflammatory demyelinating polyneuropathies: clinical and electrodiagnostic features. *Muscle Nerve* 1989;**12**:435–51.
11 Thomas PK. The Guillain-Barré syndrome: no longer a simple concept. *J Neurol* 1992;**239**:361–2.
12 Hughes RAC, Atkinson P, Coates P, Hall S, Leibowitz S. Sural nerve biopsies in Guillain–Barré syndrome: axonal degeneration and macrophage-mediated demyelination and absence of cytomegalovirus genome. *Muscle Nerve* 1992;**15**:568–75.
13 Hall SM, Hughes RAC, Payan J, Atkinson PF, McColl I, Gale A. Motor nerve biopsy in severe Guillain-Barré syndrome. *Ann Neurol* 1992;**31**:441-4.
14 Zochodne DW, Bolton CF, Wells AG, *et al* Critical illness polyneuropathy. A complication of sepsis and multiple organ failure. *Brain* 1987;**110**:819–42.
15 Bolton CF, Gilbert JJ, Hahn AF, Sibbald WJ. Polyneuropathy in critically ill patients. *J Neurol Neurosurg Psychiatry* 1984;**47**:1223–31.
16 Cavanagh JB, Fuller NH, Johnson HRM, Rudge P. The effects of thallium salts, with particular reference to the nervous system changes. *Q J Med* 1974;**43**:293–319.
17 Donofrio PD, Wilbourne AJ, Albers JW, Rogers L, Salanga V, Greenberg HS. Acute arsenic intoxication presenting as Guillain–Barré like syndrome. *Muscle Nerve* 1987;**10**:114–20.
18 Rappuoli R, Perugini M, Falsen E. Molecular epidemiology of the 1984–1986 outbreak of diphtheria in Sweden. *N Engl J Med* 1988;**318**:12–14.
19 Swift TR, Rivener MH. Infectious diseases of nerve. In: Matthews WB, ed. *Handbook of clinical neurology*. Amsterdam: Elsevier, 1987:179–84.
20 Calderon-Gonzalez R, Rizzi-Hernandez H. Buckthorn neuropathy. *N Engl J Med* 1967;**277**:69–71.

21 Norman M, Elinder G, Finkel Y. Vincristine neuropathy and a Guillain-Barré syndrome: a case with acute lymphatic leukemia and quadriparesis. *Eur J Haematol* 1987;**39**:75–6.
22 Wilder-Smith E, Roelcke U. Meningopolyradiculitis (Bannwarth syndrome) as a primary manifestation of a centrocytic-centroblastic lymphoma. *J Neurol* 1989;**236**:168–9.
23 Vital C, Vital A, Julien J, et al. Peripheral neuropathies and lymphoma without monoclonal gammopathy: a new classification. *J Neurol* 1990;**237**:177–85.
24 Krendel DA, Stahl RL, Chan WC. Lymphomatous polyneuropathy: Biopsy of clinically involved nerve and successful treatment. *Arch Neurol* 1991;**48**:330–2.
25 Ridley A. Porphyric Neuropathy. In: Dyck PJ, *et al*, eds. *Peripheral neuropathy*. Philadelphia: Saunders, 1984:1704–16.
26 Mitchell G, Larochelle J, Lambert M, *et al* Neurologic crises in hereditary tyrosinemia. *New Engl J Med* 1990;**322**:432–7.
27 Newsom-Davis J. Diseases of the neuromuscular junction. In: Asbury AK, *et al*, eds. *Diseases of the nervous system. Clinical neurobiology*. Philadelphia: W B Saunders, 1992: 197–212.
28 Hughes JM, Blumenthal JR, Merson MH, Lombard GL, Dowell VR, Gangarosa EJ. Clinical features of type A and B food-borne botulism. *Ann Intern Med* 1981;**95**: 442–5.
29 Swift TR. Weakness from magnesium-containing cathartics: electrophysiologic studies. *Muscle Nerve* 1979;**2**:295–8.
30 Argov Z, Mastaglia FL. Drug-induced neuromuscular disorders in man. In: Walton J, ed. *Disorders of voluntary muscle*. Edinburgh: Churchill Livingstone, 1988:981–1014.
31 Lindesmith LA, Baines RD, Bigelow DD, Petty TL. Reversible respiratory paralysis associated with polymyxin therapy. *Ann Intern Med* 1968;**68**:318–27.
32 Senanayake N, Román GC. Disorders of neuromuscular transmission due to natural environmental toxins. *J Neurol Sci* 1992;**107**:1–13.
33 Mills AR, Passmore R. Pelagic paralysis. *Lancet* 1988;**1**:161–4.
34 Donat JR, Donat JF. Tick paralysis with persistent weakness and electromyographic abnormalities. *Arch Neurol* 1981;**38**:59–62.
35 Braun NM, Arora NS, Rochester DF. Respiratory muscle and pulmonary function in polymyositis and other proximal myopathies. *Thorax* 1983;**38**:616–23.
36 Keunen RWM, Lambregts PCLA, Op de Coul AAW, Joosten EMG. Respiratory failure as initial symptom of acid maltase deficiency. *J Neurol Neurosurg Psychiatry* 1984;**47**: 549–52.
37 Trend P, Wiles CM, Spencer GT. Acid maltase deficiency in adults: diagnosis and management in 5 cases. *Brain* 1985;**108**:845–60.
38 Mohamed SD, Chapman RS, Crooks J. Hypokalaemia, flaccid quadruparesis, and myoglobinuria with carbenoxolone. *BMJ* 1966;**1**:1581–2.
39 Newman JH, Neff TA, Ziporin P. Acute respiratory failure associated with hypophosphatemia. *N Engl J Med* 1977;**296**:1101–3.
40 Mastaglia FL, Ojeda VJ. Inflammatory myopathies. *Ann Neurol* 1985;**17**:215–27, 2317–23.
41 Sitwell LD, Weinshenker BG, Monpetit V, Reid D. Complete ophthalmoplegia as a complication of acute corticosteroid- and pancuronium-associated myopathy. *Neurology* 1991; **41**:921–2.
42 De Vere R, Bradley WG. Polymyositis: its presentation, morbidity and mortality. *Brain* 1975;**98**:637–66.
43 Pendersen J. The effect of nasotracheal intubation on the paranasal sinuses. *Acta Anaesthesiol Scand* 1991;**35**:11–13.
44 Azar I. The response of patients with neuromuscular disorders to muscle relaxants—a review. *Anaesthesiology* 1984;**61**:173–87.
45 Dalos NP. Cardiovascular autonomic dysfunction in Guillain-Barré syndrome. *Arch Neurol* 1988;**45**:115–17.
46 Grover ER. The role of tracheostomy in the intensive care unit. *Postgrad Med J* 1992; **68**:313–17.
47 Ciaglia P. Percutaneous dilational tracheostomy—results and long term follow-up. *Chest* 1992;**101**:464–7.
48 Maynard N. Post-operative feeding. *BMJ* 1991;**303**:1007–8.
49 Wilmore DW. Catabolic illness—strategies for enhancing recovery. *New Engl J Med* 1992; **325**:695–702.
50 Pingleton S. Nutritional management of acute respiratory failure. *JAMA* 1987;**257**: 3094–9.

51 Deitch EA. The role of intestinal barrier failure and bacterial translocation in the development of systemic infection and multiple organ failure. *Arch Surg* 1990;**125**:403–4.

52 Freeman J. Association of intravenous lipd emulsion and coagulase negative Staphylococcal bacteremia in neonatal intensive care units. *New Engl J Med* 1990;**323**: 301–8.

53 Detsky AS. Parenteral nutrition—is it helpful? *New Engl J Med* 1991;**325**:573–5.

54 Bihari D. Nosocomial infections in the intensive care unit. *Hospital update* 1992;**18**: 266–71. *Am Rev Respir Dis* 1992.

55 Fagon J-Y. Nosocomial pneumonia in patients receiving continuous machanical ventilation. *Intensive Care Med* 1989;**139**:877–84.

56 Loirat PH. Selective digestive decontamination in intensive care unit patients. *Intensive Care Med* 1992;**18**:182–8.

57 Lichtenfeld P. Autonomic dysfunction in the Guillain-Barré syndrome. *Am J Med* 1971;**50**:772–80.

58 Winer JB, Hughes RAC. Identification of patients at risk of arrhythmia in the Guillain-Barre syndrome. *Q J Med* 1988;**68**:735–9.

59 Tuck RR, McLeod JG. Autonomic dysfunction in Guillain-Barre syndrome. *J Neurol Neurosurg Psychiatry* 1981;**44**:983–90.

60 The Guillain-Barré Syndrome Study Group. Plasmapheresis and acute Guillain-Barré syndrome. *Neurology* 1985;**35**:1096–104.

61 French Cooperative group in plasma exchange in Guillain-Barré syndrome. Efficiency of plasma exchange in Guillain-Barré syndrome: role of replacement fluids. *Ann Neurol* 1987;**22**:753–61.

62 McKhann GM, Griffin JW, Cornblath DR, *et al* Plasmapheresis and Guillain-Barré Syndrome: analysis of prognostic factors and the effect of plasmapheresis. *Ann Neurol* 1988;**23**:347–53.

63 Osterman PO, Fagius J, Safwenberg J, Daniellson BG, Wikstrom B. Early relapses after plasma exchange in acute inflammatory polyradiculoneuropathy. *Lancet* 1986;**2**:1161.

64 Ropper AH, Albers JW, Addison R. Limited relapse in Guillain-Barré syndrome after plasma exchange. *Arch Neurol* 1988;**45**:314–15.

65 Hughes RAC, Newsom-Davis JM, Perkin GD, Pierce JM. Controlled trial of prednisolone in acute polyneuropathy. *Lancet* 1978;**2**:750–3.

66 Hughes RAC. Ineffectiveness of high-dose intravenous methylprednisolone in Guillain-Barré syndrome. *Lancet* 1991;**338**:1142.

67 Van der Meché FGA, Schmitz PIM, Dutch Guillain-Barré Study Group. A randomized trial comparing intravenous immune globulin and plasma exchange in Guillain-Barré syndrome. *New Engl J Med* 1992;**326**:1123–9.

68 The Plasma Exchange/Sandoglobulin Guillain-Barré Syndrome Trial Group. Comparison of Plasma Exchange, Intravenous Immunoglobulin, and Plasma Exchange followed by Intravenous Immunoglobulin in the treatment of Guillain-Barré Syndrome. *Ann Neurol* 1995;**38**:972.

69 Cosi V, Lombardi M, Piccolo G, Erbetta A. Treatment of myasthenia gravis with high dose intravenous immunoglobulin. *Acta Neurol Scand* 1991;**84**:81–4.

70 Arsura EL, Bick A, Brunner NG, Namba T, Grob D. High dose intravenous immunoglobulin in the management of myasthenia gravis. *Arch Intern Med* 1986;**146**:1365–8.

71 Arsura E, Bick A, Brunner NG, Grob D. Effects of repeated doses of intravenous immunoglobulin in myasthenia gravis. *Am J Med Sci* 1988;**295**:438–43.

72 Panegyres P, Squier M, Mills KR, Newsom-Davis J. Acute myopathy associated with large parenteral corticosteroid dosage in myasthenia gravis. *J Neurol Neurosurg Psychiatry* 1993;**56**:702–4.

73 Dau PC. Plasmapheresis in idiopathic inflammatory myopathy. Experience with 35 patients. *Arch Neurol* 1981;**38**:544–52.

74 Miller FW, Leitman SF, Cronin ME, *et al.* Controlled trial of plasma exchange and leukapheresis in polymyositis and dermatomyositis. *New Engl J Med* 1992;**326**:1380–4.

75 Jann S, Beretta S, Moggio M, Adobbati L, Pellegrini G. High-dose intravenous human immunoglobulin in polymyositis resistant to treatment. *J Neurol Neurosurg Psychiatry* 1992;**55**:60–2.

76 Borel CO. Diaphragmatic performance during recovery from acute ventilatory failure in Guillain-Barré syndrome and myasthenia gravis. *Chest* 1991;**99**:444–51.

77 Senanayave N, Johnson MK. Acute polyneuropathy after poisoning by a new organophosphate insecticide. *New Engl J Med* 1982;**306**:155–7.

318

78 Greenberg C, Davies S, McGowan T, Schorer A, Drage C. Acute respiratory failure following severe arsenic poisoning. *Chest* 1979;**76**:596–8.

79 Graziano JH. 2,3-dimercaptosuccinic acid (DMSA). In: Goldfranks LR, *et al*, eds. *Toxicological emergencies*. Norwalk, Ct: Appleton and Lange, 1990:638–40.

80 Watt G, Theakston RDG, Hayes CG, *et al*. Positive response to edrophonium in patients with neurotoxic envenoming by cobras (Naja Naja Philippinensis) A placebo controlled study. *N Engl J Med* 1986;**315**:1444–8.

81 Vernay D, Dubost JJ, Thevent JP, Sauvezie B, Rampon S. "Choreé fibrillaire de Morvan" followed by Guillain-Barré syndrome in a patient receiving gold therapy. *Arthritis Rheum* 1986;**29**:1413–14.

82 Brust JCM, Hammer JS, Challenor Y, Healton EB, Lesser R. Acute generalized polyneuropathy accompanying lithium poisoning. *Ann Neurol* 1979;**6**:360–2.

83 Hughes RAC, Cameron JS, Hall SM, Heaton J, Payan JA, Teoh R. Multiple mononeuropathy as the initial presentation of systemic lupus erythematosus—nerve biopsy and response to plasma exchange. *J Neurol* 1982;**228**:239–47.

84 Christie AB. Diphtheria. In: Weatherall DJ, *et al*, eds. *Oxford textbook of medicine*. Oxford: Oxford University Press, 1987;**5**:164–5.

85 Calderon-Gonzalez R, Gonzalez-Cantu N, Rissi-Hernandez H. Recurrent polyneuropathy with pregnancy and oral contraceptives. *N Engl J Med* 1970;**282**:1307–8.

86 Senanayake N, Roman GC. Toxic neuropathies in the tropics. *J Trop Geogr Neurol* 1991; **1**:3–15.

87 Danon MJ, Carpenter S. Myopathy with thick filament (myosin) loss following prolonged paralysis with vecuronium during steroid treatment. *Muscle Nerve* 1991;**14**:1131–9.

88 Gould DB, Sorrell MR, Lupariello AD. Barium sulfide poisoning. *Arch Intern Med* 1973; **132**:891–4.

319

12 Acute visual failure

SHIRLEY H WRAY

Acute visual failure is the presenting symptom of an ocular stroke. Ocular strokes are due to a central retinal artery occlusion, branch retinal artery occlusion, or anterior ischaemic optic neuropathy which is the result of infarction of the optic nerve.

Central retinal artery occlusion

Clinical signs and symptoms

Sudden blindness is the major symptom in central retinal artery occlusion unless a cilioretinal artery is present to supply circulation to the macula. Eye pain is atypical, but when present suggests involvement of the ophthalmic artery.

Blindness is confirmed by failure of the pupil to react to direct light, but what is seen ophthalmoscopically depends on how soon after the occlusion the examination is made. If the fundus is examined within the first few minutes while the occlusion persists, the striking finding is the presence of segmentation of the blood column, boxcar segmentation, with slow "streaming" of flow in the retinal veins. Blood in the arterial branches is dark and a few arterioles may show segmentation (clear areas alternating with areas where the cells appear clumped together), but this is nowhere so obvious as in the veins.

Ophthalmoscopy is not often performed within the first hour, however, and later inspection of the fundus will show surprisingly little. Typically the disc will show no more than mild pallor whereas the arteries may be only slightly attenuated. Gentle digital pressure on the globe during ophthalmoscopy may nevertheless elicit segmentation of the blood column, indicating the presence of a slow but not completely arrested circulation. Total obstruction posterior to the lamina should be suspected when the retinal arteries on the disc start to pulsate at a touch indicating very low retinal diastolic pressure. When the signs of central retinal artery occlusion are secondary to an ophthalmic artery occlusion, the intraocular pressure in the eye is low.

With the passage of time, typically after an hour or more, the characteristic fundus changes are seen. The ischaemic retina takes on a white ground glass appearance and the normal red colour of the choroid showing through at the fovea accentuates the central cherry-red spot at the macula (fig 1). Within days of the acute event, the retinal opacification, the cherry-red spot, and the nerve fibre layer disappear and optic atrophy of the primary type develops.

Pathogenesis

There are five principal causes of occlusion of central retinal artery (box 1).

The cause may be evident if examination shows: a retinal embolus, hypertension, atrial fibrillation and/or disease of other

---

Box 1—Principal causes of occlusion of the central retinal artery

● Embolic obstruction

● Occlusion in situ in association with atheromatous disease when the narrowed arterial lumen becomes obliterated by superimposed thrombosis or haemorrhage

● Inflammatory endarteritis, such as temporal arteritis,[1] thromboangiitis obliterans,[2] and polyarteritis nodosa with involvement of the choroidal and retinal arteries[3]

● Simple angiospasm, a rare cause that may be the mechanism of central retinal artery occlusion associated with Raynaud's disease[4] or with migraine[5]

● Arterial occlusion that occurs hydrostatically with the high intraocular pressure of glaucoma, the low retinal blood pressure of carotid stenosis or the aortic arch syndrome, or severe hypotension

---

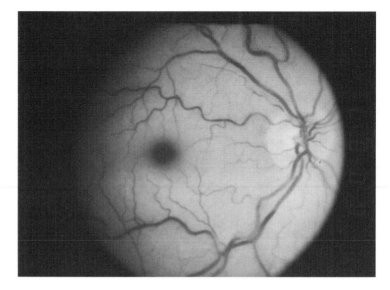

Figure 1—Central retinal artery occlusion with opacification of the retina and a macula cherry-red spot.

arteries, notably the ophthalmic or temporal artery, or the internal carotid artery in the neck. Even in cases of embolic genesis, however, an embolus may not be seen because emboli frequently impact behind the lamina cribrosa.

Transient monocular blindness (type I or II, table I) as a premonitory symptom suggests an embolic cause or temporal arteritis.[6] In patients under the age of 40, the heart is the leading source of emboli[7 8] because of rheumatic valvular disease, bacterial endocarditis, or cardiac myxoma (table II).[9] In older patients, the source of the embolus may be cardiac[10] or intra-arterial from atheromatous ulceration of the aorta or the ipsilateral internal carotid artery.

Trauma is also an important cause. Compression of the globe may be self inflicted in circumstances involving heavy alcohol use with or without drug consumption followed by stupor.[11] Iatrogenic central retinal artery occlusion has been reported in patients undergoing surgery where prolonged pressure to the orbit has occurred inadvertently in association with a period of hypotension during anaesthesia.[12 13]

322

TABLE I—Types of amaurosis fugax*

	Type I	*Type II*	*Type III*	*Type IV*
Onset	Abrupt	Less rapid	Abrupt	Abrupt
Visual loss	All or partial	All or partial	Total or progressive contraction of visual fields	Resembles type I or II
Length	Seconds or minutes	Minutes or hours	Minutes	Any length
Recovery	Complete	Complete	Usually complete	Complete
Pain	No	Rare	Often	No
Mechanism	Embolus Arteritis	Hypoperfused carotid/ ophthalmic occlusive disease	Vasospasm (migraine) of ophthalmic artery or central retinal artery	Anticardiolipid antibodies or idiopathic
Unusual features	Vision may black out completely	Loss of contrast vision; photopsias; sunlight provoked	Visual loss may spare fixation	Alternating between eyes

*Based on 850 personal cases.

Diagnosis

Diagnosis is usually straightforward; however, the differential diagnosis of acute persistent monocular visual failure includes a number of ophthalmic emergencies, that is, anterior ischaemic optic neuropathy, acute occlusion of the central retinal vein, detachment of the macula, acute closed-angle glaucoma, sudden vitreous or macular haemorrhage, as well as factitious visual loss.

Management

Bock *et al* [14] and Hayreh *et al* [15] suggest that the retina suffers irreparable damage after a central retinal artery occlusion of 105 minutes but may recover well within 97 minutes of the ictus. By the time most central retinal artery occlusions are seen, however, there is usually a longer lapse of time and there is no effective treatment available for the restoration of normal vision. Nonetheless, every case deserves referral for urgent treatment as restoration of an area of peripheral visual field may be achieved.

Therapy for acute visual loss due to a central retinal artery occlusion or ophthalmic artery occlusion is often unsatisfactory.

TABLE II—Sources of emboli

	Type	Patient age
Cardiac valves		
Rheumatic disease	Platelet/calcium⋆	Any age
Lupus	Platelet	Young women
Acute or subacute endocarditis	Marasmic	Damaged heart
Floppy mitral valve	Platelet	Any age; mostly women
Cardiac chamber		
Myxoma	Myxoma	
Mural thrombus	Platelet/clot	Older adult
Carotid artery		
Ulcerated plaque	Platelet/cholesterol ester	Older adult
Stenosis	Platelet	
Fibromuscular dysplasia	Platelet	Young woman
Other		
Amniotic	Debris?⋆	Young woman
Long bone fractures	Fat⋆	Any age
Chronic intravenous drug users	Talc⋆	Any age
Disseminated intravascular coagulopathy⋆	??	??
Antiphospholipid antibody(s)	??	Young adult

⋆Produces retinal infarction; no amaurosis fugax. (Reproduced from Burde[9] with modification, courtesy of the publishers, *J Clin Neuro-ophthal.*)

Ocular massage using digital pressure or a Goldmann contact lens has been advocated as an initial treatment to dislodge an obstructive embolus and improve flow.[16] Some success has been reported with sublingual nitroglycerin, which has a vasodilator effect.

Immediately following the initial therapy, and within 24 hours of the acute onset of blindness, patients should be referred on an urgent basis to an ophthalmologist for an anterior paracentesis. Anterior paracentesis in conjunction with breathing carbogen (a mixture of 95% oxygen and 5% carbon dioxide) for 10 minutes every 2 hours for 24 to 48 hours has improved visual acuity by three Snellen gradations in about 35% of eyes with obstruction of the central retinal artery. In an acute situation, a hyperbaric chamber, if available, should be considered.

Recently, because of the beneficial results of intra-arterial fibrinolysis in the carotid and vertebrobasilar systems, micro-catheter urokinase infusion has been introduced as a treatment for central retinal artery occlusion. To avoid fatal cerebral complications and to obtain a high local concentration of fibrinolytic activity, urokinase is injected directly into the ophthalmic artery through a transfemorally introduced catheter. The urokinase is injected by hand at a speed of 1 ml/minute (10 000 IU of urokinase) through a microcatheter introduced through the diagnostic catheter. In one study the first 2 patients of 14 consecutive patients treated were given 5000 IU/minute. The injection of urokinase was discontinued in 3 patients when clinical signs of improvement in visual acuity were apparent. In patients who did not show clinical improvement, the fibrinolytic treatment was stopped as soon as ophthalmoscopic and catheter-angiographic evidence of improved profusion of the retinal arteries was seen. To prevent systemic reaction, the total amount of urokinase was limited to 800 000 to 900 000 IU. In all patients fibrinolysis was succeeded by heparinisation for 2 to 3 days with doses between 20 000 and 25 000 IU per day. All patients were subjected to superselective angiography of the ophthalmic artery before and after treatment. Fluorescein angiography was performed in most patients pre and post the infusion to study retinal perfusion. Fluorescein angiography disclosed hypoperfusion of the choroid in addition to the decreased retinal circulation in 6 patients, implying that these cases had occlusion of the ophthalmic artery. In 3 patients, tissue plasminogen activator was used instead of urokinase. Overall, the results showed that vision improved markedly in 4 of the 14 treated patients. Five of the 14 patients had slight improvement of visual acuity, visual field, or both and in 5 no improvement occurred. In these 5 patients, visual acuity was impaired pre-operatively for more than 7 to 8 hours.

Clearly, the window of opportunity is short for fibrinolytic therapy to be effective, but in centres using this therapy for hemispheric stroke, microcatheter urokinase infusion might be expected to restore vision following a central retinal artery occlusion from 20/200 to 20/40 or better if infused within 4–6 hours.[17] The authors of the study caution, however, that fibrinolytic treatment should not be performed in every patient with central retinal artery occlusion. Intra-arterial fibrinolysis is contraindicated in patients with severe general systemic disease, after myocardial infarction, or in patients with cardiac insufficiency, endocarditis, aneurysm of the heart wall, or auricular fibrillation, haemorrhagic diathesis, cirrhosis of the liver, hypertension (unless the blood pressure has first been reduced) and in patients treated with oral anticoagulants.

In the late stage of central retinal artery occlusion, where a cherry-red spot is present, an anterior paracentesis may be of little benefit because the infarcted retina is probably already damaged beyond recovery.[17] Nevertheless, in eyes that have been blind for several hours, heroic measures can be undertaken if less than 24 hours have elapsed as gratifying recovery of vision has been reported in eyes treated six, eight, and 12 hours after the event.[18]

Heparin anticoagulation is useful in the treatment of an impending occlusion. High dose systemic corticosteroids are essential in the therapy of suspected inflammatory arteritis.

Management of patients with central retinal artery occlusion must also include an evaluation for associated hypertension, cardiac disorders, arterial vascular disease (ophthalmic, temporal, and internal carotid artery), and the presence of antiphospholipid antibodies.

Hypertension is an important factor in the genesis of all strokes. The early detection of hypertension, its vigorous treatment, and close surveillance may be expected to reduce the increasing prevalence of central retinal artery occlusion.

Heart disease is frequently present in patients with central retinal artery occlusion. In a retrospective study, Appen et al[8] found that 30% of younger and 23% of older patients had associated cardiac valvular disease. In a prospective study,[19] 56% of patients under the age of 50 had a potential cardiac source of embolus, compared with 24% in the older age group. Aortic stenosis was the most frequent lesion but mitral leaflet prolapse was an isolated finding in 10 patients. Transthoracic echocardiogram has contributed significantly to visualising cardiac findings associated with stroke including intracardiac thrombi, mitral valve prolapse, and mitral annular calcification, but the aortic arch is essentially impossible to evaluate with transthoracic imaging. Because of the proximity of the esophagus to the aorta clear views of the aortic arch are obtained using transesophageal echocardiography. Atheromatous plaques can form in the aortic arch and may cause ischemic stroke if pieces of atheroma or thrombus formed on them break off and go to the brain or to the eye. In one study 26% of 239 patients with cerebrovascular disease had ulcerated aortic arch plaque compared to only 5% of the 261 patients with other neurologic diseases. Among the cryptogenic stroke patients, this number reached 61%.[20]

There is also an association between patent foramen ovale,

paradoxical embolism, and stroke, not only in the young but also in the elderly. In one study, patients with cryptogenic stroke had a higher prevalence of patent foramen ovale in patients with stroke of determined cause in all age groups, even after correcting for the presence of recognised stroke risk factors.[21] This identifies patent foramen ovale as a risk factor for cryptogenic stroke. Regardless of patient's age, contrast echocardiography should be considered when the cause of stroke is unknown. Patent foramen ovale can also be detected by transcranial Doppler with agitated saline injection which demonstrates that embolic material can be delivered to the brain via a patent foramen ovale.[22]

Ophthalmic artery occlusion mimics a central retinal artery occlusion clinically and produces opacification of the infarcted retina. But the typical cherry-red spot may be absent or extremely indistinct due to coexisting infarction of the choroid. Optic atrophy and retinal pigment epithelial changes develop subsequently and are present funduscopically.[20-22] A timed fundus fluorescein angiogram is the test of choice to diagnose ophthalmic artery occlusion. The fundus fluorescein angiogram in a central retinal artery occlusion will show a normal arm to eye circulation time and choroidal phase, and a delay in filling of the branches of the central retinal artery. The fundus fluorescein angiogram in an ophthalmic artery occlusion will show a delayed arm to eye circulation time and simultaneous delayed flow in both the choroidal and central retinal artery circulation. The flash electroretinogram is also valuable and shows absence of both the a and b waves.[23] Ophthalmic artery occlusion carries a very poor prognosis for vision;[21] in two isolated cases, however, vision recovered from light perception vision to 20/30[22] and from an acuity of counting fingers at 15 cm to 20/50 with the restoration of normal retinal and choroidal blood flow.

An occlusion of the central retinal artery may be the only symptom of giant cell arteritis in 5–10% of elderly patients and the risk of blindness in the fellow eye is extremely high. Diagnostically, giant cell arteritis is characterised by an elevation of the erythrocyte sedimentation rate (ESR) and the fibrinogen level, and an inflammatory arteritis with giant cells on histopathological examination of an affected artery. A high index of suspicion clinically, with or without an abnormal ESR and fibrinogen level, is, however, an indication for immediate high dose corticosteroid therapy (prednisone 80 mg daily until ESR starts to fall,

327

tapering to 15 mg daily as soon as ESR is normal), pending a temporal artery biopsy.

Ipsilateral internal carotid artery dissection, occlusion, or stenosis with or without ulceration may be the cause of a central retinal artery occlusion and auscultation of the neck, eyes, and head for a bruit is important.

When a bruit at the bifurcation is also audible over the ipsilateral eye, the physician can be confident that the bruit is of internal carotid artery origin and that the artery is patent. An ipsilateral ocular bruit alone may indicate stenosis of the intracavernous segment of the internal carotid artery. When flow in the internal carotid is severely diminished, no bruit may be audible.

Anisocoria with normal pupil reflexes is an important sign of internal carotid artery dissection. Meiosis and partial ptosis in the ipsilateral eye indicate an oculosympathetic palsy, Horner's syndrome. Horner's syndrome results from damage to the autonomic nerve fibres in the internal carotid artery sheath in the neck. The presenting symptom of internal carotid artery dissection is pain. Ipsilateral neck pain, headache, pain in the face or retro-orbital pain may occur. After a latent interval the patient may have a transient ischemic attack, an episode of transient monocular blindness or a central retinal artery occlusion. Neck tenderness and bruit are inconstant features and less common symptoms are pulsatile tinnitus or hypoglossal palsy.

Carotid non-invasive studies are indicated in all patients with a bruit and the entire carotid-ophthalmic system must be evaluated in the symptomatic patient with or without a bruit. The goal is to identify patients at high risk for stroke, and stenosis of the internal carotid artery in the neck is the vascular change we most need to identify with diagnostic tests. For this purpose, the battery of carotid non-invasive studies should include at least one direct and one indirect test. But, to optimize the reliability of the non-invasive studies, several of each should be performed. Direct tests examine the common carotid bifurcation itself. These tests include B-mode real time ultrasound imaging to demonstrate vessel wall configuration, continuous and/or pulsed wave Doppler to assess rheological change (from which one interpolates degree of stenosis) and colourflow techniques to show the contours of the blood column in velocity encoded colours. When B-mode and pulsed-Doppler information are integrated, the combination is called duplex imaging. Duplex techniques permit simultaneous demonstration of the vessel walls, velocity data and the site in the lumen from which the Doppler data are being generated. Indirect tests monitor bifurcation events by assessing hemodynamic change in distal circulatory beds. Some carotid lesions that put a patient at risk for ocular or hemispheric stroke may be associated with normal direct but abnormal indirect tests. The most common indirect tests used today are periorbital directional Doppler ultrasonography and oculoplethysmography. The former monitors the superficial and the latter the deep orbital circulation. Periorbital directional Doppler for ultrasonography detects changes in internal carotid artery flow and pressure by detecting reversal of flow direction in the supratrochlear and supraorbital branches of the ophthalmic artery. Periorbital studies can be done essentially in 100% of patients. Oculoplethysmography detects changes in the filling characteristics of ocular vessels as a result of impaired flow or pressure in the carotid/ophthalmic system. One type of oculoplethysmography examines the differential arrival time of the ocular pulse wave in each eye. A delay of greater than 20 msec is significant. Oculoplethysmography, however, requires placing a cup on the sclera and elevating intraocular pressure above systolic ophthalmic artery pressure. A rare patient will have a subconjunctival hemorrhage. Oculoplethysmography cannot be done in patients with glaucoma, recent laser therapy, cataract surgery or lens implantation, a history of retinal hemorrhage, an eye infection, or an allergy to novocaine. In all patients who present with transient monocular blindness, or an acute central retinal artery occlusion, who do not have tight carotids, we recommend transcranial Doppler testing of the ophthalmic arteries and the siphons; if the siphon results are positive, a full transcranial Doppler study to include both anterior and posterior circulations is indicated.

If carotid non-invasive and transcranial Doppler studies are normal, the search for the etiology of an embolic stroke to the eye can focus more comfortably on the heart and great vessels. If the carotid studies are negative, and the transcranial Doppler positive for an intracranial obstructive lesion, the findings can help accelerate the decision for arteriography and/or anticoagulation. If the carotid non-invasive studies are positive (in symptomatic or asymptomatic patients), transcranial Doppler can assess the adequacy of collateral flow. At present, transcranial Doppler is useful and sometimes complementary to magnetic resonance angiography (MRA) of the brain. At this time, MRA cannot provide precise information on the degree of carotid or intracranial stenosis. MRA basically images physiology and the MRA should be interpreted in conjunction with carotid non-invasive and transcranial Doppler studies. If the MRA and ultrasound studies disagree and the latter are of good quality and definitely abnormal, they should be given greater weight. MRA alone cannot yet replace conventional angiography in routine assessment of the extra and intracranial vessels in patients who are considered medically suitable for carotid endarterectomy. Spiral CT angiography is an important new non-invasive tool in assessing carotid disease arteriographically and it can provide complementary information. Of all the non-invasive tools it is most analogous to conventional angiography and may replace MRA in the future (for a complete review see ref. 24).

Data correlating the incidence of significant internal carotid artery disease in patients with central retinal artery occlusion predates the era of non-invasive testing and is based on standard x-ray angiography. In one study of 62 patients with central retinal artery occlusion,[25] 25 patients had carotid angiography and 56% of these had ipsilateral extracranial internal carotid artery disease. Somewhat surprisingly these patients generally did not have carotid bruits and had normal findings on non-invasive carotid tests. Ten of 14 had ipsilateral carotid endarterectomy and were found to have either an embologenic ulcerated plaque or tight internal carotid artery stenosis. In this study 11 of 62 patients had normal angiograms and 13 who did not have angiography had clinical evidence of other "aetiological" factors. The remaining 24 patients had no diagnostic work up.

Occlusion of the central retinal artery in association with a complete occlusion of the ipsilateral internal carotid artery may be due to propagation of thrombus from the carotid siphon into the ophthalmic artery.[26] Combined data[5 24 27 28] suggest that, if no cause is apparent clinically for the retinal stroke, and no alternative cause is evident, it is likely that the ipsilateral carotid artery is occluded, stenosed, or ulcerated and that one patient in seven will go on to have a stroke.

Central retinal artery occlusion has also been shown to be associated with elevated levels of antiphospholipid antibodies (anticardiolipin antibody and lupus anticoagulant).[29–32] Clotting studies (prothrombin time, partial thromboplastin time, and platelet count) and tests for systemic lupus erythematosus including antiphospholipid antibodies are indicated in young adults, especially women with central retinal artery occlusion and retinal vascular disease.[33] [34]

Prognosis

The prognosis for visual recovery in central retinal artery occlusion is extremely poor. A total of 58% of eyes are blind, and only 21% of eyes retain useful vision.

Branch retinal artery occlusion

Clinical signs and symptoms

The lodging of a calcific embolus in a branch of the central retinal artery, usually at a first or second order bifurcation, produces sudden and permanent loss of a sector of the visual field with retinal infarction corresponding to the vascular territory of the arteriole (fig 2). Transient cerebral ischaemic attacks and a stroke are rare preceding symptoms in patients with branch retinal artery occlusion unless large numbers of calcific emboli are released at the time of aortic or mitral valve surgery. Amaurosis fugax is the most common preceding visual symptom (table III).

Pathogenesis

The ophthalmoscopic appearance of a retinal embolus can provide specific information about the embolic material and its possible source (table II). Bright, yellowish, glinting, lipid emboli (Hollenhorst's plaques) are the most common emboli seen in the eye (fig 2). They have been confirmed to be cholesterol and they are associated with atheromatous changes of the ipsilateral carotid artery or aortic arch disease.[35] [36] Calcific emboli, in contrast, are characteristically matt-white, non-scintillating, and somewhat wider than the blood column. Calcific emboli may be dislodged by the surgical manipulation of calcified heart valves at the time of valvulotomy or may occur spontaneously from rheumatic valvular vegetation. Some of the circulating microemboli that pass through the retina, so called migrant pale emboli, are believed to be composed of platelets and their occurrence is associated with thrombocytosis. The emboli that occur after myocardial infarction fall into the category of fibrin plugs. They are especially frequent in patients who have neurological complications after open heart surgery.

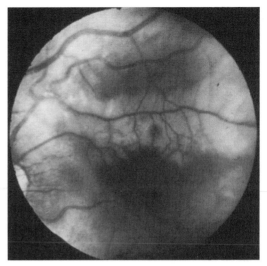

Figure 2—Branch retinal artery occlusion with imputation of two emboli in the artery. The retina shows an arcuate band of infarction.

Potential sources of emboli are: mitral annulus calcification causing cerebral and retinal emboli in the elderly,[37-39] and a prolapsed mitral valve causing similar problems in younger patients.[40-42] In the case of embolic seeding from a myxoma of the heart, the embolus shares the histopathology of the original tumour.[7]

Diffuse disseminated atheroembolism from disease of the aorta is a rare condition closely related to atherosclerosis. Cholesterol rich atheromatous emboli break off from unusually fragile plaques

TABLE III—Preceding vascular events in occlusion of branch and central retinal arteries*

	Retinal artery occlusion	
Preceding event	*Branch†* *n = 68*	*Central‡* *n = 35*
Amaurosis fugax	12 (18)	4 (11)
Transient cerebral ischaemia	8 (12)	1 (3)
Stroke	2 (3)	4 (11)
Ischaemic heart disease	15 (22)	2 (6)
Claudication	5 (7)	2 (6)

*Based on data in ref. 19. †43 male, 25 female patients; mean age 55.
Numbers in parentheses are percentages.
‡23 male, 12 female patients; mean age 36.

in the aorta and its major branches and occlude arteries in the brain, retina, kidney, bowel, and other organs. The diagnosis of diffuse disseminated atheroembolism deserves serious consideration in all patients in middle age or late life with headache, stroke, transient monocular blindness, elevated ESR, hypertension, or cholesterol emboli in the retina. Early diagnosis is important because anticoagulation seems to increase the risk for serious, even fatal embolisation in these patients.

Diagnosis

A patient with a visible retinal embolus, even though suffering no visual loss, should be investigated urgently because of the risk of a stroke. Each case warrants a general physical examination with emphasis on the cardiovascular and neurovascular systems.[43]

In patients with retinal emboli, especially calcific emboli, the investigative work up should focus on the heart (table IV).

Management

The management of an embolic branch retinal artery occlusion is dictated by the patient's vascular status. A carotid endarterectomy is the treatment of choice in a patient with a high-grade carotid artery stenosis with or without severe atheromatous ulceration. Anticoagulation with coumadin or aspirin is a conservative alternative for carotid occlusion without significant stenosis or ulceration.

Surgical treatment of a cardiac source of emboli, that is, aortic or mitral valve disease, or both, is only warranted if the patient also has significant cardiac symptoms. Subsequent retinal embolisation from another calcific embolus is rare and a patient with an isolated calcific retinal embolus can usually be followed without treatment. Anticoagulation is advisable, however, in patients with atrial fibrillation. No treatment is recommended in patients with idiopathic emboli and a normal cardiac rhythm.

Prognosis

Savino et al[28] reported that patients with retinal infarcts and visible emboli showed a shortened survival compared with age- and sex-matched controls (59% v 75%, over nine years) and that a visible retinal embolus predicted a dramatic reduction in survival (44%). When no embolus was visible, more patients survived. Death was related in most cases to cardiac infarction.

333

TABLE IV—Clinical findings in occlusion of branch and central retinal arteries*

| Clinical finding | Retinal artery occlusion | |
	Branch n = 68	Central n = 35
Hypertension	17 (25)	20 (57)
Carotid bruit	12 (18)	5 (14)
Visible retinal embolus	46 (68)	4 (11)
Cardiac valvular abnormality	23 (34)	6 (17)

*Based on data in ref. 19.
Numbers in brackets are percentages.

Anterior ischaemic optic neuropathy

Anterior ischaemic optic neuropathy due to acute infarction of the optic nerve head is a common cause of sudden persistent visual failure in patients past middle age.[44]

The blood supply of the optic nerve head is primarily derived from choroidal and posterior ciliary branches of the ophthalmic artery. The posterior ciliary arteries arise from the ophthalmic artery as independent branches, or in common with other branches of the ophthalmic artery, and may number two (in 48%), three (in 39%), or four branches (in 8%). There are usually only two posterior ciliary arteries, a medial posterior ciliary artery and a lateral posterior ciliary artery. These vessels are end arteries, so that the border zone between the areas of the supply of the medial posterior ciliary artery and the area of supply of the lateral posterior ciliary artery is a watershed zone. The lateral and medial posterior ciliary arteries supply the corresponding half of the choroid. In humans the watershed zone may be located anywhere between the fovea and the nasal border of the optic disc (fig 3).[45] The position of the watershed zone is of great clinical significance because it determines the extent of involvement of the optic nerve head by ischaemia following an occlusion of one of the two main posterior ciliary arteries.[45 46–48]

Clinical signs and symptoms

Anterior ischaemic optic neuropathy occurs most often in patients over the age of 40. Typically, sudden painless visual field

334

loss, an altitudinal field defect, and pallor and swelling of the optic disc occur. Rarely, optic disc changes precede visual loss. Occasionally, visual loss may progress over 1–7 days.

The ischaemic optic disc has a characteristic appearance on funduscopic examination. Usually there is no significant hyperaemia, and even in the early stages the disc tends to be pale. Both the swelling and the pallor may be sectorial, affecting only the superior or inferior half of the disc head. Superficial flame shaped haemorrhages are frequently present, mainly along the peripapillary capillaries (fig 4). When the disc oedema begins to subside, optic atrophy develops and optic disc cupping, similar to that seen in glaucoma, may occur.

In rare cases, embolic ischaemic optic neuropathy can be diagnosed funduscopically by the presence of ischaemic disc swelling and emboli in the branches of the central retinal artery.

Pathogenesis

Anterior ischaemic optic neuropathy occurs in two forms: (a) non-arteritic (median age 56 years) in which the risk factors are diabetes mellitus in younger patients and hypertension in older patients;[49-53] and (b) an arteritic variety due to giant cell arteritis (median age 74 years). Symptoms of giant cell arteritis, anorexia, malaise, proximal arthralgia, myalgia, headache, jaw claudication, and an elevated ESR or fibrinogen level, or both, are indications for prompt systemic corticosteroid therapy and a temporal artery biopsy. Arteritic ischaemic optic neuropathy may affect the contralateral eye and cause blindness in 40% of cases.

Non-arteritic anterior ischemic optic neuropathy is the most common cause of sudden visual loss from optic nerve disease among individuals older than 50 years. Visual loss from non-arteritic anterior ischemic optic neuropathy is often severe with 45% of affected eyes having visual acuity of 20/200 or worse. For individuals with visual loss from non-arteritic anterior ischemic optic neuropathy in one eye, the fellow eye is affected within 3 years in 25% of patients, and in just over 50% by 10 years.

Systemic conditions in association with non-arteritic disease include collagen vascular diseases, such as systemic lupus erythematosus and polyarteritis nodosa, arterial hypotension during surgical procedures, renal haemodialysis or massive haemorrhage, and haematological disorders such as sickle cell trait, polycythaemia, thrombocytopenic purpura, leukaemia, and various

335

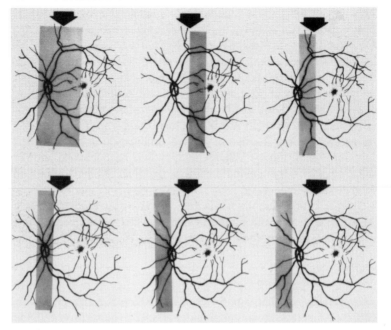

Figure 3—Diagrammatic representation of the locations of the watershed zone (arrows and shaded areas) between the medial and lateral posterior ciliary arteries in human eyes. In the upper left illustration, the shaded area represents the location where the watershed zone may be situated anywhere within this area. The remaining five illustrations are examples of the variations in the location. (From reference 45, with permission.)

types of anaemia. Ocular factors include no cup or only a small cup in the optic disc,[53][54] raised intraocular pressure, and marked optic disc oedema.

Embolism has not been thought to be a major factor in the pathogenesis until relatively recently. Eagling et al[55] studied 40 patients (56 eyes) and found only two patients with retinal emboli. Liberman et al[56] published one of the early reports demonstrating multiple emboli occluding small vessels that had led to retrolaminar infarction of the optic nerve. Burde et al[20] described a patient with metastatic chondrosarcoma with clinical findings of anterior ischaemic optic neuropathy and compromised retinal blood flow. Histological sections of the eye revealed emboli in the short posterior ciliary arteries as well as in the choroidal vessels and central retinal artery. Portnoy et al[57] described a man

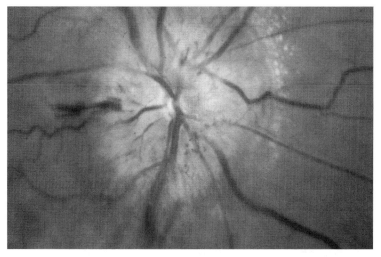

Figure 4—Anterior ischaemic optic neuropathy with pale swelling of the optic disc and flame shaped peripapillary haemorrhages.

with cholesterol emboli within the retinal vasculature combined with a clinical picture of anterior ischaemic optic neuropathy and choroidal non-perfusion demonstrated by fundus fluorescein angiography. In this patient the source of the multiple emboli was an ulcerating plaque in the ipsilateral left carotid artery. I have seen three cases of anterior ischaemic optic neuropathy combined with retinal and posterior ciliary artery emboli, post coronary artery bypass surgery. Choroidal infarction was detected in each case by fluorescein angiography (unpublished data).

Diagnosis

The diagnosis is based on the presence of an altitudinal or complex nerve fibre bundle field defect, ischaemic swelling of the optic disc, and peripapillary haemorrhages. In non-apoplectic anterior ischaemic optic neuropathy with progressive visual loss, compression of the nerve by a mass lesion must be ruled out by a gadolinium MRI of the optic nerve and chiasm.

Management

Diagnostic studies are urgently required in all cases. They include a complete blood count, ESR, fibrinogen level, ausculta-

337

tion of the heart, neck, eyes, and head and carotid non-invasive studies. A temporal artery biopsy is indicated when there is a high index of clinical suspicion of temporal arteritis. A cardiac work up and MRA of the neck and brain are indicated when anterior ischaemic optic neuropathy is thought to be embolic. In non-arteritic disease, tests should also be directed towards the detection of hypertension, diabetes mellitus, and hyperlipidaemia.

Urgent high dose corticosteroids pending a temporal artery biopsy are the treatment of choice in arteritic anterior ischaemic optic neuropathy. Embolic disease, when symptomatic of ipsilateral carotid atheroma should be managed according to the severity of the carotid disease.

There is no effective treatment for non-arteritic disease. Optic nerve sheath decompression for treatment of progressive non-arteritic anterior ischemic optic neuropathy[58 59] is not advised, and corticosteroids are of questionable value, although they are frequently used when the second eye becomes involved. The efficacy of levodopa and carbidopa in promoting visual recovery in eyes with non-arteritic anterior ischemic optic neuropathy has recently been reported but confirmation of this observation is awaited from larger population studies.[60]

Prognosis

The prognosis for recovery of vision is poor, particularly in patients with the arteritic variety due to giant cell arteritis.

The long term clinical course is not well documented. In one follow up study of 205 patients with non-arteritic anterior ischaemic optic neuropathy, there was a slightly greater incidence of stroke and myocardial infarction than expected but no greater mortality.[61] In a retrospective study of 71 patients with non-arteritic disease, the data showed a two- to three-fold higher myocardial and cerebral infarction mortality than expected.[62]

Management of acute visual failure

The diagnostic process for each patient with ocular stroke requires meticulous attention to:

● Blood pressure, heart rate and rhythm, palpation of the temporal arteries, and auscultation of the heart, neck, eyes, and head.

● Dilated funduscopic examination.

● Immediate blood tests: complete blood count, prothrombin time, partial thromboplastin time, platelet count, ESR, fibrinogen level, fasting blood sugar, cholesterol, triglyceride, and blood lipids. A test for antiphospholipid antibodies (anticardiolipin antibody and lupus anticoagulant) is recommended in unexplained cases of central retinal artery occlusion.

Non-invasive investigations should use a battery of tests:

● Carotid non-invasive studies; the useful tests give information about the presence of a hemodynamic lesion (Doppler ultrasonography and oculoplethysmography), and the site of stenosis and residual lumen diameter (B-mode real time ultrasound and continuous and/or pulsed wave Doppler) of the internal carotid artery in the neck.

● Transthoracic and transesophageal echocardiogram.

Invasive investigations are required in selected patients:

● A temporal artery biopsy.

● A carotid arteriogram if the patient is a candidate for endarterectomy. The patient can be screened first with a non-invasive MRA of the neck and brain and/or a spiral CT of the neck.

● A timed fundus fluorescein angiography, particularly in cases of central retinal artery occlusion when occlusion of the ophthalmic artery is suspected, in cases of anterior ischaemic optic neuropathy of possible embolic origin, or in anterior ischaemic optic neuropathy to document the position of the watershed zone of the choroidal circulation and its relation to the optic nerve head.

Emergency treatment in central retinal artery occlusion is designed to lower intraocular pressure and dislodge the embolus. In impending central retinal artery occlusion heparin is useful. Urgent systemic corticosteroids are needed when central retinal artery occlusion or anterior ischaemic optic neuropathy is due to arteritis. In other situations treatment is directed towards preventing recurrence or involvement of the other eye by reducing or eliminating identified risk factors.

1 Cullen JF. Occult temporal arteritis. *Trans Ophthalmol Soc UK* 1963;**83**:725.
2 Gresser EB. Partial occlusion of retinal vessels in a case of thromboangitis obliterans. *Am J Ophthalmol* 1932;**15**:235.
3 Goldsmith J. Periarteritis nodosa with involvement of the choroidal and retinal arteries. *Am J Ophthalmol* 1946;**29**:435.
4 Anderson RG and Gray EB Spasm of the central retinal artery in Raynaud's disease. *Arch Ophthalmol* 1937;**17**:662.
5 Katz B. Migrainous central retinal artery occlusion. *J Clin Neuro-Ophthalmol* 1986;**6**:69-75.
6 Wray SH. Extracranial internal carotid artery disease. In: Bernstein EF, ed. *Amaurosis fugax.* New York: Springer-Verlag, 1988:72–80.
7 Cogan DG, Wray SH. Vascular occlusions in the eye from cardiac myxomas. *Am J Ophthalmol* 1975;**80**:396–403.
8 Appen RE, Wray SH and Cogan DG. Central retinal artery occlusion. *Am J Ophthalmol* 1975;**79**:374.
9 Burde RM. Amaurosis fugax, an overview. *J Clin Neuro-ophthalmol* 1989;**9(3)**:185–9.
10 Zimmerman LE. Embolism of central retinal artery; secondary to myocardial infarction with mural thrombosis. *Arch Ophthalmol* 1965;**73**:822.
11 Jayam AV, Hass WK, Carr RE and Kumar AJ. Saturday night retinopathy. *J Neurol Sci* 1974;**22**:413.
12 Givner I, Jaffe N. Occlusion of the central retinal artery following anesthesia. *Arch Ophthalmol* 1950;**43**:197.
13 Hollenhorst RW, Svien HJ and Benoit CF. Unilateral blindness occurring during anesthesia for neurosurgical operation. *Arch Ophthalmol* 1954;**52**:819.
14 Bock J, Bornschein H, Hommer K. The recuperative time of the human retina. An electroretinographic study. Albrecht von Graefes. *Arch Klin Exp Ophthalmol* 1963;**165**:437–51.
15 Hayreh SS, Kolder HE, Weingeist TA: Central retinal artery occlusion and retinal tolerance time. *Ophthalmology* 1980;**87**:75–8.
16 Sfytche TJ, Bulpitt CJ, Kohner EM, *et al.* Effect of changes in intraocular pressure on the retinal microcirculation. *Br J Ophthalmol* 1974;**58**:514–22.
17 Schmidt D, Schumacher M, Wakhloo AK. Microcatheter urokinase infusion in central retinal artery occlusion. *Am J of Ophthalmol* 1992;**113**:429–34.
18 Stone R, Zink H, Klingele T, Burde RM. Visual recovery after central retinal artery occlusion: Two cases. *Ann Ophthalmol* 1977;**9**:445.
19 Wilson IA, Warlow CP, Ross Russell RW. Cardiovascular disease in patients with retinal arterial occlusion. *Lancet* 1979;**1**:1292–4.
20 Amarenco P, Duyckaerts C, Tzourio C, Hénin D, Bousser M-G, Hauw J-J. The prevalence of ulcerated plaques in the aortic arch in patients with stroke. *N Eng J of Med* 1992;**326**:221–5.
21 Di Tullio M, Sacco RL, Gopal A, Mohr JP, Homma S. Patent foramen ovale as a risk factor for cryptogenic stroke. *Ann Int Med* 1992;**117**:461–5.
22 Teague SM, Sharma MK. Detection of paradoxical cerebral echo contrast embolization by transcranial doppler ultrasound. *Stroke* 1991;**22**:740–5.
23 Henkes HE. Electroretinography in circulatory disturbances of the retina. II. The electroretinogram in cases of occlusion of the central retinal artery or of one of its branches. *Arch Ophthalmol* 1954;**51**:42.
24 Ackerman RH. Neurovascular non-invasive evaluation. In Taveras, Ferruci, eds. *Radiology.* Philadelphia: Lippincott, 1995;**3**:1–29.
25 Sheng FC, Quinones-Baldrich W, Machleder HI, *et al.* Relationship of extracranial carotid occlusion disease and central retinal artery occlusion. *Am J Surg* 1986;**152**:175–8.
26 Ross Russell RW. Observations on the retinal blood vessels in monocular blindness. *Lancet* 1961;**2**:1422–8.
27 Kearns TP, Hollenhorst RW. Venous stasis retinopathy of occlusive disease of the carotid artery. *Mayo Clin Proc* 1963;**38**:304–12.
28 Savino PJ, Glaser JS, Cassady J. Retinal Stroke: Is the patient at risk. *Arch Ophthalmol* 1977;**95**:1185–9.
29 Englert H, Hawkes CH, Boey ML, *et al.* Dego's disease: Association with anticardiolipin antibodies and the lupus anticoagulant. *BMJ* 1984;**289**:576.
30 Glueck HI, Kant KS, Weiss MA, *et al.* Thrombosis in systemic lupus erythematosus: relation to the presence of circulatory anticoagulants. *Arch Intern Med* 1985;**145**:1389–95.
31 Shalev Y, Green L, Pollack A, *et al.* Myocardial infarction with central retinal artery occlusion in a patient with antinuclear antibody—negative systemic lupus erythematosus. *Arthritis Rheum* 1985;**28**:1185–7.

32 Jonas J, Kolbe K, Volcker HE, *et al.* Central retinal artery occlusion in Sneddon's disease: association with antiphospholipid antibodies. *Am J Ophthalmol* 1986;**102**:37–40.

33 Pulido JS, Ward LM, Fishman GA, *et al.* Antiphospholipid antibodies associated with retinal vascular disease. *Retina* 1987;**7**:215–18.

34 Silverman M, Lubeck MJ, Briney WG. Central retinal vein occlusion complicating systemic lupus erythematosus. *Arthritis Rheum* 1978;**21**:839–43.

35 Hollenhorst RW. The ocular manifestations of internal carotidarterial thrombosis. *Med Clin North Am* 1960;**4**:897–908.

36 Hollenhorst RW. Significance of bright plaques in the retinal arterioles. *JAMA* 1961;**178**:123–9.

37 D'Cruz IA, Cohen HC, Prabhu R, *et al.* Clinical manifestations of mitral-annulus calcification, with emphasis on its echocardiographic features. *Am Heart J* 1977;**94**:367–7.

38 Guthrie J, Fairgrieve J. Aortic embolism due to myxoid tumor associated with myocardial calcification. *Br Heart J* 1963;**25**:137–40.

39 diBono DP, Warlow CP. Mitral-annulus calcification and cerebral or retinal ischemia. *Lancet* 1979;**2**:383–5.

40 Barnett HJM. Transient cerebral ischemia pathogenesis, prognosis and management. *Ann R Coll Physicians Surg Canada* 1974;**7**:153–73.

41 Barnett HJM. Delayed cerebral ischemic episodes distal to occlusion of major cerebral arteries. *Neurology* 1978;**28**:769–74.

42 Barnett HJM., Boughner DR, Wayne Taylor D, *et al.* Further evidence relating mitral valve prolapse to cerebral ischemic events. *N Engl J Med* 1980;**302**:139–44.

43 Younge BR. The significance of retinal emboli. *J Clin Neuro-ophthalmol* 1989;**9(3)**:190-4.

44 Boghen DR, Glaser JS. Ischemic optic neuropathy. The clinical profile and natural history. *Brain* 1975;**98**:689–708.

45 Hayreh SS. *Arterial blood supply of the eye in amaurosis fugax.* In: Bernstein EF, ed. New York: Springer-Verlag, 1988:1–23.

46 Hayreh SS. *Anterior ischemic optic neuropathy.* Berlin: Springer-Verlag, 1975:3–23.

47 Hayreh SS. Anterior ischemic optic neuropathy. I. Terminology and pathogenesis. *Br J Ophthalmol* 1974;**58**:955–63.

48 Hayreh SS. Anterior ischaemic optic neuropathy. II. Fundus on ophthalmoscopy and fluorescein angiography. Manifestations. *Br J Ophthalmol* 1974;**58**:964–80.

49 Ellenberger C Jr, Keltner JL, Burde RM. Acute optic neuropathy in older patients. *Arch Neurol* 1973;**28**:182–5.

50 Repka MX, Savino PJ, Schatz NJ, Sergott RC. Clinical profile and long-term implications of anterior ischemic optic neuropathy. *Am J Ophthalmol* 1983;**96**:478–83.

51 Beri M, Klugman MR, Kohler JA, Hayreh SS. Anterior ischemic optic neuropathy. VII. Incidence of bilaterality and various influence factors. *Ophthalmology* 1987;**94**:1020–8.

52 Ellenberger C Jr. Ischemic optic neuropathy as a possible early complication of vascular hypertension. *Am J Ophthalmol* 1979;**88**:1045–51.

53 Beck RW, Savino PJ, Repka MX, Schatz NJ, Sergott RC. Optic disc structure in anterior ischemic optic neuropathy. *Ophthalmology* 1984;**91**:1334–6.

54 Doro S, Lessell S. Cup-disc ratio and ischemic optic neuropathy. *Arch Ophthalmol* 1985;**103**:1143–4.

55 Eagling EM, Sanders MD, Miller SJH. Ischemic papillopathy. Clinical and fluorescein angiographic review of forty cases. *Br J Ophthalmol* 1974;**58**:990–1008.

56 Lieberman MF, Shahi A, Green WR. Embolic ischemic optic neuropathy. *Am J Ophthalmol* 1978;**86**:206–10.

57 Portnoy SL, Beer PM, Packer AJ, *et al.* Embolic anterior ischemic optic neuropathy. *J Clinic Neuro-ophthalmol* 1989;**9(1)**:21–5.

58 Sergott RC, Cohen MS, Bosley TM, Savino PJ. Optic nerve decompression may improve the progressive form of nonarteritic ischemic optic neuropathy. *Arch Ophthalmol* 1989;**107**:1743–54.

59 Letter to Editor. *Arch Ophthalmol* 1990;**108**:1063–8.

60 Johnson LN, Gould TJ, Krohel GB. Effect of levodopa and carbidopa on recovery of visual function in patients with non-arteritic anterior ischemic optic neuropathy of longer than six months' duration. *Am J Ophthalmol* 1996;**121**:77–83.

61 Guyer DR, Miller NR, Auer CL, *et al.* The risk of cerebrovascular and cardiovascular disease in patients with anterior ischemic optic neuropathy. *Arch Ophthalmol* 1985;**103**:1136–42.

62 Sawle GV, James CB, Ross-Russell RW. The natural history of non-arteritic anterior ischaemic optic neuropathy. *J Neurol Neurosurg Psychiatry* 1990;**53**:830–3.

341

13 Criteria for diagnosing brainstem death

M D O'BRIEN

The traditional criteria of cardiac and respiratory arrest for the certification of death are appropriately used in the huge majority of cases, but the development and widespread use of cardiac resuscitation and artifical ventilation in the late 1960s created a need to redefine the criteria of death in the very small numbers of patients in apnoeic coma, who could be maintained on a ventilator for days or weeks, a need made more pressing by the demand for organs for transplantation.[1]

Twenty years ago, many such patients were ventilated until asystole supervened, by which time the brain had often liquefied. Over several years the concept that deep apnoeic coma, caused by irreversible destruction of the brainstem, was incompatible with life led to the establishment of criteria to diagnose brainstem death. Brainstem death equates with death of the brain as a whole but not, of course, with death of the whole brain. Brainstem death can be ascertained clinically at the bedside with absolute reliability and without the use of special techniques such as EEG, evoked responses, or blood flow measurements, provided that the appropriate protocol is rigorously followed. If these criteria are met, life support systems may be withdrawn with the confidence that recovery cannot occur. Organs may then be removed for transplantation and better use made of intensive care facilities. Relatives should be kept fully informed at each stage in this process.

The diagnosis of brainstem death requires preconditions that are of critical importance. Most of the examples in the medical literature claiming survival after brainstem death have failed to fulfil the preconditions. Only when the cause of the brain damage has been established and is known to be irreversible, should the tests of brainstem function be carried out. These are tests of reflex function of the brainstem. Although the oculocephalic reflex (doll's head eye movement) was not part of the United Kingdom code,[1] it is worth doing because it is a simple and easy test to elicit. If the oculocephalic reflex is present, there is no need to proceed further. The pupil light reflex should be elicited with a bright light: the light from an ophthalmoscope is not sufficient. Similarly, the corneal and gag reflexes should be sought with adequate stimuli, which need to be relatively coarse compared with those used in a conscious patient. In addition motor responses should be sought by adequate stimulation in the trigeminal nerve territory, and in the limbs. Ice cold water irrigation of the tympanic membrane should not elicit any eye movement. Tonic deviation of either eye during this test indicates some residual brainstem function. These are all straightforward bedside tests and should not create any difficulties. The test for spontaneous ventilation is usually carried out by an anaesthetist with blood gas analysis, which should be available in all intensive care units where these problems are likely to arise.

The criteria have been set out in a form suitable for reproduction and inclusion in a patient's notes (see pages 336–7).[2] The background to the concept of brainstem death, the historical aspects, and its validation has been fully discussed by Pallis.[3 4]

1 Conference of Medical Royal Colleges and the Faculties in the United Kingdom. Diagnosis of brain death. *BMJ* 1976;2:1187–8.
2 O'Brien MD. Criteria for diagnosing brain stem death. *BMJ* 1990;**301**:108–9.
3 Pallis C. *ABC of brain stem death*. London: British Medical Association, 1983.
4 Pallis C. Brain stem death. In: Vinken PJ, Bruyn GW, Klawans HL, eds. *Handbook of clinical neurology*. New York: Elsevier 1990;57:441–96.

CRITERIA FOR DIAGNOSING BRAINSTEM DEATH

Patient's name.. Ward..

Date of birth... Hospital number.......................

	Assessor A	Assessor B	Assessor A	Assessor B
Name				
Status				

If a patient in deep coma, requiring mechanical ventilation, is thought to be dead because of irreversible brain damage of known cause, an assessment of brainstem function should be made according to the following guidelines. These follow the Department of Health recommendations in "Cadaveric organs for transplantation—a code of practice, including the diagnosis of brain death", 1983 (London: HMSO).

Two assessments should be made by two doctors once the preconditions have been met. Diagnosis should not normally be considered until at least six hours after the onset of coma or, if anoxia or cardiac arrest was the cause of the coma, particularly in children, until 24 hours after the circulation has been restored, and then only if the preconditions have been satisfied.

(1) Two medical practitioners, who have expertise in this field, should assure themselves that the preconditions have been met before the examination.
(2) It is often convenient for the examination to be performed by one assessor and witnessed by the other.
(3) The respirator disconnection test is usually performed by an anaesthetist and witnessed by one of the assessors.

What is the cause of the irremediable brain damage?..

Why is it irremediable?..

Start of coma: Time.......................................Date..

Preconditions (All answers must be "No")   Time..

Date..

1   Could primary hypothermia, drugs, or metabolic/ endocrine abnormalities be contributing significantly to the apnoeic coma? (Where appropriate, check plasma and urine for drugs, and plasma pH, glucose, sodium, and calcium.)

2   Have any neuromuscular blocking drugs been administered during the preceding 12 hours?

3   Is the rectal temperature below 35°C? (If so, warm the patient and reassess.)

CRITERIA FOR DIAGNOSING BRAINSTEM DEATH

Examination
Do not proceed until the preconditions have been met.
The answer to all questions must be "No".

			1st		2nd	
			A	B	A	B
		Time Date				
1	When the head is gently, but fully rotated to either side is there conjugate deviation of the eyes in the opposite direction (Doll's head eye movement)?					
2	Do the pupils react to light?					
3	Is there any response to corneal stimulation on either side?					
4	Do the eyes deviate when either ear is irrigated with 50 ml of ice cold water for 30 s? (First confirm tympanic membranes visible and intact)					
5	Is there a gag reflex?					
6	Is there a cough reflex following bronchial stimulation by a suction catheter?					
7	Are there any motor responses within the cranial nerve distribution following adequate stimulation of any somatic area? (Supraorbital and nail bed pressure)					
8	*Tests for spontaneous ventilation* Are there any spontaneous respiratory movements?					
			CO_2	O_2	CO_2	O_2
	Pre-oxygenate the patient for 10 min with 100% oxygen. Record blood gases ($PaCO_2$ before disconnection must exceed 5·3 kPa. If not, slow ventilation until $PaCO_2$ rises to this level) Ventilation with 95% O_2 and 5% CO_2 is an alternative					
	Disconnect the patient from the ventilator and give oxygen at 6 litres per minute via a suction catheter in the trachea. Wait approximately 10 minutes, then measure blood gases ($PaCO_2$ must exceed 6·65 kPa at the end of the disconnection period)					
	Is there any spontaneous respiratory movement?					
	Assessor's signature					

Index

347